Medieval Military Medicine

Front cover: Knight with a missing leg using a crutch and pointing his sword. Last quarter of the thirteenth century. (With the kind permission of General Collection, Beinecke Rare Book and Manuscript Library, Yale University MS 229 (Lancelot Prose Cycle), 257v); *Back cover*: Lancelot and the wounded knight in a litter, carried between two horses. Last quarter of the thirteenth century. (With the kind permission of the General Collection, Beinecke Rare Book & Manuscript Library, Yale University, MS 229 (Lancelot Prose Cycle), 100v); *Inside flap*: Dominican doctor examining a patient's urine. (With the kind permission of Kislak Center for Special Collections, Rare Books and Manuscripts, University of Pennsylvania, LJS 24, f. 121v)

Medieval Military Medicine

From the Vikings to the High Middle Ages

Brian Burfield

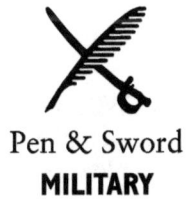

Pen & Sword
MILITARY

First published in Great Britain in 2022 by
Pen & Sword Military
An imprint of
Pen & Sword Books Ltd
Yorkshire – Philadelphia

Copyright © Brian Burfield 2022

ISBN 978 1 52675 474 5

The right of Brian Burfield to be identified as Author of this work has been asserted by him in accordance with the Copyright, Designs and Patents Act 1988.

A CIP catalogue record for this book is
available from the British Library.

All rights reserved. No part of this book may be reproduced or transmitted in any form or by any means, electronic or mechanical including photocopying, recording or by any information storage and retrieval system, without permission from the Publisher in writing.

Typeset by Mac Style
Printed and bound in the UK by CPI Group (UK) Ltd,
Croydon, CR0 4YY.

Pen & Sword Books Limited incorporates the imprints of Atlas, Archaeology, Aviation, Discovery, Family History, Fiction, History, Maritime, Military, Military Classics, Politics, Select, Transport, True Crime, Air World, Frontline Publishing, Leo Cooper, Remember When, Seaforth Publishing, The Praetorian Press, Wharncliffe Local History, Wharncliffe Transport, Wharncliffe True Crime and White Owl.

For a complete list of Pen & Sword titles please contact

PEN & SWORD BOOKS LIMITED
47 Church Street, Barnsley, South Yorkshire, S70 2AS, England
E-mail: enquiries@pen-and-sword.co.uk
Website: www.pen-and-sword.co.uk

Or

PEN AND SWORD BOOKS
1950 Lawrence Rd, Havertown, PA 19083, USA
E-mail: Uspen-and-sword@casematepublishers.com
Website: www.penandswordbooks.com

Contents

Preface vii
Acknowledgements viii

Chapter 1   Leechbooks and Surgeries   1
Chapter 2   Chronicles, Songs and Saints   14
Chapter 3   Soldiers, Smiths and Safety   29
Chapter 4   Wounds and Surgery   43
Chapter 5   Broken Bones and Fractured Skulls   59
Chapter 6   Disfigured and Disabled   75
Chapter 7   Illness and Infection   93
Chapter 8   Tormented Minds   111

Conclusion 129
Glossary of Chroniclers, Surgeons and Miracle Collections 131
Notes 138
Bibliography 190
Index 203

For Catarina

Preface

> Dear God, the standards of the knights
> hovered like birds round your enemies!
> The spears punctuated what the swords wrote;
> the dust of battle was the sand that dried
> the writing; and blood perfumed it.
>
> 'The Battle' by Ben Said Al-Magribi (1214–74),
> translated by Lysander Kemp[1]

The strange eloquence of this thirteenth-century poem called 'The Battle' hides so much of the brutality and violence of war in the Middle Ages. The turbulence and grim reality of the battlefield are there but buried just beneath the calm of the writer's five short lines and oddly seductive style. Savagery, wounds, filth, disease and psychological trauma are all waiting to be uncovered by pulling at the threads of this verse, words like *spears* and *blood*.

This book aspires to do just that, pick away at these strands to find the terror felt by those medieval warriors caught in the middle of the fighting crying *Dear God* and unearth the ghastly injuries caused by the arrows and axes of *battle*. Attached to the *swords* of those that wielded them are the casualties who were left disabled and disfigured by their wounds. Dysentery and infections are among the invisible enemies, which were hidden in the *dust*, regularly causing more harm than the wars themselves. The psychological trauma of combat is slightly more difficult to find, but it is there in what the nightmares and suicides of the knights and soldiers *wrote*. Significant for this study are those who *hovered* close to the victims of war, treating, comforting and safeguarding them, they too are secreted right below the surface of this poem's few words.

Acknowledgements

It gives me such pleasure to be able to acknowledge my gratitude to so many people and institutions for their guidance, knowledge and assistance in making this book a reality. To begin, this project is in part the natural collaboration of influences in my life made up of my Father's love for history and my Mother's years spent in the medical field. Both have supported me so strongly through so much and I could never say a 'Thank You' large enough to either of them for all their encouragement, inspiration and love.

There have been many others who have impacted me along the way, the researchers, writers and translators of history, medicine and disability, whose books and papers have sparked such curiosity in me to understand more about these subjects, especially as they relate to the soldiers of the Middle Ages. I am so thankful for their work. The British Library, The Wellcome Library, The National Archives at Kew and St Bart's Hospital, London have all been enormous resources throughout the process of compiling this study. The librarians and experts at these facilities have been so generous with their time and knowledge and I am forever grateful. These places and those who work there ask so little in return for the tremendous benefit they provide for so many.

There have indeed been others without whom this volume simply would not have been achievable. I could never adequately express my appreciation to D. Goldring who spent many hours reading most of the early drafts and many of the later versions, providing frank and valuable feedback and helping to steer the text in a much more positive and readable direction. Maureen Lee and Tyler Mort both read some of the early drafts and provided useful and important notes on the material. I am forever grateful to both. There is a large group of others, especially Steph, Ruth, Steve, Andrew, Alison, Emma-Rae, Grace, Lauren, Harri, Norm, Kelly, Quinn and Emma to whom I owe so much. Quinn and Emma, thank you for all the equine information. Thanks also to Alex for the laptops and to those others who have been so helpful and supportive along the way.

Pen & Sword Books, particularly commissioning editor Rupert Harding, have been very understanding and patient during the time of COVID-19 when this book was written, and I greatly appreciate all of their help. Alison Flowers, the copy editor on this project, did a tremendous amount of meticulous editing work to prepare this text for publication and I am so thankful for her help.

Without question my biggest debt of gratitude belongs to Catarina who has supported me in this project from its conception. Her incredible inspiration, imagination, encouragement and love have enabled me to overcome so much to write this book. You have all my love and appreciation.

Chapter 1

Leechbooks and Surgeries

> There you would have seen so many armed knights fall, their good shields split apart and their sides opened up, some had broken legs and severed arms, others had their chests opened up, helmets were broken and heads were split apart, flesh was torn and buttocks were sliced away, blood had been spilled everywhere; and the men were either busy fighting or attempting to remove the wounded from the field of battle.
>
> *La chanson de la croisade contre les Albigeois*[1]

The epigraph above, from the thirteenth-century poem known as *La chanson de la croisade contre les Albigeois*, or *The Song of the Crusade Against the Albigensians*, relates so much about the kinds of wounds a soldier of the Middle Ages might have expected to see or even worse experience on the battlefield. Thankfully, the hideous soundtrack of shouts, screams and cries belonging to the wounded and those soon to expire cannot be heard and the sickening stench of sweat, blood, flesh and faeces cannot be sensed, but still the violence and horror are made abundantly clear as they are throughout this poem. This savage campaign, known as the Albigensian Crusade, took place in Southern France nearer to the end of the 500-year period covered by this book, but the brutality of war had changed little since the ninth century when Scandinavian warriors began to terrorize much of Europe. Axes and swords sliced through unprotected flesh with gruesome ease, arrows and spears were made to puncture both armour and the wearer and even more sinister weapons caused severe burns and crush injuries. Wounds like these that damaged soldiers of Northern and Western Europe between the ninth and thirteenth centuries are indeed the focus of this study, but they are just a portion of this story with disease, disability, disfigurement, damaged minds and the practitioners of medicine all playing their parts in this awful reality.

The tournaments and games of these five centuries were another place where serious injury and death were a very real possibility for knights and soldiers alike. The mock battles of our imaginations, the sort with knights separated by a barrier and riding at one another with lances raised and well aimed, belong to the later centuries of the Middle Ages.[2] Known also as tourneys or mêlées, many of the tournaments of the twelfth and thirteenth centuries contained little that was 'mock' about them. These events became the de facto school for the bellicose, preparing young warriors for the chaos and bloodshed of armed combat, while keeping sharp the skills of those more experienced in the art of war.[3] Not only were they a place where warriors were regularly wounded and lives were taken, but armour, horses and large sums of money were also won and lost.[4] The distant cousins of these tournaments can be found in the games and contests of the Vikings and other Germanic peoples of earlier centuries.[5] They were a combination of the physical and mental and had the same purpose of preparing a warrior for battle.[6] Sports and contests included violent games and proficiency with weapons all intended to improve strength, endurance and skill.[7] Those who participated 'often came home blue and bloody', as *Kormak's Saga* described it.[8] A ball game in the saga of *Bosi and Herraud* highlights this brutality, as Bosi put out a player's eye with the ball and then broke the neck of another when he knocked him to the floor.[9] Once again with *Kormak's Saga*, during a spring assembly, feelings ran high between two men, leading to a duel with swords and shields. Ahead of the fight, during a swimming race, they attacked one another in the water only fuelling the bad feelings.[10] On the day of the duel the loser received a deep sword cut that went through his buttocks and down the back of his legs. He had to be carried away to have his painful wounds treated before being taken home to begin a lengthy recovery.[11]

This investigation into the casualties of wars and tournaments during this period frequently features contemporary individuals to help highlight different types of wounds and illnesses, alongside the associated procedures and medicines that might have been used to treat them. Extracting their stories of injury, sickness and death from doctor's casebooks, miracle collections, government records, chronicles and other documents helps to make the medicine of the medieval soldier a more three-dimensional topic. The prose, poetry and literature of these centuries are also of great value in bringing these themes to life, as are present-day reports and records from archaeological, historical and scientific books and journals. They all help to provide further evidence of who the wounded were and how they were looked after during this time. Occasionally, examples from elsewhere, the Islamic world, the Crusades or the years before and after the ninth and thirteenth centuries respectively, spill over into the discussion, but hopefully with a view to better understanding the questions or issues being explored.

The sort of person that can be found in the extant materials and collections from this period is Hugh de Gundeville (also Gondeville), a knight close to the court of Henry II of England. He was a man who can frequently be found in Henry's presence between the 1150s and 1170s and was a part of the king's forces that invaded Ireland, being left in charge of Waterford, along with two others.[12] Hugh also turns up among the assemblage of miracles from the abbey of Rocamadour in France, a place of pilgrimage that was often visited by sick and wounded knights and soldiers. According to the record Hugh suffered from an illness while he was in Ireland, one that took his speech, which is what makes him of interest to this discussion.[13] Many other names in these sources belong to minor knights and ordinary soldiers who were also wounded or became sick, men like Bernard from Auvergne who suffered from a serious illness and depression.[14] The medieval scribes and chroniclers left us with varying amounts of information about men like these. Frequently it is just a name and where they came from or the castle they defended, making fully identifiable individuals like Hugh de Gundeville all the more important in helping to affirm the lives of those about whom less is known. A more thorough evaluation of sources like these is made in the chapter that follows.

Along the way we will also come across several of those who looked after the casualties of war. As with the knights and soldiers, a fair bit is known about a few practitioners of medicine, such as Hugo de Lucca and William of Saliceto, surgeons who were experienced in treating the war wounded. All that is left for many others is just a name and a line or two of detail, men like Roger Causcy who treated soldiers in the army of Edward I of England. There were a large number who were women, but very sadly most of their names have been erased by history. However, as evidenced by the poems and stories of the time it is clear they not only treated the war wounded but could frequently be found all too close to the violence. To account for the need for more advanced skills or just more manpower the group of those who looked after these casualties could expand to include monks and nuns, bonesetters, barber-surgeons and one or two other rather unexpected groups of individuals who will be explained in a later chapter.

Unquestionably, the various examples of wounds and illnesses that can be found throughout the chapters that follow are in no way intended to be exhaustive, but rather a representation of what might have been expected to be found on the battlefield and other places where violence and cruelty existed. War has always held an uneasy place in the history and evolution of medicine, with its dreadful necessity regularly becoming the hopeful mother of invention.[15] During the Second World War, for instance, when the Royal Air Force found many of its pilots and airmen suffering terrible burn injuries this led to major advancements being made in this field by those like Sir Archibald McIndoe and his team who developed new methods to help reconstruct the damaged bodies and minds.[16] At times, the Middle Ages were no different as evidenced by the new methods and devices continually being developed to better extract arrows from the bodies of soldiers, since they were such prolific weapons.[17] This book hopes to tell the wider story of the treatment of injuries, including advancements like these, but also many procedures and remedies that will likely seem quite *medieval* to modern minds. Broken and dislocated bones are given their own chapter, which includes damaged teeth and fractured skulls. Disfiguring scars and disabling injuries are examined as are the contemporary attitudes towards them. Illnesses like dysentery and leprosy are also investigated, as they were often more deadly than the arrows and swords of the enemy. Finally, a chapter on the psychological trauma caused by war is included, which contains a significant focus on the world of the Vikings.

Certainly, this book is not meant to be an attempt to write a history of medieval medicine. There are already many excellent works on the subject penned by those far more qualified to do so. The intention is to unite available treatments of the time to the injuries and illnesses of those who fought the battles. This is not to say that one specific remedy or procedure was necessarily that which was practised on a particular individual, but more generally what was available at that time. This volume relies, in the main, on a small group of medical texts from across the period, being the Anglo-Saxon leechbooks from the early centuries of this study, Roger Frugard's surgery of the twelfth century, Theodoric's text and the work of William of Saliceto, both from the thirteenth century. The balance of this short chapter will be spent on some of the background of these books and their importance to the field of medicine at the time. These texts and the names of those who compiled them will no doubt become quite familiar as the chapters unfold. Also found dotted throughout are those who wrote and assembled other surgeries, herbals and manuscripts, adding to the knowledge of medieval medicine relating to warfare during these five centuries.

Anglo-Saxon Leechbooks

> Here are wound salves for all wounds and drinks and cleansings of every sort.
>
> *Bald's Leechbook* – Book I[18]

The word *Viking* is one of those evocative words, which when inserted into a title or headline tends to catch the eye, but when sat alongside the word *medicine* it is often the brow that becomes furrowed in question or puzzlement. What do we really know about the medicine of the Vikings or other Germanic peoples for that matter? The answer is probably quite a bit more than we may think. Just focusing on the Viking world for the moment, their sagas and poems tell us a fair bit about their own medicine and healers. While a lot of these texts were written down after the Viking Age, they existed as oral versions, passed down from one generation to the next, making them very worthy of investigation. The chapter which follows this one will examine the value of some of this material in a little more detail and many extracts from the sagas can be found throughout the chapters of this volume.

There are also a few useful clues in the archaeological evidence such as the Viking Age surgical instrument excavated at a village near Skanderborg, Denmark. It is a decorated bronze implement combining a scalpel at one end and tweezers at the other.[19] A small number of similar objects relating to medicine and the age of the Vikings have been found elsewhere in Denmark, as well as in Sweden.[20] Finds like these often tend to pose as many questions as they answer, such as who owned these tools, native physicians or others from a foreign land? It is just not possible to know at this point, but at the very least they help to confirm what must have been true, which is that physicians and healers existed in Viking society.

Medical knowledge was of great value across Europe in the Middle Ages, especially to those with a warlike nature, because once the fighting was done lacerations needed to be sutured and broken bones required fixing. There can be little doubt that those identified as being able to treat battle casualties and illnesses would have been extremely valuable individuals both as healers and instructors.[21] One way of gaining this kind of expertise was by capturing those individuals who possessed it. Although it comes from beyond the Viking Age, this can be seen in the twelfth-century Georgian epic poem by Shot'ha Rust'haveli, called *The Man (or Knight) in the Panther's Skin*:

> One of my slaves was a surgeon, he bound up the wounds,
> he drew out the arrowheads so that the wounds hurt not.[22]

When the Vikings began their assaults on Britain in the late eighth century it was not just gold and silver that they were after. They also sought human plunder as the chronicler Simeon of Durham noted about the initial raid on Lindisfarne in 793, 'Some of the brethren they killed; some they carried off in chains.'[23] The chronicler says that they returned the next year attacking another monastery and so it would continue, the plundering, killing and capturing.[24] These religious centres contained a great deal of knowledge in many areas, including medicine, making those monks and nuns with skills and expertise in this area very valuable. There were also healers who existed outside of the church to consider, as well. As the territories of the Vikings expanded the numbers of individuals who were enslaved and the networks through which they were bought and sold grew ever larger. Captured from Ireland, Britain and all across Europe, they were traded at places like Hedeby and Birka and funnelled across the Viking world and to places beyond. An entry in the *Annals of Ulster* for the year 870 highlights the large numbers of those who were enslaved and exploited: 'Amhlaigh and Imhar [Ivar] came again to Atl-cliath [Dublin] from Alba [Scotland] with two hundred ships; and a great multitude of men, English, Britons and Picts, were brought by them to Ireland in captivity.'[25] Dublin was another major Viking centre with a grim but thriving slave trade. The chronicler includes many from right across Britain among those who had been captured by Viking slave poachers. Although we are likely dealing with exaggerated figures here, if there were anything like 200 ships arriving at Dublin on that single day then it only takes some quick maths to arrive at a shocking number of captured individuals, well into the thousands.[26]

Through raiding and trading the Vikings also had significant contact with the Arab world from Spain to Byzantium and North Africa to the Middle East and at a time when Islamic medicine was at its peak. It was not all one-way traffic, either.[27] Arab travellers and explorers made the journey northwards, men like Ibrahim ibn Yacoub at-Tartushi who travelled to the large trading centre at Hedeby.²⁸ This terrible trade in people from all over would have presented a huge opportunity to find those who had specialist medical knowledge and who could offer skills and expertise alongside the homegrown Scandinavian healers.²⁹

What about the medicine that was practised by these physicians, especially those from Northern Europe, how were wounds dressed and diseases treated? At this point we can switch gears and begin to consider the Anglo-Saxon medical texts or leechbooks, which are referred to throughout this study. They are of interest for a few reasons including the fact that they were texts that were written in the middle of the Viking Age and in a place where the Northmen were beginning to settle, England. Just how much influence they had is impossible to say, but in both books we can find the medicine of Northern Europe.

The word *leech* is derived from the Old English word *læce* or the Old Danish word *læke* and means physician or healer with leechbooks being the texts that provided instructions and remedies for the treatment of injuries, ailments and diseases. The books up for consideration within this study are *Bald's Leechbook*, which is actually two books, and the less evocatively named *Leechbook III*. Coming from the same manuscript, they make up the oldest surviving medical book written in Old English and the only one that remains from Europe, before 1100, in a language that is not Greek or Latin. Transcribed at Winchester in around 950, it was likely derived from an earlier text that existed at the end of the ninth century. The fact that they appear in the same manuscript is the only thing that seems to connect *Bald's* and *Leechbook III*, so they are worth examining separately.³⁰

As the name indicates, *Bald's Leechbook* belonged to a man called Bald who was almost certainly a physician, as it seems unlikely that a book like this would have appealed to many others. There is another name in the text, Cild, who was the one instructed by Bald to either copy or compile the information, the translation is not definitive on this point. Nothing further is known about either Bald or Cild, but there are two further names Oxa and Dun that are also recorded, both of whom were presumably doctors themselves. Phrases such as, 'Oxa taught us this leechdom' and '… a leechdom; Dun taught it …' appear in a few places, providing clues about their occupations.³¹ Oxa and Dun were clearly the sources for some of the information contained within *Bald's*, but there is also a fair bit that can be identified from Graeco-Roman medical texts all the way from the Mediterranean at a time when the light of Salerno had only just begun to burn. The exotic ingredients found in the treatments and remedies of the original Greek and Latin texts, which were not available in England at that time, were substituted by the author for ones more locally obtainable.³² There are other influences that can be found in the text, as well including those from Scandinavia and Ireland.³³

The treatments and remedies found within *Bald's* cover a wide range of ailments and injuries, things like broken bones, sore teeth and dysentery, many of which will be seen later in this book. In 2015, an experiment was undertaken to faithfully recreate one of the salves from *Bald's Leechbook* meant to treat an eye infection.[34] Ingredients like those that were available in tenth-century England were carefully sourced and combined. When tested it was discovered that this salve not only had the antibacterial properties ascribed to it in *Bald's*, but it was also found to be powerful enough to kill the modern MRSA superbug.[35] This is not to say that all the treatments found in *Bald's* would have worked so successfully, but it is interesting to see the effectiveness of some like this eye salve.

Leechbook III is a much different work than *Bald's* in that it probably represents the most northern of these early works, in the sense that it is the one least influenced by the ideas of medicine from the Mediterranean. As Cameron notes, it is '… as close as we can get to ancient Northern European medicine'.[36]

In terms of treatments it is ordered from head to foot and contains an array of remedies and fixes to care for wounds and afflictions. Take for instance this remedy for a sore knee: 'If a knee be sore, pound henbane and hemlock, foment therewith and lay on.'[37] Quite a simple and useful analgesic mixture and hemlock is something that continues to be used today in natural medicine as a topical pain reliever. This entry is indicative of most entries in *Leechbook III*, being short and straightforward. There are, however, others that are perhaps more indicative of what comes to mind when we think of this earlier medicine of Northern Europe: 'Work thus a salve against the elfin race and nocturnal goblin visitors, and for the women with whom the devil hath carnal commerce.'[38] The text goes on to recommend quite a complex remedy for such matters. There are other charms and spells like these that are included in this book. In fact, it is fair to say that *Leechbook III* contains considerably more of these sorts of strange-sounding medical treatments and charms than are found in *Bald's*, but they are part of what make it such an interesting and unusual text.

As we will see in the chapters that follow, it is not unusual for these Anglo-Saxon texts to have little in the way of detailed instructions for what must have been seen as common procedures like setting broken bones. A few written directives were perhaps all that was necessary for the leech who was experienced in the practical side of medicine, stretching a point made by the influential Lanfranchi of Milan near the end of the thirteenth century that a surgeon must be '… aware of the fact that all that belongs in Surgery cannot be found in books'.[39] There is of course the possibility that other contemporary volumes did exist, long since lost to history, which may have explained such operations. However, with that said, throughout *Bald's Leechbook* there are phrases such as, '… after the manner which leeches well know …', meaning the leech must have understood what was necessary for a particular treatment without it being written down.[40] The same seems to have been true for the dosing of remedies and medications, as the amounts are not always indicated within these texts. It appears that leeches kept in their heads or elsewhere knowledge of the correct quantities that were to have been administered, likely being based on the individual being treated.[41] An example from *Bald's Leechbook* contains just such a remedy for liver disease, with no instructions given for the amounts of each constituent that was to be ground up and provided to the patient: '... let one work for drinks for a liversick man, seed of marche, of dill, of wormwood, rub these fine into water in the manner *in which leeches ken how*, and give to drink.'[42]

These leeches were clearly no backwoods healers but learned people of medicine who relied on a wide variety of sources to gain their knowledge. In addition, they possessed an expansive understanding of plants and medicines. Their names, where they were taught and a whole host of other questions will likely remain forever unanswered, but in *Bald's* and *Leechbook III* we have an idea of the state of medicine from this time, not just in England, but also Northern Europe at the time of the Vikings. The treatments and remedies found in these Anglo-Saxon texts are used to represent the earlier centuries of this volume, while understanding that there were certainly other medical texts being relied upon elsewhere in Europe at this time, some from the Mediterranean and others which are perhaps less well understood.[43]

Salerno to Saliceto

> Everlasting praise is the meed of distant Salerno,
> Thither from every land come the sick in throngs unnumbered,
> Never to be contemned is the skill of its lofty teaching.
>
> Twelfth-century Rhineland poet[44]

The so-called Twelfth Century Renaissance of Western Europe began in around 1050 and would last into the early decades of the thirteenth century. Not to be confused with the resurgence of art and learning later in the Middle Ages, this explosion of scientific, social and cultural ideas and improvements helped to bring about advancements in many areas, including medical knowledge and practice.[45] In the early years, the most significant centre of medicine was at Salerno, along the west coast of what is Italy today. It had begun to emerge as the seat of medical innovation and learning in the mists of the ninth century, however, by the eleventh and twelfth centuries it had well and truly earned that reputation. Situated near the Amalfi Coast, the sea and warm climate worked to aid those in need of healing. Salerno's central location in the Mediterranean and its large market meant that exotic spices and drugs could be brought in from places like Constantinople and Asia with great ease.[46]

Knowledge and ideas also flowed in and out of Salerno by these same routes allowing it to become a place where medicine could be taught and learned, although somewhat informally to start with. The thriving medical community was bolstered by the many women who also practised there.[47] A clearer picture of the knowledge available at Salerno began to develop with an eleventh-century physician called Gariopontus. Unhappy with the terrible state of the available Latin medical texts, he managed to pull them together into one usable treatise called the *Passionarius*, which became popular with physicians in many places. Not long after Gariopontus, another physician at Salerno, called Alfanus, began translating and creating medical texts of his own, but more importantly he would sponsor one of the most interesting and influential men of medicine, Constantine the African. Likely born in North Africa, his early life is something of an enigma, but he seems to have been a man who travelled extensively before making his way to Salerno in around 1070. He likely arrived there already knowledgeable about medicine, meaning it is quite possible that he had at one time been involved in the medical field in some capacity.[48] He was soon convinced by Alfanus to move to the Benedictine abbey at nearby Monte Cassino where he would become a monk. What Constantine added to the lexicon of European medicine were Latin translations of a large number of important and previously unavailable Arabic and Greek medical texts. One of the most significant and comprehensive of these Latin conversions was a large Arabic work on some of the general themes of medicine, in both theoretical and practical terms, called the *Pantegni*. Constantine managed to translate a substantial part of this text. By converting works like these into a language that could be understood they became extremely useful to the medical community that was at nearby Salerno and to those much further afield.[49] Constantine died sometime near the end of the eleventh century, but what he brought to the European medical community would continue to be relied upon by doctors and writers long after he had gone.

Practical medicine was also being performed at Salerno with what seems like a steady stream of patients making their way there for help and healing, including soldiers like Bohemond I. The Anglo-Norman monk and chronicler Orderic Vitalis (1075–c. 1142), noted how the great Norman warrior was cared for after being wounded in 1084 during a battle with the Byzantine navy: 'Bohemond, who had been wounded in the battle, was sent for his cure to the surgeons of Salerno, whose reputation for skill in medicine was established throughout the world.'[50] About fifteen years later, as the First Crusade came to an end, many soldiers stopped at Salerno on their way back home to Europe. Those who were wounded had their injuries treated and the sick were likewise looked after by those who practised medicine.[51] Salerno would become famous far and wide for its physicians, teaching and care, being mentioned in chronicles and stories across Europe in the twelfth century.[52]

Ultimately, later in that same century Salerno would start to give way to other towns and cities such as Parma, Bologna, Paris and especially Montpellier, which were becoming important centres of medical teaching and knowledge. Experts, masters and students migrated from all across Europe to the schools and universities in places like these.[53] An early reference from the first half of the twelfth century indicates that the medical fame of Montpellier began quite early:

> Dear old Montpellier, whose real middle name is Live-well-aye,
> Where medical science is granted a seat and appliance.
> Here, too, sound doctrine, practical precepts of medicine,
> By doctors are stated who have truly mediated
> On giving advice to the well, to the sick a poultice.[54]

Having begun to risk defaulting on the commitment to not write a poor man's history of medieval medicine this cursory introduction is just about as far as we need to go. It offers a good place to begin looking at some of the practitioners of medicine appearing in the twelfth and thirteenth centuries who are important to the subject at hand and who were themselves influenced by the long shadows cast by those like Gariopontus and Constantine the African. Each of them produced their own text or *surgery*, although there was a fair bit of borrowing going on from earlier works, as well as from each other. These surgeries did not just involve the cutting of the body, but provided instructions on the treatment of various injuries, illnesses and conditions, many of which were the result of violence. Significantly, at least a couple of these men had seen and treated, first-hand, the damage that the weapons of the battlefield had caused to the bodies and minds of soldiers. Some of them were also clerics and most were teachers, as well, meaning that their ideas and methods were passed along to others who would also look after the casualties of war. The list below takes these men in order of the date that their surgeries were produced:[55]

- Roger Frugard, or Roger of Parma as he is also known – his surgery was compiled and published between 1170 and 1180.
- Roland of Parma – written after 1240 and published in around 1250, Roland's work was more or less a direct copy of Roger's text with a few additions of his own included.
- Bruno da Longoburgo of Calabria – heavily influenced by the earlier Arabic writers, Bruno produced his volume in 1252.
- Theodoric of Bologna – the son of the famous Bolognese surgeon called Hugo de Lucca (also known as Master Hugo and Ugo de Lucca), Theodoric composed his work in 1265, which relied heavily on his father's teaching and experience.
- William of Saliceto – he assembled his surgery in around 1275, including, unusually, a rudimentary section on anatomy.
- Lanfranchi of Milan – a student of William of Saliceto, his surgery was written in 1295.

Roland, Bruno and Lanfranchi are only minor characters in this book, which is not to diminish their work, but there is simply not enough room on the page or patience on behalf of the reader to include the ideas of everyone. Additionally, there were other men and women of medicine, many of them shining lights like Hildegard of Bingen, Taddeo Alderotti and Henry de Mondeville who are also deserving of a share of the ink and paper from time to time.

The three most important surgeons from the list, as they relate to this volume, are Roger Frugard, Theodoric (along with his father) and William of Saliceto. Beginning with Roger Frugard or Roger of Parma, his work was collected and published by his students, being led by a man called Guido II of Arezzo some time between 1170 and 1180.[56] Much of Roger's life and experiences are a mystery and there is no evidence that he even practised medicine on the battlefield.[57] What makes him of such importance is his surgery, a work clearly influenced by earlier volumes such as the so-called *Bamberg Surgery*, but nevertheless Roger's would quickly become one of the most significant medical texts in the history of Western Europe.[58] His volume includes a considerable focus on the treatment of wounds, such as the removal of arrows, fixing dislocated bones and the proper methods for suturing lacerations, all with clear and concise instructions. Beginning with the head and moving down the body, the text describes the types of injuries that commonly occurred to each part of the anatomy along with the associated treatments. Choosing an example from the first part of this surgery, the repair of a facial laceration caused by a sharp-bladed weapon, the details are easy to follow. Injuries caused by the same blade stroke that cut through the nose and lips were to be carefully fitted back into position and stitched closed. Sutures were to be done using a sharp needle and silk thread, making sure to keep them continuous and close together. Pads were then to be set over the damaged area and held in place by a bandage shaped like a 'horse's halter', which also served to keep everything aligned. Drains for pus were to be placed in the nostril and at the bottom of the laceration.[59] Roger's often suggested 'red powder' was to be applied to the wound for the following nine days of healing. Made from iron oxide rich clay and mixed with mastic, greek tar, sangdragon, frankincense and comfrey, this remedy was meant to stop the bleeding and promote healing.[60]

Being copied and translated it was not long before Roger's surgery became a successful and distinguished text at Salerno and elsewhere around Europe.[61] There are about twenty copies that still survive, with the earliest dating from around 1200. Importantly, the first translation of Roger's work from Latin into another language may well have been in about 1209 in Southern France when a portion of it was translated into Occitan prose by Raimon of Avignon.[62] This truncated version was fine-tuned by Raimon, who added some military specific additions to the text.[63] Other early translations of Roger's work include French and Anglo-Norman versions made during the thirteenth century.[64]

There were those armies that carried with them their own surgeons who were of immense value, as the early thirteenth-century German poem *The Lay of the Nibelungs* spells out quite clearly:

> To all well skilled in leechcraft no guerdon [reward] was denied.
> Unstinted store of silver and shining gold beside,
> If they could heal the heroes, who wounded were in fight
> To load his guests with presents was eke this king's delight.[65]

One such practitioner and teacher was Hugo de Lucca, the city surgeon for Bologna, being appointed to the role in around 1214. He was also attached to the Bolognese army in the same capacity during the Fifth Crusade, between 1218 and 1221.[66] Exposure to battlefield injuries continually provided surgeons like Master Hugo with the opportunity of refining existing ideas of medicine, adding their own thoughts and experiences. It was one of his sons, Theodoric, who would compose a surgical text in around 1265, drawing heavily on his father's ideas and teachings along with a whole host of other influences. Within this surgery Theodoric was not afraid to credit and challenge the work of the early Greek and Roman physicians such as Galen, as well those from the Islamic world such as Abulcasis and even more contemporary Europeans such as Roland of Parma.[67] Theodoric's text includes specific examples of his father's work that serve to enhance the volume.[68] Hugo had two other sons who were also involved in the medical field, with his son Franciscus taking over his father's role as Bologna's city surgeon.[69] However, it is Theodoric's work that is relied upon throughout this study, in large part for its close ties to the medieval battlefield thanks to his father Master Hugo.

The third of these professional surgeons, William of Saliceto, was additionally both teacher and cleric. William practised medicine throughout the area now considered Northern Italy where he looked after soldiers, monks and others.[70] Within his surgery, composed in around 1275, William provided clues that may point to his own military involvement when he was young:[71]

> J'ai vu encore un certain soldat de Bergame qui fut frappé dans quelque armée, où j'étais moi aussi, et j'étais assez jeune, par une grande flèche qui entra dans la gorge ...[72]

> I helped a soldier from Bergamo who was in the same army where I was also when I was quite young. He was hit by a big arrow that entered his throat ...

This first-hand knowledge of soldier's injuries is obvious from the many anecdotes William included within his text. They paint an intimate and vivid picture of the treatment of these wounds, details that are usually absent from what is known about so many doctors and casualties of the time. Continuing with the soldier from Bergamo, William treated him successfully, using his hands to discover that the arrow had lodged itself by his left shoulder blade. He was able to remove the arrow and heal the resulting injury.[73] While sharing his successes, William was not afraid to note his failures too. One such account involved a man referred to as Mr Boniface, the nephew of Sir Hubert the Marquis of Palavicino. He was hit in the neck by a small arrow, which sliced through his jugular vein. The arrow cut the vein in such a manner that it neither plugged it nor allowed for clotting to occur and as a result his blood flooded out like rain from a roof-gutter, according to William. Sadly, he was unable to stem the flow of blood and Mr Boniface died within an hour. Initially, William felt that the arrow must have been poisoned, but after investigating the injury further he changed his opinion. The case seems to have weighed on William's mind as he reflected on his own failings and the precious little time he had to treat the wound.[74]

These three texts belonging to Roger, Theodoric and William progressed in size and complexity, with William's being the most exhaustive and at times exhausting, because of his repetitiveness, but more about that later. Along with the Anglo-Saxon leechbooks, these texts help to build up a picture of the treatment of the casualties of war during this 500-year period and will be used time and again throughout this book. Each offers a different point of view and progress in medicine can regularly be seen being made over the decades and centuries, but occasionally there are some techniques and procedures that do not appear to change much at all.

Herbals, or collections of plants and their uses, were another type of medical text produced during the Middle Ages. They too are relied upon within this book, but to a much lesser extent than the leechbooks and surgeries. Taking just a brief look at a few of them, they include the *Herbarium*, or *Old English Herbarium*, the only illustrated assemblage that survives in Old English.[75] The *Lacnunga* is another of the few Anglo-Saxon texts that have come down to us. It is a collection of about 200 herbal recipes, folk remedies and charms, with influences from the Mediterranean and Northern Europe. The highly influential French herbal known as *Macer Floridus De Viribus Herbarum*, or just *Macer Floridus*, is a later text containing seventy-seven plants and their many uses. Taking frankincense as an example, it is a constituent of Roger's 'red powder' above and likely familiar to many of us from the Nativity play. It has many uses in *Macer Floridus*, everything from the treatment of wounds and staunching the flow of blood to being part of remedies intended for problems of the mouth and stomach.[76] The herbal of *Macer Floridus* is noted numerous times in the surgery written by Theodoric proving their value as references to medieval physicians and surgeons.[77] A further text known as *An Old Icelandic Medical Miscellany*, or MS Royal Irish Academy 23 D43, is a manuscript that combines an array of Scandinavian charms and remedies in one place. It was compiled in the late fifteenth century, with much of the material being gleaned from earlier texts. It includes within it *The Book of Simples*, a herbal based on information derived from the works of *Macer Floridus* and Constantine the African, by way of a Danish medical writer called Henrik Harpestræng (d. 1244).[78] These works and others like them will be found sprinkled across the chapters on the care of injuries and illnesses.

We can bring this section to a close having come full circle with Constantine the African, from his arrival at Salerno to the influence of his work in later texts like Roger Frugard's surgery and the Danish herbal of Henrik Harpestræng.[79] The impact of his translations will be seen in a few other examples, later in the book. Leaving the leechbooks, surgeries, herbals and Constantine for now we can look to other sources, the chronicles, sagas, poems and miracle collections of these five centuries for more on the subject of the medicine of the medieval battlefield.

Chapter 2

Chronicles, Songs and Saints

> Like a skilful physician who at one time makes use of fomentations, at another of the instrument of incision, and at another of cauterizing instrument.
>
> Matthew Paris[1]

In 1243 Henry III of England and his army were in France trying to regain control of lands lost by his father King John. In the early part of the year he and his men attempted to besiege the monastery at Vérines, which had been turned into a fortress by a group of Gascon rebels. The fighting was fierce and Henry's men struggled to gain any ground in the siege. Among the English was a man called John Mansel, a councillor and clerk of Henry III and an especially fearless soldier.[2] Mansel took it upon himself to try and rally the troops, but as did so he became exposed to one of the heavy weapons employed by the rebels. He was struck by a large stone that was hurled from within the monastery. His leg was badly crushed, leaving him with a compound fracture and incapable of moving. Fortunately, others quickly came to his rescue using their bodies and large shields to protect him from further injury as more projectiles were aimed at Mansel. He was finally able to be extricated, but the damage done was severe and he was left in poor condition. It was only through the skill of the surgeons who treated Mansel that he was saved, later being promoted by Henry III for his bravery.[3]

There is a fair bit of information useful to the study of medieval military medicine that can be gleaned from such a passage. First, this episode stresses quite clearly the importance of being able to offer protection to the wounded on the battlefield, a subject that will be studied in a little more detail in the chapter that follows. Clearly, had Mansel not been safeguarded in the way he was he would have lost his life to more of the projectiles aimed toward him. We also gain some understanding about the potential lethality or life-changing nature of a compound or open fracture during this period, again a topic that is examined in more detail later on. It would have been a skilled surgeon indeed who could have fixed such a wound and in this case Mansel appears to have been treated by Henry's own medical men.

We know about this event and the details that go with it because of the contemporary chronicler Matthew Paris (*c.* 1200–59), a well-known English monk and writer who composed a few texts during his lifetime. His accounts help to bring us closer to events like this one and much of life during the thirteenth century. In fact, so many of the casualties of war in the Middle Ages, those who were left injured, disabled or sick, can be found in sources such as this one and the same is true of some of the cures and therapies used to treat them. It was not just the chronicles and annals from across this 500-year period that documented such facts, as the sagas, poems and miracle accounts from places like Ireland, Germany, France and Iceland all contain similar sorts of information important to the subjects of warfare and medicine. The details contained within these records add so much to the knowledge base of this complex field of study. These histories and verses also offer information about many of the peripheral issues around military medicine such as protection for the wounded, as we have seen already.

This chapter picks up where the previous one left off, taking the opportunity to explore some of the various sources that are relied upon throughout this volume to illustrate and expand on a wide range of themes and subjects. Chronicles and annals, such as the one written by Matthew Paris, are among the most accessible sources for this kind of detail, as they typically relate to a specific war, campaign or era. Like Matthew Paris, many who created these historical records tended to be clerics and monks, in part because of their ability to read and write. Humour, both intended and otherwise, their own likes, prejudices and foibles, all come out in their writing styles and the things they recorded, making some of these texts very engaging to the modern reader.[4]

Abbot Suger of St Denis (1081–1151) is another such chronicler who provided a useful insider's view of the violent world of the first half of the twelfth century, especially as it related to King Louis VI of France, sometimes referred to as Louis the Fat (1081–1137). Suger was a close associate of the French monarch, both professionally and personally, which meant that occasionally the truth was stretched just a little.[5] During the siege of the castle of Livry near Paris, Suger noted how Louis was struck by a projectile thrown from a catapult that caused 'severe injury' to his leg, even though no medical attention seems to have been required. He went on to say that it was his regal strength and constitution that allowed him to simply shake it off, endure the pain and keep fighting as if it were nothing.[6] Embellishments aside, first-hand accounts of wounds, mutilations, torture, disease and other subjects are all contained within Suger's words.[7] This sort of 'backstage access' to a particular conflict or era adds so much to studies of the medieval world. It is worth exploring a few more of the chronicles found within this work, in a cross-section of these centuries, to gain a flavour for just what it is that they have to offer to this examination of medieval medicine associated with the battlefield.

The Royal Frankish Annals, *The Annals of St Bertin* and *The Annals of Fulda* are three chronicles that bring to life the world of ninth-century Europe, especially as it relates to the Frankish Empire under Carolingian rule. Set out year by year, they provide frequent reports about the length and severity of a particular winter, unusual events such as the delivery of an elephant to Charlemagne and entry after entry describing the Viking raids that were occurring all over.[8]

While the information incorporates everything from the mundane to the fascinating and at times even entertaining, the notes pertaining to armies and their soldiers are the ones that pique the interest, as the entry for the year 877 in *The Annals of Fulda* demonstrates, '... a terrible malady followed Carloman's army on its return from Italy, so that many coughed up their lives'.[9] Accounts like this are more general reminders of the spread of disease through a military force of the Middle Ages, but in doing so they speak to medieval soldiers living and fighting so closely together, quite commonly in less than healthy conditions.

The Islamic world includes similar texts describing a view of the Middle Ages through a different lens. Reports on the Vikings in both the West and East were written by several philosophers, historians and travellers, such as Miskawayh (932–1030) who used eyewitness reports to enhance a vivid description of the Swedish or Rūs Viking attacks on Azerbaijan in 943. Disease and suicide were among the issues that he wrote about, providing details relating to the subjects within this book.[10] Usāmah ibn Munqidh (1095–1188) is another who provided a first-hand account of European (Frankish) crusaders and some of the early crusader era. Conflict, friendly interaction and even the sharing of medical information are all a part of this chronicle.[11]

One annal that described a specific campaign is that of the monk Peter of les Vaux-de-Cernay who recorded much of the Albigensian Crusade during the early part of the thirteenth century. This was a large-scale attack sanctioned by Pope Innocent III, which sent a Catholic army to annihilate the Cathars of Southern France, a dualist religious sect that had become unacceptable to the papacy. Peter, who was writing very much from a Catholic perspective, included detailed notes on many things related to medieval warfare, such as the use of heavy military equipment and mining to destabilize the fortifications of Carcassonne in 1209.[12] While this chronicle has little to say in the way of specific medical information, Peter's work does offer insights on topics such as weapon injuries and torture, which in turn provide the opportunity to examine how these sorts of wounds might have been treated, based upon available medical texts and treatises.[13]

There are many more chronicles and histories that exist from these 500 years, written by those with exotic sounding names like Ahmad ibn Fadlān, who recorded the customs of the Rūs Vikings in the 920s, and the chronicle of Orderic Vitalis, which detailed much of the eleventh and twelfth centuries in Normandy, France and England. The annals of others with more pedestrian sounding names such as Gerald of Wales and Roger of Wendover are no less valuable. As with Ibn Fadlān and Orderic Vitalis, they are relied upon time and again throughout this study for their accounts of those soldiers who were the casualties of warfare.

Sagas and Troubadour's Songs

> King Arthur, who loved them well, had them
> both brought before him, and summoned a
> surgeon whose knowledge of surgery was supreme.
> *The Knight with the Lion, Yvain*[14]

Like the chronicles and annals described already, the sagas, poetry and songs of this 500-year period are filled with references to war and its casualties, including much about the care of wounds and illnesses. The authors of this literature came from a variety of backgrounds and vocations and included women, as well. There were of course clerics and monks, but knights too turned to songs and poetry to describe their experiences of war. Sagas, epic Arthurian romances, plus shorter songs and lyrics at times described factual events or told stories of fiction with occasional elements of truth added in, many recording the ways in which soldiers were looked after when they became the victims of war. This section samples the kinds of literary sources that appear in this book and the sort of details they have to offer to the discussion.

Beginning in the ninth century, the monk called Abbo of Saint-Germandes-Prés used an epic poem to relate his eyewitness account of the Viking attacks on Paris, which contains clues about the victims of battle, including one man who apparently had a metal prosthesis where his hand had once been.[15] Another ninth-century writer, Torbjørn Hornklove, a court poet of Harold Fairhair, explained how the wounded were protected from further injury onboard ships by being placed head-first under the rowing benches with their backs covered by their shields.[16] In keeping with these earlier works, the author of the fictional Anglo-Saxon poem *Beowulf* wrote how Wulf, the brother of Eofor, was treated for his wounds of battle with bandages and the care of many of his men.[17]

Perhaps most well known in all of this are the oral traditions of the Vikings, their sagas and poems, where we find tales with descriptions of extreme violence and the most gruesome wounds. A few of these works were committed to vellum in the tenth and eleventh centuries and many others would be transcribed later, such as *The Story of Burnt Njal*, a saga full of grisly scenes from skirmishes and battles: 'Wolf the quarrelsome cut open his belly, and led him round and round the trunk of a tree, and so wound all his entrails out of him, and he did not die before they were all drawn out of him.'[18] Along with the horror contained within the saga's many lines is an example of a female healer called Hildigunna the Leech, something not at all unusual in these stories.[19] It also provided some understanding of the limits of medicine at that time. King Hacon was killed in battle when he was struck in the shoulder by an arrow, a wound that nicked an artery. The author explained that the blood simply could not be staunched because of the 'rude leechcraft' that was available to treat him, meaning that he bled to death.[20]

The lesser known Icelandic saga *The Vapnfjord Men*, or *Vápnfirðinga Saga*, includes a successful healer known as Thorvard Leech, widely regarded as one of Iceland's best physicians.[21] Thorvard was clearly a skilled doctor, able to look after just about anything that came his way. In one incident he was sent to set a leg fracture that had occurred on a farm.[22] Later, he was called upon to care for the men who had been injured in battle while under the leadership of a man called Bjarni.[23] Thorvard treated the casualties, looking after them until they were well enough to take care of themselves. As the warriors reached a point of wellness, Bjarni sent Thorvard to look after Thorkell, the leader of those who had fought against him. Thorkell was clearly unwell, but within a short time Thorvard had him on the mend, being paid handsomely for his good care with a horse and a silver bracelet.[24]

Spells, charms and magic also played their part in healing within these Viking tales. In *Kormak's Saga*, Thordis the Prophetess recommended to Thorvard, whose broken ribs were healing slowly, that he appease the elves in order that he might recover more quickly. She suggested that he take the blood of a bull and spread it onto a hill to make a feast for them, advice that worked for Thorvard.[25] In other texts, such as *Eirik the Red's Saga*, the occult can be found in a seeress named Thorbjorg (also called the 'Little Prophetess') and in *Egil and Asmund* it was an old hag who healed Egil's hand with the use of magic.[26]

A rich Viking Age grave discovered at the ringfort of Fyrkat, near Hobro in Denmark offers more on the subject of magic and healing. It contained a female buried with luxury goods and items associated with a seeress, a spit, wand and a purse of henbane seeds among other things.[27] She helps to show that those like Thordis the Prophetess and Thorbjorg the Little Prophetess formed a genuine and important part of Norse society.[28] The henbane seeds are interesting, because when burned the smoke would have produced a mild hallucinogenic reaction, which she may have used in religious practices or for medical purposes. Henbane was used in many pain-relieving treatments found in the English medical texts that parallel the Viking Age, including *Bald's Leechbook* and the *Old English Herbarium*.[29]

While there can be a good deal of fantasy within these sagas and poems there is a lot that is genuine.[30] Perhaps without the veracity of the *The Saga of the Greenlanders* and *Eirik the Red's Saga* the Viking Age settlement in North America, from around the year 1000, would never have been discovered and established by archaeology.[31] Lacking *Egil's Saga* we would understand much less about Egil Skallagrímsson, a warrior and poet of the tenth century. The same can also be said for the medicine of the Vikings included among these tales, particularly as it relates to battlefield injuries.

In the twelfth century, writers such as Marie de France and Chrétien de Troyes commonly interspersed details relating to medicine throughout their *lais* (shorter verses of romance and chivalry) and epic poems. Marie de France included female healers in some of her verses. The *lai Les Deus Amanz* features a successful physician who practised medicine at Salerno, where she had been for more than thirty years.[32] In another known as *Guigemar* a woman clearly versed in the healing arts can be found treating the arrow wound in her lover's leg.[33] Chrétien de Troyes especially seems to have had an interest in the world of medicine, including brief references and elaborate scenes involving the treatment of injuries in his tales of Arthur and his knights. Little is known about de Troyes' personal history beyond what he wrote, so just why he appears to have had an appreciation for medicine is not certain. Taking an example from the epic poem *The Knight of the Cart (Lancelot)* it contains a lacerated and bloodied Lancelot whose wounds were treated with an unusual sounding remedy called 'the ointment of the Three Marys'.[34] Looking a little closer at this salve its name implies the three Marys who can be found in the gospels of the New Testament Bible. They are a combination of women with that same name who were meant to have anointed Christ's body after he died to make it ready for burial.[35] Other medieval works also mention this ointment that had the power to heal wounds, including *Fierabras*, a poem written by an unknown author around the same time as de Troyes' *Lancelot*. The title character is a Saracen of giant proportions whose father captured Rome, grabbing hold of a few sacred Christian relics including the crown of thorns that had been placed on Christ's head and the balm used to anoint him after his death. This second precious item was said to be able to heal any wound, no matter how severe.[36]

The make-up of this ointment of the three Marys may be partially explained by the Gospel of John where aloes and myrrh were to be used to consecrate the body of Christ.[37] Both elements were employed in medieval medicine, so there was likely something of substance in this medieval balm. Myrrh is known to have analgesic properties and aloes was recommended for stopping the flow of blood and healing injuries. They can be found separately and together in many ointments throughout the major surgical works and herbals of this time.[38]

One of the most explicit accounts of the violence of war in the thirteenth century is *La chanson de la croisade contre les Albigeois*, or *The Song of the Crusade Against the Albigensians*, a work already referenced and one that is often looked to within this book. Written in two parts, this chronicle-style song recalls the many sieges and battles of the Albigensian Crusade. The first portion was compiled by William of Tudela, a fairly dependable writer who made use of eyewitness accounts when he could, but who also had a tendency to record things in favour of the crusaders.[39] The larger second part of the poem was completed by an anonymous writer who, while not in favour of the heretical Cathars, seems to have understood the plight of the people of Southern France who were under attack.[40] This account of war in the Middle Ages contains several references to the practitioners of medicine who looked after the wounded:

> Cependant le comte de Montfort mande les médecins
> savants pour faire des emplâtres et des onguents,
> et ramener à la vie les blessés;[41]

> However, the Count de Montfort summoned the doctors,
> who understood their science, to make plasters and ointments,
> and bring the wounded back to life;

A different sort of literature also offers a realistic and intimate look at the terror and casualties of war. These are the poems and songs written by knights and soldiers, such as those penned by the baron and warrior turned troubadour Bertran de Born, who recalled the details of battle with an explicit and direct style. His work, which thrived in the 1180s, includes the song *Miei sirventes vuolh far dels reis amdos*, or *About Two Kings I'll Write Half-a-Poem*, that listed the armour and equipment of war strewn across the battlefield, along with the torn and damaged bodies of the dead and wounded.[42] In another of these songs, *Leu m'escondisc, domna, que mal no mier*, or *I Apologise, My Lady, Though Guiltless*, de Born grouped physicians alongside others who were an essential part of any castle and warfare:

> May my castle be divided
> With four owners to one tower
> May they never live in friendship
> And always need their bowmen
> Doctors, soldiers, gatemen, guards,
> If I ever longed to love another lady.[43]

A German knight called Wolfram von Eschenbach wrote *Parzival*, a version of the Arthurian tale of Perceval, which is full of the wounds received by knights and soldiers in combat and at tournaments. Having been so close to the field of battle himself, many of von Eschenbach's references seem to ring true, like this brief description of the procedure to remove a spear from a wound:

> Then a leech stretched his hand to the spear-wound, and the iron he found fast within,
> With the hilt, wrought of reed, and hollow, and the twain from the wound he drew.[44]

Lastly, some of the more tedious things related to the casualties of war are also found in these sources, such as the anonymous thirteenth-century Arthurian tale *The Knight of the Two Swords* which provides a representation of a litter, the sort used to carry the wounded of the knightly classes from the battlefield.[45] Hartmann von Aue or von Ouwe (*c*. 1165–*c*. 1215), another German knight and poet, wrote *Der Arma Heinrich* providing a comparison of the two great medieval medical centres of Salerno and Montpellier, with the former being described as a more scientific and learned place of medicine.[46]

In the same poem he claimed to relate the description of a doctor's room at Salerno, a workplace containing a large, tall table with straps so that patients could be forcibly held down. It was an elaborately fitted room, well stocked with medicines, ointments and the tools of the doctor's trade such as knives for cutting and whetstones for sharpening his surgical instruments.[47]

The information taken from the sagas of the Vikings, the epic poems of the Arthurian writers and the songs of the troubadours provides another point of view and reference for the subjects covered in this volume, even if at times the details must be tested for evidence of their truth. Occasionally, a passage or verse from a more modern war poet such as Siegfried Sassoon or Wilfred Owen is also offered, hopefully adding perspective and understanding to sensitive matters such as disability or the damage that combat trauma can cause to the mental health of a soldier.

Miracles

> Unable to find a doctor who could cure him, the knight resolved to come to the church of the Blessed Mary of Rocamadour.
> *Les miracles de Notre-Dame de Roc-Amadour*[48]

One of the richest sources of knowledge describing the injuries, healing and lives of medieval warriors is found among the collections of miracles documented at some of the many pilgrim sites throughout Europe, particularly those in France and England. It may be the area that seems the least familiar to most of us, but there is great benefit in these accounts thanks to the social history and details that they provide for those knights and soldiers who suffered in some way because of war.[49] They present identifiable places, individuals, medical knowledge, surgical methods, folk remedies and occasionally even elements of sieges and battles. The group of twelfth-century miracles of St Ivo in England is an ideal example as it includes the nobleman called Pagan Peverel, a fighting man who is known to have taken part in the First Crusade alongside Duke Robert of Normandy, while another record provides a useful inventory of the armour and equipment of a knight of that period.[50]

The twelfth-century collection of miracles from Rocamadour in South-Central France is one that features knights and soldiers in many of its entries. One account that shows the elaborate nature of some of them is that of a soldier called William Goirans, an experienced and skilled warrior from Montpellier, fighting on the side of King Alphonso II of Aragon in the war against Raymond V, Count of Toulouse.[51] A part of the record describes how he and eleven other men fought against twenty-two enemy soldiers. Pulling themselves into a tight formation, they seemed to fend off the larger force, but after some vicious hand-to-hand fighting William and his men were soon drawn into a trap:

En fuyant comme des vaincus, tantôt ils se retournaient pour résister, tantôt ils couraient comme s'ils eussent eu des ailes; mais ils entrainaient derrière eux leurs imprudents adversaires du côté du gros de leurs troupes. Près de quatre cent hommes d'armes étaient cachés en embuscade, prêts à lancer leurs flèches sur les gens de bien.[52]

They (the twenty-two) turned away as if defeated, at times mounting a rearguard action and at others appearing to flee quickly in retreat. In doing so they managed to pull them (William and his men) into an ambush where four hundred men were hiding, ready to shoot their arrows.

William was nearly drowned by the strong currents of a river when he leapt into it to try and escape the ambush, only to then be pierced by one of the enemy's arrows. He managed to survive both the water and the arrow, in the end claiming that it was the Virgin Mary who had saved him.

Trying to comprehend the miracle portion of these accounts in the twenty-first century can be difficult and to be sure the interest for this study lies in the other information contained within these records that pertains to individual knights and soldiers. A thorough and lengthy investigation around what constituted this type of divine intervention centuries ago would be well beyond the scope of this book, but a short discussion of what may have been involved in some of these cases is worthy of the few remaining pages of this chapter.[53]

Generally, these collections involve the healing of wounds and diseases, although other events such as being freed from captivity or finding something that had been lost are also included among the records.[54] These things were said to have been the result of God or more exactly a saint looking after the individual. As with William Goirans above, the healing or event could take place almost anywhere prompting a later visit to an abbey or shrine devoted to that saint to give thanks and relate the story of the miracle. There were others who were seemingly cured once they had made a pilgrimage to one of these holy places where relics of a saint, in the form of bones or other special items associated with them, were often kept. Lastly and perhaps least convincingly were those who had gone on pilgrimage and received no relief only to become well some time after they had returned home.[55]

When a miracle was said to have occurred the recipient of the healing or someone close to them would report the event to the religious centre associated with the saint, initially to a group of monks so that the details could be massaged and the story put into its best light. They would then tell the revised version to a notary, who was not usually a monk, but whose job it was to record the particulars. Also present to hear the specifics would have been other pilgrims, plus some of the monks. The recorded information would then pass back to the monks who would revise, polish and arrange the miracle accounts as they saw fit.[56] The first two books of miracles from St Foy at Conques in South-Western France, for instance, were taken down by a man called Bernard of Angers who arrived there in the early part of the eleventh century. Initially, he had been interested in the miracles that were said to have been occurring at St Foy and wanted to know more about them before becoming the scribe who recorded the first couple of books.[57] As time moved forward, more regularly a council or panel was expected to investigate and validate the legitimacy of these blessed events.[58] The miracles of St Hugh of Lincoln were tested in such a way during the second half of 1219, being investigated by a papal commission, consisting of the Abbot of Fountains and Stephen Langton, the Archbishop of Canterbury.[59]

It seems that there could have been many things at play when it came to miraculous events and venerated sites in the Middle Ages. The word *miracle* is of course one that still exists in modern language, used regularly as a figure of speech to exaggerate a point or explain away something we do not completely understand: 'He left a blanket near the fire, it was a miracle he didn't burn the house down' or 'It was a miracle that I didn't hit the camper van', that sort of thing. Exaggeration and the explaining away of things not understood by citizens of the Middle Ages were probably two factors quite close to some examples of what have come down to us as miracles. Additionally, it is important to keep in mind that embellished or not many of these records represented the unusual, those individuals who survived the odds when so many others did not. There would have been a multitude who did not make it through their injuries and illnesses, being left instead among the numberless who have not been remembered by history.

The first record under examination may involve all three of these elements, exaggeration, misunderstanding and a warrior who managed to beat the odds. It comes from around 1020 and was recorded by Bernard of Angers, being first reported by a man called Peter, a cleric from an eminent family in Auvergne, who had himself spent time at St Foy.[60] The entry is that of a warrior called Raymond from Valières, a vassal of Peter's family, who received the most grievous facial injuries while leading fifty men against a rebellion. During the fight he was struck in the face by a rebel who possessed superior sword skills:

> … il fut atteint d'un furieux coup d'épée d'une violence telle qu'il eut le nez coupé en deux, sur le milieu des joues, l'une des mâchoires entièrement partagée, l'autre à demi tranchée, et la racine de la langue détachée de la gorge. Sa face n'offrait plus qu'une ouverture béante au-dessous des yeux, ouverture si énorme que les os de la moitié inférieure du visage pendaient horriblement.[61]

> … he was struck violently by a sword blow that cut through his nose and along the middle of his cheeks, one side of his jaw was sliced through completely, the other side was damaged too, and his tongue was cut out at the root. He was left with a gaping hole below his eyes and the bones of his face could be seen hanging down in a horrible manner.

According to the account it was only through the kindness of his close friends that he was able to stay alive for nearly three months. They fed him some thick nourishing liquids, dripping them into the huge hole that had once been his mouth. Unable to even speak, he used signs and gestures to request that he be carried to the abbey at St Foy, but before he could be taken there, he fell into a deep sleep dreaming of the good saint herself, seeming to see her repair the damage to his mouth and face. When he awoke, he put his hands to his face to find that it had been restored to its proper form and he discovered that he could even speak.[62] Later and more than once, he took himself to the abbey at St Foy to show the monks how he had been healed, being left with a thin red scar that marked the path where the sword had cut him across his face.[63]

Raymond's case has all the hallmarks of a repair done by a doctor, scar and all. It always seems convenient that these cicatrices were left to prove the existence of a miracle and in this case the word 'thin' seems to have been included if only to make the scar sound less sinister. If we consider the possibility that the injuries to his face were somewhat exaggerated to begin with and repaired by a female physician, then perhaps we are getting closer to the truth here. Henbane, the juice of the poppy plant or something similar used to dull the pain or put him to sleep during the procedure would have caused euphoric effects and an altered sense of reality perhaps even hallucinations, quite possibly making him believe that it was the young saint herself who had done the work.[64] Claiming to have seen St Foy would have been like gold dust to the monks of the abbey, something to be included in the final version of Raymond's entry into their collection of miracles. As for exaggerating the severity of the damage he suffered, it is the kind of thing that many of us do, it is just human nature. Something that begins as an accidental cut or gash to a leg or arm can become a near miss amputation after the story has been told a few times. These tales can then take on a life of their own as time goes by, becoming almost lethal events had we not been seen by a doctor when we did. Those living a thousand years ago, such as Raymond and his friends and even the monks at St Foy, were likely no different. Here again, it certainly would have suited the abbey, because the worse the wound had sounded then the more divine his healing would have seemed.

Miracles that occurred at a religious centre, after a pilgrimage had been undertaken, may also have involved a combination of things including the power of the individual's own mind. Call it faith, belief in a higher power, superstition or simply the *placebo effect*, the mind has tremendous power to heal the body. This phenomenon, known as the placebo effect, is a person's ability to heal themselves or improve their health because they are being treated by something or by someone in whom they believe. Numerous studies have been done to show that the placebo effect does have a positive and genuine therapeutic impact on a certain percentage of the population. The Program in Placebo Studies & Therapeutic Encounter, or PiPS, at the Harvard Medical School is one modern medical facility that has been researching and using this phenomenon for years to treat patients with medical problems of many different types.[65] There are other universities and hospitals applying this same principle, giving credibility to some of those individuals in the Middle Ages who were said to have been miraculously cured at the many sites of pilgrimage in Europe. Their faith in God or a saint would have had a significant impact on their ability to be healed.

These centres of religion did more than just house holy relics, they were also places of great learning, which included being at the literal cutting edge of medicine.[66] They kept important books on medicine, which were rare enough in themselves. During the twelfth century, St Evroult, where Orderic Vitalis spent most of his monastic life, was known to have had a copy of the works of Hippocrates, the great and ancient Greek physician.[67] As well as these precious volumes were those who understood and practised medicine, some of whom were very skilled physicians and surgeons. At Bath Abbey, in the latter part of the eleventh century a well-respected physician, John of Tours, became Bishop of Wells. He had made a great deal of money in the world outside the church by practising medicine before deciding on the monastic life at Bath.[68] In the early twelfth century, at the Abbey of Jervaulx in Yorkshire, a monk called Peter de Quincy from Savigny was said to be '... expert in the art of medicine ...'. It was because of his superior skills in dealing with wounds and diseases that he was asked to stay with Alan, Duke of Richmond in Yorkshire, eventually being given a piece of land for the monastery in thanks for his fine service in medicine.[69]

The medical and surgical skills of these men and women of religion were extremely important to medieval society. At times their work must have seemed miraculous to those who were treated by them. They may have been simple things, such as boosting the power of faith in those pilgrims suffering from something quite curable by providing them with medicine or a cure. In his translation of the miracles of St Thomas of Canterbury, Edwin Abbott suggested something similar: 'While the monks were mixing the blood with water might they not think themselves justified in blending the water with some medicinal drug?'[70]

At the other end of the scale, their skills could be quite remarkable as shown by an example from Nidaros in Norway, the medieval name for what is now Trondheim. Being one of Europe's most northerly sites of pilgrimage in the Middle Ages, due to the burial place and shrine of St Olaf (also Olav), it was a place recorded by the German chronicler Adam of Bremen as the capital of Norway where there were '... very great miraculous cures'.[71] Crowds of people flocked there hoping to be healed of what had ailed them, including one young man who was treated using an elaborate surgical procedure. A recent examination of a thirteenth-century skeleton excavated during the mid-1980s has highlighted the work of a very highly skilled surgeon working at Nidaros. The skeleton, recovered from a local cemetery, was that of a young man who died in his late twenties or perhaps early thirties.[72] It appears that this individual was born and lived not far from Nidaros and what sets him apart is the almost completely healed hole in his skull where a trepanation procedure had been performed.[73] Trepanation involves surgically peeling back the scalp and drilling a hole through an individual's skull. The operation was done to relieve pressure on the brain, remove bone fragments from a wound or to treat disease and mental illness, as will be seen later in other examples. There were any number of things that could have gone wrong during such a procedure, including infection, damage to the brain and of course death. Incredibly, this case represents the only known medieval example of trepanation from Norway and, in fact, it is one of only a handful that come from Scandinavia in the Middle Ages.[74] While trauma could have been the reason for the operation, disease may be more likely. This man survived the ordeal and lived for a considerable time after the operation as evidenced by the significant healing of his skull around the site where the hole was drilled. Even as far north as Trondheim, Norway such expertise as this was available at religious houses and shrines.[75] It is easy to see how a complicated procedure like this, done successfully, would have appeared to many as a miraculous cure. The term *miracle* is still commonly used by many to describe such healing, even if only casually. In serious cases like these, medieval nuns and monks would have had even more control over the miracle narrative with the patient recovering in their infirmary. If a pilgrim and his family and friends were going to shout 'miracle' to everyone that would hear it, as was common, those at the priory or monastery were certainly not going to complain.

At other times, these miracle accounts were far from miraculous, being just short-lived remedies, coincidences and incidents turned into morality tales or left as someone unhealed or even an odd mix of many things.[76] Less than miraculous was one thing, but worse than that were the complete frauds. These healing shrines were big business in the Middle Ages, bringing in huge sums of money and where there are riches to be had there are almost always fraudsters and cheats. The French monk Guibert of Nogent (c. 1055–c. 1125) described some of these contemporary tricksters in his text *On Saints and Relics*. He noted a situation that he himself had witnessed involving a young knight's squire who passed away a couple of days before Easter. He had lived near Beauvais in Northern France, dying on land belonging to a well-known abbot. Having expired on a holy day, some peasants began falsely attributing miracles to the young squire and before too long the lad's grave was covered with candles and other offerings from '… nearby ignorant country folk …', as Guibert put it bluntly.[77] A building was soon erected over the spot where he had been buried and many pilgrims began to arrive from as far away as Brittany. There were a lot who were fooled by these so-called miracles, venerating the shrine and bringing money and gifts in hopes of their own miracles. Lured by the offerings being brought to the site, the abbot and his monks encouraged fake miracles, people pretending to be deaf or mad, lame or crippled before being 'healed' at the grave of the knight's squire.[78] This only motivated more who really needed help to arrive with their money, hoping for a similar outcome.

One last area of note regarding these miracle accounts are the offerings of wax or silver that were given to a venerated saint or place of pilgrimage by those hoping to be healed or who had become well again.[79] These were often formed into the part or area of the body that was of concern, teeth, legs, ears, hands or even the entire physique, at times being life-sized.[80] These sorts of offerings hark back to more ancient times when stone, bronze and terracotta gifts, again in the shape of bodies or body parts, were left as offerings at temples in the hope of healing from injury or disease or as thanks for the same.[81] In 1672 Richard Strange published a book on the life and miracles of St Thomas, Bishop of Hereford, England (1218–82) in which he explained the findings of the papal commissioners who had examined the saint's shrine in 1307. They found a huge quantity of wax and silver figures of complete bodies, along with various parts of the human form.[82] There were also assorted gifts and mementos that had been left at the shrine for a similar purpose, jewels, gold, silk, crutches, carts and of particular interest to this subject were the quantity of weapons found, arrows, swords, spears and other items of war and violence.[83]

An example that may combine these wax offerings and potential trickery comes from Rocamadour. The account involves a man who stopped at the abbey, a knight called Senorez from Dordogne in South-Western France. It is important to note that in the early years Rocamadour lacked any famous relics that would seem to have attracted many devotees.[84] It was also a very difficult place to get to, being that it was located off the beaten track and required a steep climb up a mountain and yet still the pilgrims flocked there.[85] The entry seems to explain why they came so eagerly:

> Il vit là suspendues de nombreuses images de cire transpercées d'armes diverses, les unes d'une façon, les autres de l'autre; non seulement il n'y ajouta pas foi, mais mème il prétendit que c'etait pure tromperie, que ces images n'avaient pas été apportées par les pèlerins et qu'elles avaient été placées là par les gens du monastère.[86]

> He saw hanging there numerous wax images that had been pierced with various weapons, some in one way, others in another; not only did he not believe, but he claimed that it was pure deception, these offerings had not been brought there by the pilgrims, but they had been put there by the people of the monastery.

Senorez refused to believe that the offerings were genuine, so when the knight returned home, he was very vocal in his protests against the abbey telling anyone who would listen about the goings on there. He told people that he had not seen this practice anywhere and he had visited many other sites of pilgrimage.[87] Being more of a morality tale than a miracle, as some of these records from Rocamadour tend to be, Senorez was later paralysed by an unidentified illness. Of course, the entry blamed the coincidence of the malady on his blasphemous behaviour when he spoke out against the monks at Rocamadour. He was sick for more than two months before he was said to have repented, but still he was not cured as he was apparently not yet ready for forgiveness. Finally, as Senorez stated publicly that Rocamadour and its pierced wax figures were nothing but legitimate and sincere, he regained the use of his arms and legs.[88]

Being that this account of Senorez comes from the collection of miracles at Rocamadour, was this a way for the abbey to explain away so many of these offerings, while keeping quiet those who would question them? It is certainly true that it was a place famous for healing among knights and soldiers.[89] Presumably at least some of these offerings that Senorez witnessed were genuine and had been presented by those who had come there in search of healing.[90] Aside from their obvious illnesses and injuries, many knights and soldiers would have possessed the strength, stamina and assistance required to reach such an out of the way shrine.[91] Were some offerings added by the monks to increase their status as a centre of pilgrimage? It seems unlikely that we will ever understand the veracity of this account completely, but just maybe the good knight Senorez was on to the monks before circumstances and superstition changed his mind and allowed for the continued success of Rocamadour.

Along the way we will see a few more offerings of wax and silver and meet other warriors like Senorez from Dordogne and Raymond from Valières who turned to these saints and a Christian God in their search for healing. At times, a line or two will be devoted to the miracle portion of their accounts and in a few cases a little more time is spent on the particulars, but often it will not be mentioned, with the focus instead remaining on the warriors themselves, their problems and just how it was that they became well again after being the victims of war.

Chapter 3

Soldiers, Smiths and Safety

> The wounded must be cared for and granted quiet rest.
> *The Lay of the Nibelungs*[1]

A few of those who spent time looking after the casualties of war during the latter part of this 500-year period have already been identified in the first chapter, men such as Hugo de Lucca and William of Saliceto. Trying to pinpoint similar individuals from the earlier centuries does present a more difficult task. Some of the clues are there, such as the tenth-century law code of the Welsh king Hywel Dha, or Howel the Good, which stipulated that the royal physician was to follow the army into battle, but again names are hard to come by.[2] Moving forward, a greater number begin to come to light such as the eleventh-century Argentien, or Argentine, a surgeon and cup-bearer to William the Conqueror who appears to have been quite close to the action, being a medical officer in William's invasion forces: '… a surgeon named Argentien among a detachment of Norman knights sent to the monastery of Ely by William the Conqueror shortly after the invasion …'.[3]

There were more among William's men like Nigel the physician who would later become a part of the army of Roger of Montgomery, the Earl of Shrewsbury, for which he would receive Stanstow Manor in Shropshire for his services.[4] Quite often just a few facts like these are all that are known about many of these medieval practitioners of medicine. The surgeon called Roger Causcy is another about whom only a little is known. We know of his existence because of a request for the payment of 40*s*. made by the English Crown in 1301 in connection with his services in treating some of the soldiers in the army of Edward I of England: 'To Mr. Roger Causcy, surgeon, for his labours in healing footmen of the garrison of Stirling following the king and recently wounded near Beverley, by is own hands at Dunipace, 40s.'[5]

The details about those such as Argentien, Nigel and Roger Causcy are still of great value because their contributions add a few more pieces to the puzzle that represents the medicine of the medieval wounded. We will discover more men like them along the way, but as useful as their information is the presence of trained, male doctors looking after the ill and injured on or away from the field of battle is probably not a surprise, nor perhaps are the monks and nuns who were frequently at the forefront of medicine. The purpose of this chapter is to dig a little deeper to explore some of those who may not be the first that spring to mind when it comes to the treatment of combat casualties in the Middle Ages. Additionally, some of the methods used to keep these healers and those whom they treated safe from harm or further injury are also investigated.

Soldiers

> Hákon's men were dressing their wounds, and had been at it the whole night, beginning as soon as they landed, because so many were wounded.
> *Jomsviking Saga*[6]

Reliable casualty figures from medieval battles can at times be difficult to establish as chroniclers, poets and writers tended to exaggerate these numbers quite regularly.[7] The dead and wounded were commonly quantified using multiples of tens, hundreds and thousands, despite what the true figures might have been.[8] There are some sources though that may help to get us a little closer to the truth. The initial portion of the thirteenth-century *La chanson de la croisade contre les Albigeois*, written by William of Tudela, is one such record. He recounted the first siege of Toulouse in June 1211 when the casualty list seems to have been fairly large:

> … ils vont à leur rencontre et les frappent rudement, tellement que tant d'une part que de l'autre il y eut plus de cent tués, et bien cinq cents blessés, qui tous étaient saignants.[9]

> … they [the defenders of Toulouse] go to meet them striking hard, so much so that the fighting between the two sides caused more than a hundred to be killed, with five-hundred wounded, all of them left bleeding.

The numbers quoted are significant and while likely inaccurate to some degree we can still be reasonably certain that there were many that did not survive the violence and even more who were left damaged in some way. Certainly, there would have been a lot whose wounds were quite treatable, things such as lacerations, broken fingers and toes, muscle strains and contusions. However, a good deal of the other injuries would have been more serious and difficult to treat. This poem routinely details the terrible carnage that was apparent after many of the sieges and battles had finished, with reports of amputated limbs, entrails spilled onto the ground, burn injuries and on and on like a gruesome hit parade of medieval combat wounds.[10]

As noted earlier, this source makes it clear that there were doctors who attended to those that had been wounded in the fighting.[11] The teacher and surgeon Guillaume de Congenis was one of them, having been surgeon to Simon de Montfort, one of the leaders of the crusading forces.[12] Nevertheless, if the true count of the wounded is even close to the 500 reported by Tudela it likely represents casualty numbers that would have stretched the available medical resources to breaking point. This would have left a lot of the injured soldiers responsible for their own treatment, something that was not at all uncommon. Whether a conflict was large or small, fought with or without medical support, soldiers often had to perform first aid on themselves and each other.[13] A soldier's self care for their wounds was something that had existed prior to the Middle Ages and has continued into modern times with armies teaching their soldiers first-aid skills to make the number of injuries treated by medics and surgeons more manageable. During the Second World War Canadian soldiers were taught first-aid skills when they joined up. The training manual of 1943 shows that new recruits received twenty sessions of this kind of instruction as part of their basic education. Among the subjects taught were the care for burns and broken limbs, plus methods to control bleeding. Necessitated by this need for soldiers to look after themselves, the programme focused two of its classes on the topic entitled 'Soldier Giving First Aid to Himself'.[14] In 1982, there was similar training for British soldiers on their way to the Falklands War, which entailed intensive instruction in emergency medicine with a focus on self aid.[15]

An early reference to a warrior looking after his own injuries, if only to stabilize them, can be found in the Venerable Bede's *History of the English Church and People*. He recounted a battle in 679 between the Northumbrian King Egfrid and King Ethelred of the Mercians in which one of Egfrid's young warriors, called Imma, was hurt and knocked unconscious during the fighting. When he regained his wits the following morning, he found himself the lone survivor amid those who had perished in battle the previous day. Bede recorded that Imma had no choice but to bandage up his own wounds, rest himself and go in search of help.[16]

The authors of the Viking sagas, like Snorri Sturluson, frequently described how soldiers treated their own wounds and those of their comrades. In his *Heimskringla*, or *A History of the Norse Kings*, he famously related how King Magnus and his army fought at the Battle of Lyrskov Heath, but afterwards found themselves overwhelmed by the number of those who had been injured. Magnus had physicians, but there were just not enough of them to look after such a large number of casualties. Magnus then enlisted a dozen of his men who had 'the softest hands' to help bandage the wounded, something that sparked an interest in them to later seek further medical training.[17] In his *Gesta Danorum*, or *Danish History*, Saxo Grammaticus explained how an old soldier called Witolf gained medical knowledge through the experience of treating his own injuries, even going on to become a physician of some renown: 'Often struck himself by the missiles of the enemy, he had gained no slight skill in leechcraft by constantly tending to his own wounds.'[18]

The author of the twelfth-century French epic *La Chanson de Guillaume*, or *The Song of William*, offered more of the same do-it-yourself spirit as he outlined some of the medical skills found among a large force of injured French noblemen. Seeming to number well into the hundreds, they bound up their own wounds and assisted others in bandaging their injuries, some of which were quite serious.[19] Wine and water were also discovered and shared between the men, with those who were well enough helping the disabled to take a drink.[20] In the thirteenth-century French poem *Huon of Bordeaux* these emergency procedures were more than just temporary repairs, becoming a life and death situation according to the story. The tale features Gerard, the brother of Huon, who was stabbed in the side with a spear. He required the quick thinking and knowledge of his brother Huon who tore away a piece of his shirt to bind his brother's wound.[21] Gerard was in such pain that he collapsed twice, eventually having to be lifted onto a gentle palfrey and propped up by another knight as they rode along to safety.

It is, however, one of Chrétien de Troyes' works of the late twelfth century, *The Story of the Grail (Perceval)*, which is perhaps the most notable. Here the medical skills of the knight Gawain were described in much greater detail than any of the examples referenced above.[22] The story is another of de Troyes' that shines a light on what was apparently his own knowledge of medicine. Within this story Gawain came upon an injured knight who was later exposed as the malevolent Greoreas, an enemy of Gawain, who had suffered some severe sword wounds to his head and face.[23] Alongside Greoreas was a woman attempting to comfort him who was herself rather distraught. After quickly assessing the man's injuries Gawain left the couple but returned as fast as he could with a plant that was useful in relieving pain, something which he had managed to locate in a nearby hedgerow.[24] The woman was fearful that Greoreas had passed away in the intervening time, so Gawain quickly dismounted and began a more thorough examination of the knight. He first checked his pulse, temperature and breathing to discover that he was still very much alive. These basic steps taken by Gawain would be carried out by any modern First Responder or battlefield medic where a victim had been found so badly injured. Acting with a notable bedside manner, Gawain helped to calm the woman, reassuring her that the remedy he had found would help the injured man. He explained how '... according to the book ...' there was no better plant to place on a wound.[25] He continued to distract the woman from her grief by including her in the process of bandaging the injured man, requesting a clean wimple that could be used to make bandages. With her spirits lifted, she provided him with the one she was wearing, which Gawain soon cut into strips. Here again, in an urgent medical situation the use of clean bandages is a part of proper first-aid practice. The cloth strips were then used to bind the medicine to the knight's lacerations, with the maiden continuing to act as assistant to Gawain. According to de Troyes' own editorial comment, these last steps were the correct course of action to be taken.[26]

Far more than just fantasy, these writers were influenced by something quite genuine. Further evidence shows that many of these soldiers did possess the kind of knowledge ascribed to them, gained either through experience or training. In the middle of the fourteenth century the important French surgeon Guy de Chauliac (*c.* 1300–68), completed his work entitled *La grande chirurgie*, or *The Great Surgery*. Included within it is a history of medicine up to that point in time in which he discussed some of the noteworthy factions or sects as he called them, those who had influenced medicine and helped to push it forward. The first three were made up of medieval surgeons that included Roger Frugard, Theodoric and William of Saliceto.[27] Significantly, in the fourth sect were German knights and warriors whom he said treated their own wounds with things like herbs, wool, oil and whatever else they had to hand, using incantations to increase their efficacy.[28]

In the early part of the thirteenth century the German knight and poet Wolfram von Eschenbach wrote a version of de Troyes' *The Story of the Grail (Perceval)* entitled *Parzival*, which offers some proof of de Chauliac's claims. The knight in this case was suffering from a serious chest wound, instead of the facial injuries of de Troyes' version. When Gawain came upon the wounded knight and grieving woman the warrior's chest was quickly filling with fluid. Gawain then suggested the following:

> The wound is not all too dangerous, but the blood on his heart doth press.
> Then he stripped from a bough of the linden the bark, and did wind it round,
> (No fool he in art of healing) and he set it unto the wound,
> And he bade the maiden suck it till the blood should toward her flow –
> And strength came again and hearing, and the voice of the knight they know,[29]

A chest wound filling with blood and fluid is potentially life-threatening. What makes this procedure of drawing it out so intriguing is the fact that it was quite likely a tried and true method that von Eschenbach had witnessed or experienced. It contains the kind of rough and ready medicine Guy de Chauliac suggested was practised by German knights when he named them in his *Chirurgia Magna*. Interestingly, even the use of incantations is confirmed just a few lines after the above quoted passage, something which de Chauliac had accused them of practising:

> With the band from the maiden's tresses Gawain the wound did bind,
> And spake o'er it spells of healing, and he bade them their comfort find[30]

It was not just German knights who possessed such medical knowledge. In English law of the thirteenth century, *essoin*, or a reason for not attending court, was something that had to be proven. When the cause of the *essoin* was said to be health related the law provided for an evaluation to be carried out by a group of four knights. They were sent to the absent man's place of residence to diagnose whether he was feigning illness and injury to avoid court or truly unwell. This went even further, as part of their responsibility was to establish the degree of his disability: 'The knights should view the body of the sick man and carefully inquire about the kind of illness and the circumstances and decide accordingly whether it is a passing illness or a grave illness.'[31]

Certainly, a knight's standing in society represented part of the reason for this assignment, but doubtless there was more to it than just class. As well as wounds, these warriors would have gathered a great deal of knowledge in the recognition and treatment of diseases since armies were constantly under siege from invisible enemies like dysentery. They would have been well equipped to judge the fitness of such a person who claimed to be unable to get himself to court.

Leaving injuries and illnesses to those who were not doctors did come with some risks and problems, as Guillaume de Congenis explained to his students at Montpellier in the early part of the thirteenth century. A scholar who recorded the teachings of de Congenis revealed what could happen when a little knowledge turned out to be a dangerous thing. The injured warrior in this case had received a serious wound to his arm, which had been stitched up by other knights. Unfortunately, they failed to properly cleanse, cauterize and prepare the damaged area before doing so and gangrene soon set in resulting in the death of the unfortunate knight.[32]

Women and the Wounded

> ... as a dressing she put on his wounds
> two of the white linen bandages.
>
> *The Romance of Yder*[33]

Women too practised medicine and healing during the medieval period, including the treatment and care of the casualties of war. In fact, as Dr Faye Getz and many others have noted, '... women must have performed much if not most medical care in the Middle Ages ...'.[34] Unfortunately, we have been left with just a handful of their names, such as the twelfth-century Trota of Salerno and Hildegard of Bingen, the only known female medical authors whose works have survived.[35] Matilda and Solicita, the sisters of John, were physicians and part of a medical family in twelfth- and early thirteenth-century England.[36] In London, Katherine 'la surgiene', c. 1286, was the daughter of Thomas and brother of William, both of whom were also surgeons.[37] In thirteenth-century Lyon, Stephanie, the daughter of Etienne de Montaneis, was referred to as *medica*.[38] Margery, a leech practising in Worcestershire, England in around 1300, was thrown into a river by a man called Roger Oldrich. He was apparently trying to establish whether she was a witch. The incident ended up in court where witnesses thankfully came to Margery's aid. In the end, the court found against Roger, but the situation highlights the potential hazards of being a woman and a healer at this time.[39] There are others whose names have survived, but the list of known female doctors and healers pales in comparison with that of their male counterparts.[40] Thankfully, the contemporary literature of this period is one place that does not hide the work that these women did, especially as it pertains to the treatment of those who were injured in battle. Their voices can be heard loud and clear across the stanzas and pages of these works as they cared for the sick and wounded with great skill and expertise.

The Latin version of *Walter of Aquitaine*, known as *Waltharius*, is a good place to begin. Dating from the tenth century and written at the Abbey of St Gall, in what is today Switzerland, it was a well-known tale told right across Europe in the early centuries of the Middle Ages. Within the story a violent fight led to some rather serious casualties all of which were treated by a woman called Hiltgunt, the wife of Waltharius.[41] Unfortunately, the poem gives away little in terms of the methods used to deal with such significant wounds, but importantly it was a woman who held the role of healer. At the other end of these five centuries is Iseut or Iseult, from a thirteenth-century rendering of the *Tristan* legend, a girl who was looked upon as a great healer with her skills being key to many versions of the story. This particular account provides an especially glowing description of her medical aptitude. Before she had even reached 14 years of age the intelligent Iseut was already being described as remarkably talented with cures and remedies, understanding the potency and usefulness of plants and herbs. Whatever the type of wound or injury, '… she could deal with successfully and heal'.[42]

Female practitioners appear regularly in the Viking sagas too, like the mistress Olöf found in *Thordar's Saga*, a woman who lived in Northern Iceland in a place called Miklibær where she was described as one of the best leeches.[43] Some of these women apparently ended up close to the fighting, including the wife of Viga-Glum called Halldora, recalled in *The Saga of Viga-Glum*. Aware of a small skirmish that had broken out, she and some other women made their way to the fighting to look after the injured. The battle was still being fought when they arrived, but Halldora began attending to the wounded right away. A warrior called Thorarin had received a deep laceration to his shoulder, so bad was the damage that his lungs could be seen. The saga says that Halldora not only bound up Thorarin's injuries, but she also remained with him until the skirmish was over so she could safeguard him from any further harm.[44]

The Battle of Stiklestad is chronicled in the *Saga of Olaf Haraldson*, a part of Snorri Sturluson's *Heimskringla*. Inside the saga, Sturluson included one of the most informative passages dealing with the treatment of wounds found anywhere in the Viking sagas.[45] A barn reminiscent of the Regimental Aid Posts and Advanced Dressing Stations from the wars of the past century is recounted.[46] Near the field of battle, beside a group of houses, this shed contained a separate chamber where the pain and terror of the wounded could be heard coming from inside. Caring for these warriors were several women, some of whom tended to the fire being used to heat water and broth, while others bathed and treated wounds and dealt with the dead and those soon to be deceased.[47]

Like the Aid Posts and Dressing Stations of the First and Second World Wars, this scene in the barn points to some forethought and preparation ahead of the conflict. A suitable building close to the battle had to be located as did equipment and supplies, which then had to be readied. Most importantly were the women who were chosen for their ability to heal the wounded. Their ethnicity is not mentioned in the saga, but of course there is the strong possibility that they were not of Scandinavian origin, having been captured or traded as slaves, because of their skills in the healing arts.[48] Beyond that fact, plans and simple protocols would have been necessary to establish the inner workings of such a makeshift relief centre. As will be seen in the next chapter, something like a triage system had been set up to treat stomach wounds. There are other things not mentioned in this passage, which seemingly would have been a part of such an emergency medical set-up. Amputations, bone setting, suturing and pain management would have required skill and experience on the part of those working within such a setting. As it is today, the ability to work effectively under such conditions would have needed expertise and a personality able to deal with the screams, smells, blood and gore, plus the dangers associated with being so close to the front lines of the battle.

The sort of physician who might have treated wounds in the saga above can be found in an enticing reference to a woman who came from far afield in the manuscript called *Vita Haroldi Regis*, or *The Life of King Harold*. Written in around 1216, it describes the survival of England's King Harold at the Battle of Hastings in 1066, despite his many wounds.[49] According to this chronicle, he was taken from the battlefield to Winchester where 'he was cured by a certain woman, a Saracen, very skilled in the art of surgery'.[50] While Harold Godwinson's survival at the Battle of Hastings is highly unlikely and not supported by most other chroniclers, a surgeon described as female and from the Islamic world, living and working in Anglo-Saxon England is worth considering. It does seem to be quite a specific detail and Winchester was indeed a busy, cosmopolitan place at that time, so a skilled female physician from far away is not unexpected.[51] At a minimum it is another illustration of the movement of people, including female physicians, across the earlier medieval world either of their own accord or by more sinister means like the slave-trading networks. Another female doctor from the Islamic world, named Josain, is included in the English romance *Sir Beves of Hampton*. She was the wife of Sir Beves and was very well educated in both 'physic and surgery'. The story relates that she had studied under the great masters at both Toledo and Cologne.[52] Clearly the author intended her as a very learned woman of medicine, with skills incorporating the influences of the Islamic world from Toledo in Spain, along with those of Western Europe through Cologne in what is now Germany.

The number of poets and authors from these centuries who used female surgeons and healers in their stories involving the casualties of tournaments and war is considerable and must surely point to the fact that they existed beyond the written page. Included in de Troyes' first epic romance *Erec and Enide* are two sisters who were both surgeons: 'I have two charming and sprightly sisters who are skilful in the care of wounds; they will soon completely cure you ... First, they removed the dead flesh, then applied plaster and lint, devoting to his care all their skill, like women who knew their business well.'[53]

In *The Romance of Yder* we find Guenloie who was able to treat her lover Yder for his serious wound from a lance.[54] In the later thirteenth- or early fourteenth-century tale *The History of Fulk Fitz Warine, an Outlawed Baron in the Reign of King John* two injured knights were taken to a tower called Pendover where their wounds were looked after by the lady of the keep along with others who provided nursing care for wounded: 'And the lady and her daughters and their damsels every day comforted and solaced Sir Walter and Sir Arnald de Lys'.[55]

Throughout history when men have decided to go to war women have always responded in huge numbers to treat and comfort the sick and wounded. The two world wars of the twentieth century saw women in their tens of thousands in this capacity. In the nineteenth century, the famous American author Louisa May Alcott wrote about her brief experiences as a nurse during the American Civil War in her book *Hospital Sketches*: 'The sight of several stretchers, each with its legless, armless or desperately wounded occupant, entering my ward admonished me that I was there to work ...'.[56] The Middle Ages do not appear to have been any different in terms of women treating the war wounded. In fact, the above passage could just as easily be describing the thoughts of one of the women treating the Viking wounded at the Battle of Stiklestad in eleventh-century Norway as those of Louise May Alcott in a Union Army hospital in 1860s' America.

The Blacksmith as a Healer

> ... a red-hot iron was placed into the injured hand, causing no sensation ...
> *The Miracles of St Foy*[57]

There were others who practised medicine too like the bonesetters and barber-surgeons of these centuries, plus there was another more unusual group that can often be found hiding in plain sight, the blacksmiths or in fact metalsmiths of any type. As odd as it might seem at first blush, these metalworkers were frequently relied upon by medieval society not just for their skills at the forge, but for their perceived powers of healing as well. Evidence of their work can be found in unusual places like the miracle collections of St Foy and Rocamadour, as the examples below will show. Even beyond this period the dual role of metalworker and physician can still be seen in a man called Richard Knyght who in the mid-fifteenth century was known as a physician, surgeon, ironmonger and doctor for dogs (dogleche).[58]

Well before the period under investigation here smiths held an unusual position in society, which was both respected and feared. The notion of being able to create useful and appealing things from rocks and minerals helped to bring about this fearful reverence toward the smith. These workers in metal were thought to possess almost magical powers, being 'half-technician and half-magician'.[59] Many believed they were in league with the Devil, providing useful services to him, without paying the price of their souls.[60] This helps to explain their inclusion in the later eleventh- or early twelfth-century Irish manuscript *Liber Hymnorum*, which contains St Patrick's hymn asking for protection against women, smiths and magicians.[61] With that said, they were simply too valuable to society and the church to be excluded completely, meaning that as long as they were seen to be practising Christianity then they were nervously accepted.[62]

Sought by everyone from the sick and wounded to pregnant women who were concerned about childbirth, the metalsmith's healing touch was commonly practised in an unusual manner. The afflicted person was placed over an anvil by the smith who would then take up one of his hammers and feign a blow to the part of the body that was of concern.[63] This practised bluff, which was meant to bring about a cure by *hammering* the problem out of the ill or injured person, appears in an entry from the mid-eleventh-century records at St Foy. An unnamed soldier from Auvergne sought the guidance and help of the good saint, because he was troubled by what appears to have been an inguinal hernia, which is to say a small portion of his intestines had dropped into his scrotum. His condition caused him to lose his prestigious position as a mounted warrior, being relegated to the rank of a humble foot soldier.[64] After prostrating himself for a night in prayer at the abbey he believed St Foy herself had spoken to him. Although she was unable to cure the long-suffering man, she advised him to return home and seek out the local blacksmith for help:

> Allez le trouver au plus tôt, et priez-le de s'armer de son marteau le plus lourd, celui dont il se sert pour broyer le fer ardent qui sort de la fournaise, et de frapper de toutes ses forces sur votre mal que vous aurez étalé sur son enclume; vous serez alors subitement guéri.[65]

> Go and find him [blacksmith] as quickly as possible, and ask him to get out his heaviest hammer, the one he uses to crush the iron as it comes out of the furnace, and strike as hard as he can on that which afflicts you, which you will spread across his anvil; and suddenly you will be healed.

The smith was consulted, but at first he was said to have been very reluctant to perform the procedure. In the end all was agreed and the soldier placed his softer parts across the blacksmith's anvil and awaited his fate, but once he saw the muscular arms of the blacksmith holding the heavy hammer high in the air he fell backwards in terror. It was this backward fall that was said to have jarred everything back into place bringing about a cure for his hernia.[66]

This entry has the feel of a successful secular procedure performed by a blacksmith, perhaps made to sound fortuitous and then claimed by the church and 'Christianized' so it could be included in this collection of miracles. The addition of St Foy, her inability to cure the problem, but sending the soldier off to see a reluctant blacksmith all sound as if they have been included after the fact to legitimize this story to the church's benefit. Also unusual is the fact that this was a second-hand account, although apparently from an abbot, providing no opportunity for the abbey to question the soldier himself:

> Nous invoquons à l'appui le témoignage de Robert, abbé du monastère de Chanteuge, vieillard des plus graves et des plus vénérables. C'est de lui que nous tenons ce récit.[67]

> We have the testimony of Robert, abbot of the monastery of Chanteuge, a venerable and serious man of some age. He is the one who related this story.

Another instance shows a blacksmith using different skills to heal, as he extracted an arrow from the face of a knight after all else had failed to work. Coming from the miracle collection of Rocamadour, in the second half of the twelfth century, the entry involves a knight called Henry of Mâchecourt who had been struck in the face by an arrow close to his eye. Surgeons had been unable to locate the weapon, despite cutting a significant opening into Henry's face. The wound became badly infected making the knight very ill and causing him a great deal of discomfort. Henry reached the point where he could no longer chew his food and so he gradually deteriorated. Death seemed to him a better option than the agony he felt from the arrow and the contamination it had caused.[68] He set off on a pilgrimage to Rocamadour where he got no relief despite his devotions. On the advice of the monks he returned home, but in a much weaker state than he had been before. However, according to the account Henry did not lose faith and after apparently feeling an itch in the wound he consulted a blacksmith who successfully and painlessly extracted the arrow from the knight's face.[69] This is another case of what appears to have been a blacksmith's successful work being heavily downplayed and overshadowed in the narrative produced by the church. Rocamadour claimed the healing as their own because of Henry's faith and his earlier visit to the abbey, being ever cautious and even fearful of the blacksmith's work. However, it is clear the smith must have done far more than he is given credit for here. There was a considerable amount to be dealt with, not least of which was extracting an arrow from a very delicate part of the knight's face. In addition, there would have been healing scars from the initial surgery and the serious infection to treat. Henry is without doubt one of those lucky few who beat the massive odds against him and while his faith would have helped, it was the work of the blacksmith that seems to have saved him.

Safety

> ... the English in great trouble fell back
> upon their standard, where were collected the maimed and wounded.
>
> *Roman de Rou*[70]

The practitioners of medicine and the wounded they treated regularly found themselves in quite vulnerable positions and in need of protection from harm or further damage. The twelfth-century memoirs of the Islamic writer Usāmah ibn Munqidh contain an example of the sort of peril that was faced by both doctors and the injured. It describes the account of a Syrian bonesetter who narrowly escaped death as he fixed the lower leg bones of a soldier injured by a stone thrown from a mangonel. As he set about his work a second stone came and struck the man he was treating, killing him on the spot and just narrowly missing the bonesetter.[71] Other practitioners were not quite so fortunate, as the *Calendar of Chancery Warrants* from early fourteenth-century England recorded. An entry for 3 March 1317 at Clarendon provides some detail about Henry le Leche (or Leech): 'Henry le Leche (physician) has long stayed in Scotland attending to people who have been wounded there on the service of the king's father and the king, and has been maimed there on the king's service, and the king wishes to provide him with sustenance for life.'[72] There are a few remarkable facts contained within this entry. First, it appears that Henry le Leche had been on a mission of mercy in Scotland for quite some time. Edward II's father, Edward I, died in 1307 and had been fighting with Scotland for years before his death. Some of these men who had been 'wounded' must have been there in Scotland for a considerable period of time. Henry, who was very much in enemy territory, was then maimed while looking after these soldiers. Edward II acknowledged Henry's bravery and the work he had done as he looked to have him cared for in an 'abbey, priory, hospital or other house of religion' for the balance of his life.[73] A similar request, this time four days later, was made for a man called Ralph Russel of Keirwent who had also remained in Scotland on behalf of both Edward I and his son.[74]

The end of this chapter provides an opportunity to explore how some of these healers and those whom they treated were shielded on the battlefield and beyond. *La chanson de la croisade contre les Albigeois* relates how something as simple as the dark of night was able to bring a halt to the fighting, allowing the doctors to begin their work.[75] Similarly, things like exhaustion or an unofficial truce became ways of providing a reasonably safe opportunity to get them onto the battlefield to treat the wounded. This was the case at Beaucaire in August 1216, as the crusaders tried unsuccessfully to capture the city. A break in the fighting allowed those with medical skills, from both sides, to look after the many who were suffering from their injuries:

Quand les Français virent qu'ils n'avaient rien de plus à gagner, ils revinrent à leurs tentes, et ceux de la ville à leurs demeures. Des deux côtés les médecins et les maréchaux demandent des oeufs, de l'eau, de l'étoupe, du sel, des onguents, des emplâtres, des bandes d'étoffe pour les coups et les blessures douloureuses.[76]

Once the French saw that they had nothing further to gain they went back to their tents and those in the city returned to their homes. At this point the physicians and marshals requested eggs, water, tow, salt, ointments, plasters and cloth strips to treat those who had been wounded.

Shielding the casualties of battle could also mean just passing them back through the lines to a central point away from direct harm where they could be cared for and treated. According to Master Wace, who chronicled the Norman conquest of England in his *Roman de Rou*, this was a method employed by the English army at the Battle of Hastings in 1066.[77] Another technique apparently involved soldiers hiding among the dead to keep safe from the enemy, a tactic that is commonly depicted in modern war films. A warrior covers himself in the blood and gore of others and remains motionless on or under the dead to provide camouflage against enemy soldiers looking to slaughter those still alive. Turning again to Master Wace, he explained the concerns of the Normans after the Battle of Hastings was over:

> Many an Englishman lies bloody and mingled with the dead, but yet sound, or only wounded and besmeared with gore; tarrying of his own accord, and meaning to rise at night, and escape in the darkness ... Let a careful watch be set this night, for we know not what snares may be laid for us.[78]

The early twelfth-century Irish text *War of the Gaedhil with the Gaill* offers a few more clues about the safety of the sick and injured, along with those who were to care for them. It recalls the aftermath of the famous Irish Battle of Clontarf in April 1014 in which the great Irish leader Brian Boru fought against rival Hiberno-Norse factions. Brian was killed in the battle and soon after there were ill feelings among some of his forces, especially between the men of Dal Cais and Deas-Mumhain (Desmond). The chieftains of Desmond wanted to press their claim for dominance over the province of Munster. The Dalcassians, under the leadership of one of Brian's surviving sons, Donnchadh, coveted the same thing, but many of his men had been injured in the earlier battle. Ahead of the clash between the two sides it was Donnchadh's plan to protect his wounded soldiers by placing them in a nearby fort where they would be shielded and looked after by a third of his surviving men.[79] A sound plan to be sure, but according to the chronicle the wounded Dalcassians wanted none of it, wishing to be a part of the fight. Fortunately, the men of Desmond admired their bravery and decided not to push their advantage and the fight was called off. On their way back home the Dalcassians were once again troubled as they tried to cross through the hostile territory of the Osraighe (Ossary). It seemed clear that there would be a battle so the disabled Dalcassians secured large stakes of wood from a nearby forest and planted them into the ground. The idea was to have the wounded lean against the stakes to keep upright, allowing them to protect themselves and be of some use in the fight. Once again, the opposition decided against violence after seeing such bravery.[80] A method reminiscent of the strategy employed by the Dalcassians can be found in the twelfth-century French epic *La Chanson de Guillaume*. Within the ranks of the French were warriors that had suffered damage to their arms, but who could still make use of their shoulders. To enable them to still stick and stab with their spears they had them shortened and tied to their arms, providing at least some defence against further attack and injury.[81]

Abbot Suger of St Denis recalled something altogether different in the twelfth-century battle preparations made by the French that would enable both the physicians and casualties to be protected. Suger explained that across the field of conflict the French planned to surround their injured and exhausted soldiers with wagons and carts to form 'the defences of a castle'.[82] These portable relief centres, created by circling carts and wagons, were meant to provide a safe area for the wounded to be treated and the exhausted to be refreshed with both water and wine being made available.[83]

Lastly, hospitality, safety and a greater access to trained physicians sometimes led armies to take their wounded to the closest farm, castle or community so that they could be looked after.[84] The famous thirteenth-century poem *The Song of Dermot* explains one of these makeshift situations:

> Rather we shall go to Leighlin
> At our ease along the direct road;
> Thus we shall carry our wounded
> Who lie hurt on the battlefield …
> Towards Ferns they turned;
> With them they carry their wounded.
> When they came to the city,
> Then they severally went their ways.
> To their hostels to lodge
> The knights returned.
> They sent everywhere for physicians
> To heal the sick:
> To heal their wounded
> They sent everywhere for physicians.[85]

This common-sense approach of evacuating the injured to a populated area, away from the battlefield, was practised from the Viking era through to the latter stages of the Middle Ages. Those who were simply exhausted and in need of rest and sustenance could find food and lodging, while the wounded could be treated more safely and in greater numbers, often with more specific care for things such as fractures and dislocations.[86]

Chapter 4

Wounds and Surgery

Spreading wounds and death through their ranks by showers of arrows and bolts.

Orderic Vitalis[1]

A mid-eleventh-century entry from the miracles of St Foy provides an account of the siege of a castle, complete with battering rams, catapults and scaling ladders. This attack was led by a man called Giselfroy, a lord who had among his men a knight named Mathfred.[2] According to the record, Mathfred was struck in the face by an arrow, with the missile hitting him below the eye and plunging deep within the tissues of his face.[3] Attempts to remove the arrow caused the wooden shaft to separate from the metal tip, leaving it lost inside him:

> On arracha le bois, mais le fer demeura dans la plaie. Les médecins employèrent toutes les ressources de leur art; mais ils furent forcés de déclarer que la flèche s'était enfoncée dans les profondeurs du crane et qu'ils ne connaissaient aucun moyen de la retirer sans danger de mort.[4]

The wooden shaft came away, leaving the iron inside of the wound. The doctors tried everything within their ability, but were forced to declare that the arrow had sunk deep into the skull and that they knew of no way of removing it without danger of death.

Unusually for a miracle account, the doctors who treated Mathfred were referred to as accomplished men of medicine.[5] Even so, these doctors struggled to find a method of locating and removing the tip of the arrow. They considered a surgical procedure to try and expose it, but in the end decided against such a course of action. One of the doctors did try to find the arrow using a cautery as a probe but had no success. As the days passed the knight's wife continued to pray fervently to St Foy for her husband's safety, but his condition only worsened. Finally, as Mathfred lay unconscious one of the doctors treating him was said to have spotted the edge of the arrow, which allowed him to then remove it successfully. The knight eventually regained consciousness having survived his brush with death from this most prolific weapon of medieval warfare.[6] He made a full recovery and later travelled to the abbey to explain what had happened to him.

What separates this account from so many others is the considerable detail that makes clear the severity of such an injury and the knight's poor health in the days that followed. While the information about Mathfred's healing is vague, it seems that the physician must surely have had more involvement than just suddenly discovering an edge of the arrow and sliding it out. Did the passage of time allow the swelling to dissipate enough to enable the doctor to see it and perform the extraction or was surgery the answer that finally turned the tide and saved Mathfred?[7] Unfortunately, there is just not enough information to try and piece together the truth of what occurred.

This chapter seeks to investigate further the treatment of injuries like the one received by Mathfred, being that they were among the most common types of casualties. As well, wounds to the stomach and intestines are considered, as they could be some of the most notoriously difficult to repair followed by a discussion around limb amputations, injuries that were life-changing in nature. Lastly, methods used by medieval practitioners to aid and speed recovery in their patients are reviewed briefly. Many examples of medieval surgical treatments covered within this chapter show the skill and ingenuity of the doctors, healers and knights who performed them and of course there are one or two where quite the opposite was also true.

Before returning to injuries caused by bolts and arrows a brief examination of their construction is likely worthwhile. These were missiles that could be fired from an assortment of weapons including crossbows, bows and heavier ballistae equipment, some of which could send them with incredible force.[8] Gerald of Wales, for instance, described an arrow shot by a twelfth-century Welsh archer that went through and through the armour and leg of a mounted soldier before puncturing the saddle of his horse and mortally wounding the animal.[9] Projectiles came in a multitude of armour piercing, flesh-tearing forms and sizes, some with large heads and others fitted with smaller ones, numerous kinds of barbed arrows, as well as those made in different shapes, concave, flat, triangular and square.[10] There are even reports of unusual items like steel linen combs being used to tip the shafts of arrows.[11] Shot with some velocity they would have caused considerable damage to exposed flesh.

Some arrowheads were affixed to the wooden shaft using a pin or some similar device, but as Mathfred's case shows the tip of an arrow could also be secured using only beeswax, glue or some comparable substance. The body heat of the victim would soften the adhesive enabling the shaft to separate easily from the arrowhead, leaving a rusty piece of iron inside the individual.[12] A revealing extract from a request for payment in August 1304, during the first Scottish War of Independence, provides an idea of warfare on a large scale, including the requirements and costs necessary to produce and ship arrow components north from England to Edward I's army at Stirling in Scotland where they were then assembled with the use of glue:

> ... for 29 'balistae', 59 bows, 540 arrows, 420 staffs to make arrows, 336 goosewings, 360 feathers, 200 arrow heads, and 3 qrs. glue, bought by the King's orders to send to Stirling for the assault on the castle 119s. 11 ½d.;

small expenses, canvas rope and packing the bows, 3*s*. 10*d*.; carriage of a cask with the King's quarrels found at Newcastle, to Stirling, 30*s*.; baskets for the arrows, straw and hay to roll round the balistae, string and wax to feather the new arrows, 15 ½*d*.; for 5 hackneys carrying the above from Newcastle to Stirling and a man with them 29*s*.; wages of 4 men making arrows at 4*d*. each daily; and two boys attending them, at 2*d*. each, sent to Stirling for 8 days on 2nd June, 13*s*. 4*d*.[13]

Whether aimed directly or loosed en masse these missiles could create terrible panic and carnage among opposing soldiers. Even a less than skilled bowman, as part of a larger group of archers, could cause harm, as Snorri Sturluson rightly observed in his *Heimskringla*.[14] The Viking sagas described the arrow storms of battle in many inventive ways, with 'The twigs of the corpse' and 'The hail of the wound' being two particularly colourful representations, each telling its own five-word short story.[15] As Abbo of Saint-German-des-Prés recalled the Viking attacks on Paris, he likened their clouds of arrows to a 'swarm of bees'.[16] Norman armies used thunderstorms of arrows to great effect against the French at Varaville in 1057 and in 1066 at Hastings while fighting the English.[17] Literary sources of these centuries also made similar references to those found in the chronicles and archives. Chrétien de Troyes' twelfth-century *Cligés* compared the arrows and stones fired from crossbows and slings to being like rain mixed with hail.[18]

Caltrops, or calthrops, the static but dangerous cousins of the arrow, are also worthy of a mention here. They could be spread across the ground in large numbers to disable enemy horses and soldiers on foot. They were formed in such a way so that when dropped they landed with a sinister spike sticking straight up and while some had simple, straight points others were fashioned with barbed tips making them more difficult to extract: 'Meantime the renown of the Danish bravery spread far, and moved the Irish to strew iron calthrops on the ground, in order to make their land harder to invade, and forbid access to their shores.'[19] There were various tools and means employed to remove arrows and calthrops, everything from tongs and forceps for pulling them out, to more specialized equipment used to recover them and even less conventional methods such as the use of magnets to locate and retrieve fragments of metal.[20] Snorri Sturluson's *Heimskringla* included the use of forceps to extract an arrow at the Battle of Stiklestad in eleventh-century Norway. During the fighting a poet and warrior on the side of King Olaf, called Thormod Kolbrunarskald, was seriously wounded in his left side by an arrow. He was able to make his way to the nearby barn where the casualties were being looked after and he too was treated by one of the female healers. The swelling around his wound was such that the woman had to cut an opening into his flesh to enable her to reach the arrow with her forceps, but even so she was still unable to free the weapon.[21] 'Then Thormod took the tongs, and pulled the iron out; but on the iron there was a hook, at which there hung some morsels of flesh from the heart, some white, some red.'²² This passage makes clear the difficulty caused by trying to extract barbed arrows in this manner, tearing away flesh as they were pulled out. We are told that Thormod died of his injuries a short time later. The use of forceps to remove an arrowhead does appear elsewhere in the sagas. The *Eyrbyggja Saga* mentions the use of pincers to remove one that was lodged in the neck of a man called Snorri Thorbrandsson. He was one of two brothers who were wounded during a small battle. They were rescued by another man named Snorri, this one a temple priest and healer, who took them back to his farm where he tended to both brothers. Here again, the wooden shaft had come away from the arrowhead, but Snorri managed to locate the offending point at the base of Thorbrandsson's throat by using his hands to feel for it and then with pincers he was able to successfully draw it out.[23]

Going forward to the twelfth-century miracle collection from Rocamadour, there is a report of a man called Hubert of Pierrelatte in Burgundy who was wounded by an arrow that hit him in the chest.[24] According to the entry, the arrowhead remained lodged under his right breast for three-and-a-half years with surgeons being unable to remove it or heal the associated wound. Sending a wax effigy on ahead to Rocamadour, Hubert then made his way to the abbey in the hope of getting better. We are told that while there he was unable to convince the good Lady of Mercy that he was deserving of immediate healing.[25] Returning back home in the same poor health as when he left, Hubert summoned one of his servants to bring some tongs to try and remove the offending piece of iron. The servant was said to have been reluctant at first, but eventually he did so, being able to work the arrowhead back and forth within the rotting flesh until it finally came out.

While the account has some notes of truth, there are a few layers that likely need to be peeled away to expose what may be a more accurate reflection of what happened. First, on the matter of the tip of the arrow being lodged inside Hubert for three-and-a-half years this does seem extremely unlikely, especially with a festering wound. This record also contains strong hints that the servant who treated him could have been a metalsmith, not unlike those who treated men such as Henry of Mâchecourt and the unnamed soldier from Auvergne, described in the previous chapter.[26] Hubert had sought the assistance of the medical community and then the church, but neither were able to help him. It makes sense that he would have turned to an alternative source for help at that point, but with the church controlling the narrative they would have had every reason to want to minimize this fact, turning it instead into something more divine thanks to Hubert's earlier visit to the abbey. The so-called servant was even described in a derogatory manner, being just a rustic man, nervous and perfectly incapable of such a task.[27] It is difficult to believe that a humble, skittish attendant could manage to accomplish what surgeons had been unable to do. Instead, this man appears to have had at least some knowledge of medicine to have been able to perform the extraction and then treat the associated infection.[28]

Found in Peter of Eboli's *Liber ad Honorem Augusti* and dating from the late twelfth century is one of the earliest illustrations of the treatment of an arrow injury. It shows Count Richard of Acerra, a Norman nobleman, having been struck by an archer's arrow during the Siege of Naples in 1191.[29] The image shows how the weapon had gone through and through his face, with blood pouring out from the right cheek. In another part of the illustration Count Richard is being looked after by a man referred to as 'medic' and importantly his two female assistants, each carrying items pertaining to the treatment. The man has a hold of the shaft of the arrow, attempting to remove it from Count Richard. Such a wound must have damaged more than just his cheeks, with his teeth, tongue or palate likely to have been impacted as well. Count Richard did survive this injury, going on to live for another five years.

The selection of arrow injuries in this chapter is indicative of the wide variety of practitioners of medicine who treated wounds like these, men and women, professionals with their assistants, the less formally educated and the soldiers themselves. With that in mind we can proceed for the first time into the leechbooks and surgical texts to see what they had to offer in terms of instructions. Beginning with *Bald's Leechbook* and *Leechbook III* there are several salves included for wounds, with some that could be used specifically for those caused by iron weapons, but there is little that is well defined regarding the extraction of arrows.[30] As discussed in the initial chapter of this work, this likely points to the sort of commonplace procedure that was already understood and practised by the leech and as such required only the details for the remedies and salves that were to be used.

Roger Frugard's late twelfth-century surgery is very different, with directives to treat a variety of arrow wounds. He understood the difficulty involved in removing the heads of arrows, especially those that had disappeared into the hidden recesses of the face.[31] Roger offered some ideas, noting that each case required its own clever treatment plan before starting. If possible, he suggested a conversation with the patient to discover whether the arrow had entered from above, below or from either side. If a portion of the shaft was still tightly attached to the iron point and not buried too deeply then Roger suggested that it be rocked back and forth gently and patiently. In some cases it would allow the whole thing to be removed. If the shaft had completely detached itself from the point, then inserting a probe into the wound would help to locate it, as the doctor in Mathfred's case had done when he used a cautery to try and find the arrowhead. He went on to say that the surgeon need not worry if it could not be removed as he knew of many patients who had gone on to live with metal in their bodies. This would have been only a temporary situation until the swelling had reduced and the tissues around the arrow had become softer with infection, as had likely occurred with Hubert of Pierrelatte.[32] Once the arrow was removed Roger suggested the area be bandaged in such a way as to allow the pus to be expressed regularly.[33]

Those injuries where the arrow had gone through and through the neck or an appendage required a piece of raw bacon to be placed into the opening to permit the drainage of pus. Nothing further was to be done for the first three days or until pus began to form and then treatment was to be applied according to whether it was winter or summer, with a different approach being appropriate for each season.[34] When it came to barbed arrows, Roger offered an ingenious solution using small metal tubes or two pieces of the hollow portion of a goose's quill. They could be pushed into the wound to cover each barb of the arrow and once in place, the projectile could then be withdrawn with greater ease helping to minimize the damage to surrounding tissues.[35]

The various treatments for arrow wounds found in Theodoric's surgical text of the next century were in part the result of the large catalogue of cases that both he and his father, Master Hugo, had seen.[36] Significantly, he noted that this was an area of medicine that was forever changing, because of the number of new instruments and methods being devised by practitioners to treat this most common of battle injuries.[37] Theodoric explained the specific design of forceps that he recommended for extractions, being made of good iron that had been well tempered. The shape of the jaws was to be like that of a bird's beak and saw-toothed so that once the arrow was grasped a firm grip could be maintained on the metal. These forceps were made in different sizes to meet the needs of removing arrows of various dimensions.[38]

He also discussed extracting an arrow that had become buried within the bone of a patient, suggesting that it first be left for several days, simply pulling on it a little each day until it finally came loose from the bone. Recognizing that this was not always a successful means of treatment, Theodoric next recommended making tiny holes in the bone, all around the point of the arrow, thus creating a larger cavity so that it could be removed more easily. If these first two methods still did not shift it then a trephine, a surgical tool similar to a drill, could be employed. The trephine had to be large enough to clear the circumference of the arrowhead. Once it had been twisted into the bone the trephine and arrow could be drawn out together, but this required force. This last method needed both brains and brawn, as Theodoric noted that he had '… sometimes seen two strong men toiling at an extraction …'.[39]

Looking at William of Saliceto's casebook, he included several entries that involved arrow wounds, many of which are spread across various chapters of this volume, because of their association to other issues. In one of those not explored elsewhere William spoke of a man from Piedmont, now a part of North-Western Italy, who had received an arrow wound in his back. He was not someone that William himself had looked after, but he did have it on good authority that the man recovered from the injury, after being treated diligently using '… d'ablutions de seul vin …', or wine, to wash the wound.[40] A significant point to be sure, as the wine no doubt served to treat or halt infection in the injury, something that was a constant concern in medieval casualties, as has been seen in many of these examples already. The man from Piedmont went on to survive the damage done by the arrow, something that William said did not surprise him.

Wounds of the Stomach and Intestines

> In a stonepot she had stirred together leeks and other herbs, and boiled them, and gave the wounded men of it to eat, by which she discovered if the wounds had penetrated into the belly; for if the wound had gone so deep it would smell of leek.
>
> *Heimskringla*[41]

Stomach wounds, with entrails spilling forth from the abdominal cavities of soldiers, are commonplace in the texts of the Middle Ages. The slicing, slashing and stabbing nature of weapons like axes, swords, lances and even arrows could easily open this soft pocket of the body, especially when it was not adequately protected. Wounds to this area have long been acknowledged as some of the most complex types to repair, with the danger of infection being so alarmingly high.[42] In fact, they were so difficult that doctors like Roger Frugard and Roland of Parma deemed the treatment of injuries to the stomach, along with other major organs like the heart, lungs and liver, to be beyond the skills of a surgeon. As such, their texts strongly suggested that doctors avoid taking these cases so that no blame for a patient's death could be apportioned to them.[43] What was not on their lists though were the intestines, an area that seemingly could be operated on, at least in some cases.

The tenth-century laws of the Welsh king Hywel Dha echoed the difficulty in treating abdominal injuries where the bowels were exposed. They fell under a small group of serious wounds that entitled royal physicians to be paid extra for looking after them.[44] Looking again to the eleventh-century Battle of Stiklestad in Snorri Sturluson's *Heimskringla*, he provided specific details regarding those casualties with these types of serious wounds. Warriors inside the barn were made to drink a strong-smelling broth as part of what may have been a triage process to establish which injuries could and should be treated.[45] Understanding which soldiers were treatable versus those that were not meant that resources could be directed towards warriors with a real chance of surviving to fight another day, a sentiment that was quite common in the sagas.[46] After the broth had been consumed an absence of its pungent scent in area of the abdomen meant that the stomach and intestines were likely untouched and the tissues surrounding them could be sutured and bandaged, after a return of unfurled entrails into the stomach cavity, if necessary. However, the presence of the sharp smell of the soup would have signalled to the women treating the casualties that there were puncture wounds to that area. This sort of damage could have been looked after by someone capable of treating such injuries, but they may well have been too difficult and time consuming to treat in such an emergency setting.

The horror of these sorts of battlefield injuries was reported by the contemporary chronicler Jordan Fantosme, who recorded the war between Henry II of England and William I of Scotland during the years 1173 and 1174:

Of the unfortunate Flemings great carnage was made,
[You might see] their bowels dragged from the bodies through the fields ...[47]

The epic French poem *La Chanson de Guillaume*, reflects something similar, describing mounted riders who were forced to use their hands, not to guide the reins, but to cradle their exposed entrails so they would not get them entangled and trampled in the legs of their horses.[48]

In the miracles of St Godric of Finchale is a vivid account of a young English knight from the Lascelles family who ended up like one of the unfortunate riders noted above. Lascelles had wished to continue the battlefield achievements that had so distinguished his family and once he was old enough, he left for Normandy in search of military fame and fortune, soon finding himself in battle. Rather ill-equipped for such a fight, it was not long before he had been stabbed through the stomach by a lance, causing his intestines to spill out onto his saddle. He was saved by a small group of soldiers who recognized the severity of his plight and managed to carry him away on his shield.[49] It appeared from the serious nature of his wounds that Lascelles would not survive and so a priest was called to give the last rites to the young warrior. Notwithstanding, the same knights who had saved him from further damage during battle found that they were able to intervene, using their skills in medicine to stitch him back up before taking him into the city.[50] The ability of knights to treat themselves and each other appears to have extended to quite a high level of care if this case can be trusted. Lascelles survived his ordeal and would later return to England.

Instructions offered to treat such injuries as those outlined in the examples above can be found in the leechbooks and later surgeries, beginning with *Leechbook III*. It provides a fix for those who suffered a treatable belly wound with no punctures of the intestines: 'If a mans bowel be out, pound galluc [comfrey], wring through a cloth into milk warm from the cow, wet thy hands therein, and put back the bowel into the man, sew up with silk, then boil him for nine mornings galluc, *that is comfrey*, except need be for a longer time.'[51] Here again this passage raises many of its own questions, such as the proper procedure for fitting the bowels back inside the stomach cavity. Remarkably, it suggests another of these operations that was commonly known to those early leeches, one which required little in the way of directives, beyond the plants and medicines to be used.

Roger Frugard, on the other hand, set out quite a detailed set of instructions in his surgery that would answer many of the questions posed by such an intricate operation. The first step was to cut open the belly of a live animal and place it over the area of the wound to keep it warm while the next step was being prepared.[52] This involved a piece of thin, hollow bark from an elder tree about the same diameter as the area of the intestine that had been injured. The piece was to be cut two inches longer than the length of the damaged gut and formed into the shape of a tube and inserted into the intestine. The extra inch at each end provided some stability to the cannula, which was then to be stitched inside the gut to allow for the uninterrupted flow of faecal matter.[53] Once sutured, the exposed entrails were to be washed with warm water squeezed from a sponge until they had been cleaned of dirt and blood, both animal and human. The next steps were to place the intestines back inside the patient who was stretched over a plank of wood and bound in place. Roger noted that a larger incision into the stomach cavity might have been required in order to return the entrails to their proper place. He recommended the gentle shaking of the patient while on the board to allow the intestines to settle naturally within their place in the stomach cavity. Once it was clear that the injuries were healing properly the surgeon could close the stomach. Finally, a light and easily digestible diet was advocated during the patient's healing.[54]

The advice of surgeons in the thirteenth century would be a mix of the strange and the sane. Likely the most unusual idea came from the great man of Islamic medicine, Abulcasis (936–1013), by way of Bruno da Longoburgo. Essentially, it involved the closure of intestinal injuries using the heads of large African ants as tiny clamps. The doctor was to hold the wound closed and place an ant so that its jaws could grasp either side of the laceration. Once it had closed its jaws the doctor was to cut away the body of the ant leaving the head in place. Then a second ant's head was to be added and then another and so on until the entire length of the injury had been closed. The intestines could then be replaced safely into the abdominal cavity and sutured, leaving the heads in place.[55] Likely having had some intimate knowledge of the idea of using ants as tiny medical clamps, Theodoric completely refuted this method. He noted that they did not hold well and could be brushed away far too easily.[56] Theodoric did continue, however, to prescribe the method of using a piece of elder to form a tube that was to be fitted into and left inside the area of intestine requiring repair.[57]

Giving William of Saliceto the last word on a wooden tube being inserted into the intestines, it was his opinion that it was likely to do far more damage than good, causing discomfort, perforations and eventually death:

> Et qu'on n'écoute pas les paroles de ceux qui disent qu'une canule de sureau ou d'autre substance de ce genre doive être mise dans l'intestin avant la suture et que l'intestin blessé doive être cousu sur elle, parce que cela est faux et erroné, puisque, en effet, les intestins sont d'une grande tortuosité et que le conduit de ce genre n'est pas flexible, la nature ne pourrait pas expulser ce bois recouvert de chair et il provoquerait ainsi la douleur en la voie naturelle pour l'issue des superfluités et excréments et, dans la suite, perforerait peut-être l'intestin et, de la sorte, une plaie qui pouvait être curable deviendrait mortelle.[58]

> Do not listen to the words of those who say that a cannula made from elderberry or other such substance must be placed into the intestine before it is sutured and that the injured intestine has to be sewn onto it, because

that is false and erroneous. The intestines are in fact very flexible and full of twists and turns, whereas, a tube of this kind is stiff. Nature could not expel such a thing through the intestine and out of the anus. Such a thing would be painful and might puncture the intestine, turning a curable wound into something deadly.

One must believe that William had some experience with patients who had these wooden cannulas to form such a differing opinion. Being a student of William of Saliceto, Lanfranchi of Milan would later confirm within his own text the extreme dangers of using a wooden tube in the intestines.[59]

Catalogued in William's surgery is a detailed case involving the survival of a belly wound and the steps taken to treat the man. The account is that of a soldier called Jean de Bredella, noted elsewhere, who tried to take his own life. He stabbed himself in the stomach causing damage to his intestines. Initially, a physician from Pavia called Master Octobonus was called out and he determined that de Bredella had no hope of surviving. The injuries seemed to be too complicated with intestines nicked and spilling out, but according to William's recounting of the story both Octobonus and friends of de Bredella still sought his counsel. Initially, William concurred with Octobonus that there was little that could be done to help the soldier. However, he agreed to at least try to save the man and so he began by persistently bathing the exposed intestines with warm wine, which would have worked to keep them pliable while helping to sterilize the area as the fecal matter continued to flow out. William then sutured the damaged guts using what he called '... la suture des pelletiers ...', or the same stitch used by furriers to sew pelts together.[60] He had to increase the size of the original opening made by de Bredella's knife to get the intestines back into their proper place. Despite some very heavy bleeding William managed to close him up with everything repaired and back in place before applying various healing treatments and medicines to the area, which he later shared with Master Octobonus. According to his own words, William was able to save this soldier's life.[61]

Even if some of the surgical operations discussed above were done successfully and in time, the instances of infection would have been significant and difficult to overcome. Just how many of these intestinal injuries were survivable is hard to say for certain, but on balance it does seem likely that far more soldiers must have perished than those who managed to pull through such frightful wounds.

Loss of Limbs

> Through the great press most gallantly he strikes,
> He breaks their spears, their buckled shields doth slice,
> Their feet, their fists, their shoulders and their sides,
> Dismembers them: whoso had seen that sigh,
> *The Song of Roland*[62]

A feature of war in the Middle Ages was the ferocious life and death struggle of hand-to-hand fighting with razor sharp axes, long knives and swords slicing away limbs with dreadful efficiency. The poems and sagas of the Vikings include many of these examples, with writers giving axes names like 'The wolf of the wound' and swords too were provided with similar monikers such as 'The torch of the blood'.[63] The tales of the Vikings are far from the only source to provide confirmation of the terrible damage that medieval weapons caused to the limbs of those who fought centuries ago. The tenth-century *Waltharius* included the loss of one man's leg and the right hand of Waltharius himself during a skirmish.[64] In his early epic *Cligés*, Chrétien de Troyes likened the ease of taking off a leg with a sword to that of chopping a stalk of fennel.[65] The twelfth-century French poem *La Chanson de Guillaume* described the throng of battle where fists and feet could so easily be cut away.[66] In relating a failed siege on Toulouse by the crusading army the second author of *La chanson de la croisade contre les Albigeois* confirmed this kind of damage to the human body:

> Il y a de tels amas de pieds, de jambes, de bras;
> sur le sol il y a tant de sang et de cervelles, que
> les chemins et l'esplanade sont rouges et sanglants.[67]
>
> All over the ground were piles of feet, legs and arms,
> along with the brains and blood that made the paths
> and esplanade red and bloody.

The blood loss and shock of an arm or leg lost in battle plus the added vulnerability to further injuries would have taken the lives of many before they could receive treatment, had such care even been available. *The Saga of the People of Laxardal* recalls how Gudlaug was killed when a sword blow took off his leg.[68] Thorwald died in much the same way in *The Story of Burnt Njal* when, '… Gudleif smote him on the shoulder and hewed his arm off, and that was his death'.[69]

In addition to limbs lost directly to the battlefield were those taken by surgical intervention, because of gangrene or serious damage. Before examining some of the techniques used by medieval surgeons to treat those who required amputations or had lost limbs it is worth considering the work of the Roman writer Aulus Cornelius Celsus. He penned an encyclopedic work two millennia ago that included the subject of surgery in the first century. It contains one of the earliest written examples of an amputation procedure and in it he warned of the dangers of these surgeries, concerns that would continue to be true in the Middle Ages, '… patients often die in the operation, either by a hemorrhage, or faintings'.[70] Celsus provided detailed steps to perform the procedure, giving instructions on how to create a stump at the end of the limb. Being careful not to cut at the joint, Celsus wrote that the good flesh was to be pulled back and cut down to the bone at a point past the unhealthy tissue. With the good flesh still retracted a saw was then to be used to cut through the bone. Once the bone had been smoothed at the leading edge the good flesh could then be pulled forward providing extra muscle and skin to go over the end of the bone to create a stump. This was then to be sewn up with a sponge soaked in vinegar and wrung out, tied over the top of the wound site.[71] This operation is not terribly different from the method currently practised by modern surgeons, using skin and muscle to create a healthy stump over the end of the amputation.

It is difficult to know if the work of Celsus existed as far north as England in the ninth century, but it was not a work that was widely circulated.[72] Regardless, the instructions in *Bald's Leechbook* are based on different Latin works and suggest an operation with some important variances:[73]

> If thou must carve off or cut off an unhealthy limb off from a healthy body, then carve thou not it on the limit of the healthy body; but much more cut or carve in on the hole and quick body; thou shalt better and readier cure it. When thou settest fire on a man, then take thou leaves of tender leek and grated salt …[74]

This technique found in *Bald's* uses cauterization to close the end of the amputation site, quite unlike the procedure prescribed by Celsus. Intriguingly, when it comes to the three later surgeons only Theodoric detailed a procedure for amputation.[75] Even writing several centuries after *Bald's Leechbook* had been compiled, Theodoric relied on the same source, copying what is essentially the identical set of instructions:

> If it should be necessary for any part of the body to be amputated or cut off, you should cut down to the healthy areas and leave no part of the putrid flesh, but take away some part of the live and healthy flesh. Indeed, you will effect a cure better and more quickly in this way. And when you cauterize, you will cover the area with the leaves of young leeks ground up with salt …[76]

There were other amputation procedures known in Europe by this point, including that which had been recommended by Abulcasis, a method that made use of ligatures during the surgery, tied above and below where the limb would be cut.[77] However, it seems that Theodoric and his father still relied on this earlier method for the removal of an unhealthy or damaged limb.

There are notable omissions from both *Bald's* and Theodoric regarding the control of blood flow during the procedure, which as Cameron has pointed out may well have been managed by cauterization.[78] Nonetheless, other dangers and concerns were not addressed, not the least of which was the patient going into shock during the procedure.

In terms of pain relief, the Anglo-Saxon texts include various draughts using ingredients such as poppy, henbane and hemlock that may have helped. The *Lacnunga*, for instance, contains a recipe for a sleeping draught with both hemlock and henbane as ingredients, but as for the patient being unconscious during such an operation nothing is known for certain.[79] Significantly, in his surgery Theodoric provided his father's recipe for an anaesthetic or soporific sponge, as it is referred to quite often. A sponge, which had soaked up a mixture of opium, henbane, hemlock and mandrake, was placed under the patient's nose, '... until the subject for operation falls asleep'. Once the procedure was done vinegar was to be passed under the patient's nose to assist them in regaining consciousness.[80]

Commonly overlooked is a second section, only found in *Bald's*, which deals with the loss of a limb or appendage. The injuries within this segment resemble very closely those that were common to the battlefield: 'If a limb be smitten off a man, a finger, or a foot, or a hand, if the marrow be out, take sodden sheeps marrow, lay it on the other marrow bind it well up for a night.'[81] A salve was then recommended before the section continues with the suggestion of cauterizing the edges of the wound.[82] Being that it is so light on instructions for many elements of the process, it is a difficult one to comprehend. What is not hard to understand though is the extreme likelihood of infection caused by a treatment like this one performed on an open wound.

Taking leave of *Bald's* and Theodoric we come to the medieval hospital at Soutra Aisle, founded in the 1160s as part of the Augustinian complex of the Holy Trinity in the Scottish Borders. There the remains of amputated body parts have been discovered among the 'medical waste'. Also found were caches of black henbane seeds, opium poppy and hemlock, made up of a mixture of three parts black henbane and one each of the other two ingredients.[83] There have been a few sets of these components found together at Soutra Aisle and it seems that the monks had calculated this ratio to be used as an anaesthetic, almost certainly to perform surgical procedures. It has been suggested that when mixed as a drink or inhaled from a sponge, such as recommended in Theodoric, an individual could have remained unconscious or oblivious to pain for 48 to 72 hours.[84] Sadly, just how the amputation procedures were done is not known, but it is further evidence of the church regularly being at the leading edge of medicine. It is also of interest and certainly some relief to know that at least at times serious operations like these could have been completed while the patient was unconscious.

It is clear from both the extant documentation and archaeological evidence that there were those who survived the loss of a limb and even associated infections and multiple amputations could be overcome. As we will see later, hospitals dedicated to St Anthony became particularly adept at amputating limbs afflicted with *ignis sacer*, or St Anthony's fire. The skeleton of an adult male, dating to as early as 1250 and discovered in London, shows a healed amputation of the right lower leg below the knee. Despite signs of post-amputation infection, this individual survived for many years after losing the limb.[85] Another male, this one from Lund in Sweden, remarkably lost both hands, portions of his forearms and his left foot, but he too survived.[86]

Pulling through such terrible injuries would have just been the beginning of a much more difficult life during this period. A later chapter on disability

Recovery

> Let the seriously wounded man be careful, therefore, to observe diligently all the things which have been said about diet, for I consider this to be of first importance in every wound.
>
> Theodoric[87]

Recovery from injuries and surgical procedures is a subject that is sometimes overlooked, but clearly there was an understanding in the Middle Ages that once a wound had been stitched closed things such as diet and pain relief played an important role in the healing process, just as they do today. Looking first at nourishment, its restorative value is currently being recognized and promoted as something that is just as influential as anything else in returning the body and mind back to good health. Medical organizations and health professionals now advocate more than ever a healthy diet and proper hydration before and after surgery. In the Middle Ages medical practitioners also realized how important food and fluids could be when it came to the healing process and overall health, with some surgeries and treatises providing comprehensive instructions on the subject.[88]

Instances of food or diet being involved in recovery exist within medieval literature, as well the medical texts, with *Thordar's Saga* being an example. The story's namesake sought medical attention for his battle wounds from the previously mentioned Icelandic healer named Olöf, a woman of some renown. When she accepted him, he was taken to a separate outbuilding on her farm, but before tending to his injuries she made certain to give him food to eat. Thordar remained in her care until he had made a full recovery.[89]

In Chrétien de Troyes' *Erec and Enide* sustenance formed a large part of the treatment of the badly wounded knight called Erec. He was discovered by a man named Guivert the Little and once the two recognized one another he began to tend to Erec offering him food to eat and watered-down wine to drink:

> 'Friend', says he, 'now try a little of these cold patties, and drink some wine mixed with water. I have as much as six barrels of it, but undiluted it is not good for you; for you are injured and covered with wounds. Fair sweet friend, now try to eat; for it will do you good.'[90]

This idea of diluted wine was one that was endorsed by some medieval surgeons as part of a diet to help heal certain types of injuries and conditions.[91] Erec was next taken to the castle belonging to Guivret, as he required surgery to treat his wounds. It was Guivret's two sisters who performed the procedure before tending to Erec's recovery, which featured nourishment for the knight:

> Again and again they washed his wounds and applied the plaster. Four times or more each day they made him eat and drink, allowing him, however, no garlic or pepper.[92]

The Anglo-Saxon medical texts contain some references to diet and healing, with *Leechbook III*, for example, suggesting the consumption of '... fresh hen's flesh ...' after having intestines replaced back inside the stomach cavity.[93] Centuries later, Roger Frugard explained how some patients, especially the debilitated and elderly, might struggle to heal properly because of malnutrition, especially when it came to broken bones.[94] Theodoric included much more advice on the subject, citing the importance of diet in the healing process.[95] Throughout his surgery specific foods and fluids are recommended for healing different sorts of wounds and illnesses.[96] In many sections of his surgery William of Saliceto was on another level altogether offering copious and frequently repeated details to his students and readers on things like post surgical diets and treatments.[97]

So much of medieval medicine relied upon the doctrine of the four humours, a theory developed by the ancient Greeks and refined down the centuries by others. Its hypothesis being that the human body is a fine balance of four essential humours or fluids, namely black bile, red or yellow bile, blood and phlegm. The type of temperament that defined an individual was based on which of these four substances was thought to be the predominant one in their body. If black bile was considered primary in the person then they were thought to be Melancholic. If red or yellow bile was the principal fluid then they were deemed to be Choleric, if blood was indicated then they had a Sanguine temperament and perhaps not surprisingly phlegm pointed toward a Phlegmatic character.[98] Under this theory everyone was different. Lanfranchi of Milan offered the illustration of two men wounded in the arm by a sword, at the identical time and place, claiming only 'ignorant folk' would look after them in the same manner. According to the doctrine, their treatments should be different based on the doctor's assessment of their humours and tailored to meet those needs.[99] Bloodletting (also called phlebotomy), cupping, evacuation of the bowels and practices like these were recommended as part of a patient's treatment to assist in the adjustment of the humours of the body.[100]

Poultices and salves of many types were applied to help speed healing, with honey being one of the most common ingredients, either as a component or simply on its own. While honey's antibacterial and restorative properties were not understood by medieval doctors its obvious results meant that it was widely prescribed for wound care.[101]

As we have already seen, when it came to pain relief several plants and seeds, such as henbane, mandrake, hemlock and opium, were used by doctors and healers to provide comfort to the wounded. Henbane is one that turns up time and again from the age of the Vikings through to the beginning of the fourteenth century.[102] The analgesic qualities of cold water, cold vinegar and even snow were also valued. In the saga of *Egil and Asmund* Egil had his hand cut off during a fight with a giant. Later, in obvious pain and unable to sleep he made his way to a cold stream where he held his arm in the water, which brought him some relief.[103] Surgeons of this period suggested the use of snow for the treatment of burns, but it was also employed in other procedures such as helping to cool the water to be sponged around the eye after cauterization or the use of a painful ointment.[104] Lanfranchi of Milan included a case from the ancient physician Galen within his surgery where snow was packed around the haematoma of an injured servant. Lanfranchi was confident that this supported his own policy of cold therapy.[105] Lanfranchi's teacher, William of Saliceto, incorporated all these options into his three categories of pain relief, with each step increasing in analgesic strength. The first involved mild topical ointments, the second heat and cold therapies and lastly more powerful ointments with ingredients such as henbane and opium could be used. These topical narcotics were only to be prescribed early in the patient's recovery and not to be used for long periods of time.[106]

Chapter 5

Broken Bones and Fractured Skulls

> They broke arms, they broke knees, they
> broke legs, they broke thighs.
>
> *The Lay of Havelok the Dane*[1]

Vicious weapons, shields, heavy horses and the general crush of warfare in the Middle Ages produced countless ways for the bones, joints and teeth of soldiers to become broken or otherwise damaged. The same was true of the games and tournaments that managed to imitate the dangers of the battlefield all too well.[2] Skull fractures and the loss of teeth were common as warriors took aim at the heads of one another with everything from rocks and mailed fists to swords and maces, while falls from horses brought about dislocated shoulders and broken collarbones. Legs too were favoured targets causing incapacitating injuries that made soldiers vulnerable to even more violence and attempts to block strikes from weapons and shields put the bones of the arm at great risk of being broken.[3] Armour certainly provided some protection, but bones and teeth could still be cracked and fractured by blows from sharp and heavy weapons.[4] The leechbooks and surgeries are full of treatments claiming to '... leech his limbs that are sore, and heal his bones ...', once again making these texts worthy of investigation alongside the casualties themselves.[5]

In addition to the leeches and doctors who looked after skeletal injuries were those often referred to as *bonesetters*, specialists who worked to repair broken and dislocated bones. They would have provided a useful service at a time when daily life and work, a lack of any health and safety precautions, violence and warfare meant there would have been a lot of damaged bones and joints requiring treatment.[6] Unfortunately, trying to identify any by name from the European records of our centuries can be difficult, but by looking elsewhere a few can be pinpointed. The previously mentioned bonesetter from the memoirs of Usāmah ibn Munqidh was a man called Yahya who came from Northern Syria. He had been called upon during battle in 1138 when a soldier had his lower leg broken by a stone hurled from a siege engine. The description leaves no doubt about Yahya's expertise, confirming his position as a respected specialist: 'Another mangonel stone struck one of our men on his lower leg and broke it. They carried him to the presence of my uncle, who was then sitting in the hallway of the castle and who said, "Fetch the bonesetter". Now there was in Shayzar an artisan named Yahya who was an expert in bonesetting.'[7]

One of the earliest identifiable European bone doctors was a man called Maestro Iacopo dell'Ossa da Roma working in 1336 around the area of Florence, the 'dell'Ossa' portion of his name confirming the nature of his occupation. He was taken by the Black Death in the middle of the 1300s, but his three surviving sons carried on in the same profession.[8] While it is true that little is known about bonesetters during our centuries, by the latter part of the 1200s we begin to get an idea of their position within the medical hierarchy, which was a few rungs down the ladder.[9] Many of the well-educated medical professionals such as Taddeo Alderotti preferred to leave routine jobs to their assistants, which included the repair of broken bones. They did not wish themselves to be aligned with the lowly bonesetters and barber-surgeons who were carrying out these sorts of procedures.[10] In the fourteenth century the French physician and surgeon Guy de Chauliac confirmed that dislocations and fractures were routinely being treated by bonesetters, a practice he condemned considering it to be quite dangerous for the patient.[11]

Common Fractures and Dislocations

> ... Arnold had, in a previous tournament, broken this Roger Lemburn's leg.
> Matthew Paris[12]

Whether caused by battle, contest or daily life, predictably, the bones of the limbs were among those most susceptible to damage in the Middle Ages. Fractured arms, especially the bones of the forearm, the ulna and radius, are certainly easy to find in the archaeological record. In a major survey of the broken and damaged bones of 2,266 bodies, dating from 990 to 1536 and excavated at Lund in Sweden, Caroline Arcini found that the most frequently fractured bone among these skeletons was the ulna, with the radius also showing up in several cases.[13] Being a general burial site not all fractures were related to violence, but they certainly exist among such a large archaeological population.[14] When it came to combat it was generally a soldier's defensive position or fall from a horse that resulted in such injuries to the arm.[15] The Viking burials at Slite on the island of Gotland show that more than 30 per cent had healed fractures of the lower arm and leg bones among their wounds.[16] While battle may be the first thing that comes to mind, consider the savage nature of the ball game included in *Göngu-Hrolfs Saga*, which saw three men end up with their arms broken and many others left seriously harmed.[17]

Later excavations and studies of medieval cemeteries, such as the Augustinian Priory of St Mary Spital in London and St Helen-on-the-Walls in York, England, are also indicative of just how often these arm injuries occurred.[18] As with the Viking contests, tournaments saw the same sorts of fractures, including the one held at Cambridge in the first half of the thirteenth century where 'Arms and legs were often broken ...'.[19] Indeed, in the Arthurian tale of *The Knight of the Two Swords* there is more than one example of a broken arm resulting from a warrior tumbling off his horse during a fight.[20]

The legs and feet of opposing soldiers were regularly the aim of targeted blows, leaving victims that could then be more easily dispatched.[21] Many lower limbs would have been taken clean off by sword and axe strikes, but a good deal more left the bones of the legs and feet bashed and fractured. *The Story of Burnt Njal* features several incidents of violence in which the legs and feet of another were the immediate mark of swords, axes and spears: 'Otkell smites at Gunnar with his sword, and aims at his leg just below the knee, but Gunnar leapt up into the air and he misses him.'[22] The archaeological evidence from the mass burial of young Viking warriors discovered in Dorset in England shows that the most common area of healed injury within this group was to their feet.[23]

During early summer 1218, Sir Bernard of Cazenac directed the men of Toulouse to attack the knees of the French soldiers from the back, knowing that their bodies would be protected by double armour, while their legs would be exposed leaving them to become 'carrion' on the battlefield.[24] The mass grave from the Battle of Visby in 1361, on the Swedish island of Gotland, contains hundreds of skeletons with damage to their legs. Although this battle is several decades beyond our period of interest its significance lies in the more than 1,000 bodies that have been excavated from this site. Here again about a third of the shin bones show cut marks and other harm, the result of the technique used by the professional Danish and German soldiers to slash and swipe at the legs of their Gotland opponents to debilitate them.[25]

The collection of treatments for broken bones in the early leechbooks is surprisingly limited and many of them do of course lack the comprehensive steps that would be outlined by later surgeons. *Bald's Leechbook* offered this general treatment for broken limbs, which provides scant details for the process of applying the splint and bandages to the limb:

> For a broken limb, lay this salve on the broken limb, and overlay with elm rind, apply a splint, again, always renew these till the limb be healed; clean some elm rind, and boil it thoroughly, then remove the rind, and take linseed, grind it for a brewit or paste with the elms drink; that shall be a good salve for a broken limb.[26]

The fact that treating the bones of the arms and legs was such a common procedure would seem to validate the idea that it must have been the leeches themselves who understood how best to do it, bridging the gap in knowledge left by the leechbooks. What follows this treatment in *Bald's Leechbook* is a method for fixing a broken thigh bone, the femur, a less common type of injury. While not comprehensive by any means, intriguingly the more unusual nature of this sort of bone break may explain why at least some steps were included for both the leech and patient to aid them in realigning the bone.[27] When not realigned and set properly a broken femur can lead to a shortening of the leg, a fairly pronounced disability. One of the Viking warriors who was part of the mass grave discovered in Dorset was found to have one leg shorter than the other, the result of a broken femur that had not healed correctly.[28]

The simple nature of the treatments for broken arms and legs found in *Bald's Leechbook* differ greatly from the major surgeries of the twelfth century. The *Bamberg Surgery* certainly contains more detail for the repair of fractures and dislocations, but it is far from exhaustive.[29] Those found within Roger Frugard's text are much more instructive, providing useful steps for repairing the limbs, using the lower arm as something of a template, which could then be repeated for fractures of the leg.[30] Setting these bones required an assistant who was '... to pull on the fingers against traction on the forearm'.[31] Using cloth that was the width of four fingers the surgeon was to bandage the area to keep the bones in place. Next came cloth that had been soaked in egg white, which was to be placed over the bandaged area, followed by another round of bandaging. He warned against dressings being bound too tightly as this could induce swelling. Splints were to be used to optimize the healing, held in place with the aid of cords. The dressings were to be changed every three days for a total of nine days and on the ninth day an astringent needed to be applied to the skin before rebandaging and splinting the limb. This was to last for several days until the bones were knitted back together, with a reminder that the damaged area required protection and frequent inspection for any movement of the bones at the site of the fracture.[32]

In the thirteenth century, other surgeons like Theodoric and William of Saliceto would go on to improve upon these types of procedures, offering more information on the healing of bones within their respective surgical texts. Theodoric went into considerable detail about the things associated with the treatment of broken bones, such as diet, pain relief and the muscular atrophy a patient could expect during the healing process.[33]

It is important to note that there were other texts at the opposite end of this more sophisticated medicine, offering what might be considered more *medieval* sounding suggestions for healing broken bones. One such manuscript worth mentioning is the Leechbook portion of the *Old Icelandic Medical Miscellany*. Originating from a Scandinavian source from around 1300, it provided just a few steps for healing fractures, with nothing prior to or after these simple words:[34] 'For broken bone, take a rooster and stuff it full of feathers and bind upon whole; that heals quickly and well.'[35]

Compound or open fractures, that is when the broken bones pierce through the skin, were rightly considered to be significant injuries in the Middle Ages. Still today they have the potential to be life changing or even fatal if not treated promptly and properly. Difficult to repair, the severity of these bone breaks is highlighted by the tenth-century laws of the Welsh king Hywel Dha. These serious fractures are another in the small group of injuries that entitled Welsh royal physicians to earn extra money over and above their normal salaries.[36]

Along with the damage to the bone and soft tissues these injuries are highly susceptible to infection, which was the case for Duke Leopold V of Austria at the end of the twelfth century. He received a compound fracture when his horse fell on top of him during a tournament, breaking the bones in his lower leg and foot in a [obscured] violent manner. Attempts by the [obscured] were fruitless and his foot soon [obscured] the following day, but it was a [obscured] of the resulting infection within [obscured] de much on open fractures, except [obscured] ragments of bone from around the [obscured] odoric would offer far more on the [obscured] ork with the surgeon in repairing [obscured] ng these injuries and the correct [obscured] ompound fractures involving the [obscured] other surgeons who apparently [obscured] se cases could lead not only to a [obscured]:

[obscured] nalade mourra par le fait de la [obscured] tion ne peut pas se faire parce [obscured] t the patient will die because [obscured] nnot be regenerated, because [obscured] e use of metal splints to support [obscured] ommon, are not without their [obscured] veden and dating to as early as [obscured] e the humerus bone of a man's [obscured] or axe. This complex surgery [obscured] the bone and secured in place [obscured] metal.[41] While it would have [obscured] performed the repair, copper [obscured] properties, certainly a key factor that aided in the successful healing of the bone, which shows new growth had occurred around the site of the injury. In the Fishergate area of York a different sort of device, dating from the thirteenth or first half of the fourteenth century, was employed to support a severely injured right knee. This individual had suffered a significant twist fracture, perhaps as the result of a fall. An external device was created using copper plates covered and padded with leather and then tied around the knee to provide support for the joint.[42] This individual likely required the use of a crutch for the balance of their life, but this useful device would have provided some necessary support for what would have been a difficult type of fracture to fix in the absence of modern surgical techniques.

The collarbone or clavicle is another vulnerable bone, its placement and lack of much fleshy protection make it susceptible to fractures and dislocations.[43]

The sagas are full of these kinds of injuries, like that described in *King Gautrek*: 'Sisar hewed at Starkad's shield, gave him two nasty head wounds and broke his collarbone.'[44]

The Story of Burnt Njal too has its share of incidents involving smashed and broken clavicles, among them when Thorgeir struck Leidolf the Strong with an axe breaking his collarbone into two pieces.[45] There is archaeological evidence from the time of the Vikings which shows that the type of damage to the collarbone outlined in the sagas could be successfully repaired. The Viking cemetery at Kopparsvik on Gotland contains a warrior in grave 154 who appears to have been killed in battle, but among the healed fractures he had from incidents prior to that was one to his collarbone.[46] At Vannhög, Sweden another individual shows a fracture of the left clavicle, which had also knitted together successfully.[47]

The literature of the twelfth and thirteenth centuries continued to show just how common a broken collarbone could be, especially for mounted warriors falling from their horses or receiving a violent blow from weapons and armour. *The Song of Girart of Vienne* by French poet Bertran de Bar-sur-Aube provides an example of a fist used to break a clavicle and *The Knight of the Two Swords* contains no less than three men who were knocked from their horses, each breaking their collarbone.[48] Chrétien de Troyes highlighted the fragility of this area of the body, using it in two of his epic romances, *Erec and Enide* and *The Story of the Grail (Perceval)*.[49] The latter offers a little more value in terms of a repair to the bone. When Perceval was challenged by another of King Arthur's knights, Sir Kay, the two rode toward each other fully armed and hell-bent on knocking the other to the ground. Sir Kay struck first, but it was Perceval who hit the knight's shield so hard that it sent him to the floor, dislocating his collarbone and fracturing the humerus bone of his right arm. Concerned about Sir Kay's injuries, King Arthur '… sent him a most learned physician and three maidens trained by him, who set his collarbone …'[50]

Chrétien de Troyes' suggestion of skilled assistants being required to attend a surgeon in the treatment of damaged bones like the clavicle is corroborated by Theodoric's text, as he emphasized the level of difficulty in repairing them. To set a broken collarbone Theodoric's surgery suggested that the patient should be seated on a stool while the first assistant held his upper arm, extending the shoulder up and away from the body. A second assistant was to stretch the neck in the opposite direction to allow the doctor to realign the broken bone with his fingers.[51] Once the bone had been restored to its proper position, he offered the next steps that were to be taken; two thick round pads, one larger than the other, were to be soaked in egg white and wrung out before being rolled in a mixture of beaten egg white and fermented meal. The larger pad was to be placed beside the clavicle on the shoulder side, while the smaller one went alongside it on the chest side. A splint was to be bandaged in place and a small cushion could be tucked under the patient's armpit, with further instructions for them to sleep on their back at night. The injury was horse fell on top of him during a tournament, breaking the bones in his lower leg and forcing them through the skin in a violent manner. Attempts by the Duke's surgeons to do something about it were fruitless and his foot soon turned black. His lower leg was amputated the following day, but it was a case of too little too late and the Duke died of the resulting infection within a short time.[37]

Surprisingly, Roger Frugard did not include much on open fractures, except to emphasize the need to remove any loose fragments of bone from around the site of the wound for fear of infection.[38] Theodoric would offer far more on the subject, including the need for assistants to work with the surgeon in repairing the damage, the proper method of bandaging these injuries and the correct diet for healing.[39] In a brief discussion on compound fractures involving the upper arm, William of Saliceto chastised other surgeons who apparently believed that the loss of bone marrow in these cases could lead not only to a lack of healing, but even death for the patient:

> … et n'éconte point ceux qui disent que le malade mourra par le fait de la sortie de la moelle de l'os et que la restauration ne peut pas se faire parce que c'est faux.[40]

> … and don't listen to those who claim that the patient will die because marrow is released from the bone or that it cannot be regenerated, because they are wrong.

Evidence of specialist surgical repairs and the use of metal splints to support the bones of the arms and legs, although uncommon, are not without their examples. Discovered at Varnhem Abbey in Sweden and dating to as early as the twelfth century is an internal fix to stabilize the humerus bone of a man's left arm, which had been broken by a sword or axe. This complex surgery was done using a copper plate wrapped around the bone and secured in place with rivets or thread through three holes in the metal.[41] While it would have been unknown to the monks or surgeons who performed the repair, copper has antimicrobial properties, certainly a key factor that aided in the successful healing of the bone, which shows new growth had occurred around the site of the injury. In the Fishergate area of York a different sort of device, dating from the thirteenth or first half of the fourteenth century, was employed to support a severely injured right knee. This individual had suffered a significant twist fracture, perhaps as the result of a fall. An external device was created using copper plates covered and padded with leather and then tied around the knee to provide support for the joint.[42] This individual likely required the use of a crutch for the balance of their life, but this useful device would have provided some necessary support for what would have been a difficult type of fracture to fix in the absence of modern surgical techniques.

The collarbone or clavicle is another vulnerable bone, its placement and lack of much fleshy protection make it susceptible to fractures and dislocations.[43]

The sagas are full of these kinds of injuries, like that described in *King Gautrek*: 'Sisar hewed at Starkad's shield, gave him two nasty head wounds and broke his collarbone.'[44]

The Story of Burnt Njal too has its share of incidents involving smashed and broken clavicles, among them when Thorgeir struck Leidolf the Strong with an axe breaking his collarbone into two pieces.[45] There is archaeological evidence from the time of the Vikings which shows that the type of damage to the collarbone outlined in the sagas could be successfully repaired. The Viking cemetery at Kopparsvik on Gotland contains a warrior in grave 154 who appears to have been killed in battle, but among the healed fractures he had from incidents prior to that was one to his collarbone.[46] At Vannhög, Sweden another individual shows a fracture of the left clavicle, which had also knitted together successfully.[47]

The literature of the twelfth and thirteenth centuries continued to show just how common a broken collarbone could be, especially for mounted warriors falling from their horses or receiving a violent blow from weapons and armour. *The Song of Girart of Vienne* by French poet Bertran de Bar-sur-Aube provides an example of a fist used to break a clavicle and *The Knight of the Two Swords* contains no less than three men who were knocked from their horses, each breaking their collarbone.[48] Chrétien de Troyes highlighted the fragility of this area of the body, using it in two of his epic romances, *Erec and Enide* and *The Story of the Grail (Perceval)*.[49] The latter offers a little more value in terms of a repair to the bone. When Perceval was challenged by another of King Arthur's knights, Sir Kay, the two rode toward each other fully armed and hell-bent on knocking the other to the ground. Sir Kay struck first, but it was Perceval who hit the knight's shield so hard that it sent him to the floor, dislocating his collarbone and fracturing the humerus bone of his right arm. Concerned about Sir Kay's injuries, King Arthur '… sent him a most learned physician and three maidens trained by him, who set his collarbone …'[50]

Chrétien de Troyes' suggestion of skilled assistants being required to attend a surgeon in the treatment of damaged bones like the clavicle is corroborated by Theodoric's text, as he emphasized the level of difficulty in repairing them. To set a broken collarbone Theodoric's surgery suggested that the patient should be seated on a stool while the first assistant held his upper arm, extending the shoulder up and away from the body. A second assistant was to stretch the neck in the opposite direction to allow the doctor to realign the broken bone with his fingers.[51] Once the bone had been restored to its proper position, he offered the next steps that were to be taken; two thick round pads, one larger than the other, were to be soaked in egg white and wrung out before being rolled in a mixture of beaten egg white and fermented meal. The larger pad was to be placed beside the clavicle on the shoulder side, while the smaller one went alongside it on the chest side. A splint was to be bandaged in place and a small cushion could be tucked under the patient's armpit, with further instructions for them to sleep on their back at night. The injury was to be inspected daily and all things being equal it should have healed within a month's time.[52]

Another frequent type of skeletal injury during this period was a dislocated shoulder. In the Viking tale of *Bosi and Herraud*, Bosi managed to separate the shoulder of another player during an especially violent ballgame.[53] In *Eirik the Red's Saga* Eirik himself fell from his horse breaking some ribs and damaging his shoulder.[54] Neither of the stories manages to explain how these injuries were treated, but what does exist is the guidance found within *Leechbook III*. Here again just a salve was included with no steps for manipulating the shoulder back into place. The very painful nature of these injuries is made clear by the fact that the ointment was meant to be applied gently with the use of a feather: 'If the shoulder get up out of place, take the salve, apply a little warm with a feather, it will soon be well with the man'.[55]

The miracle collection from Rocamadour recalled the high-ranking Count Robert of Meulan who fell from his horse dislocating his right shoulder.[56] In an unusual tip of the hat to the doctors who assisted him, the scribe indicated that it was their skill that put Count Robert's shoulder back into place. He later fell again, but this second time the damage to the joint was much more severe.[57] The doctors seem to have been unable to return it to its proper position and so only poultices were applied to the area.[58] Not surprisingly, the injury left his arm hanging uselessly and the doctors without hope that he would regain mobility in the limb. As Count Robert prayed to St Mary for forgiveness and help, '… he had his arm lifted up …', which helped to slip it back into its proper position so that he was once again able to use his arm.[59] This phrase does sound rather undersold here, perhaps for the sake of the miracle story. Whatever the case, it is a prime example of the potential for recurrence with this sort of injury. It is quite likely this was something that Count Robert continued to deal with throughout his life. An excavated skeleton of a medieval male in the collections of the Museum of London shows the same type of chronic luxation probably suffered by Count Robert and many others like him. Dating to as early as the second half of the thirteenth century this individual suffered a separated shoulder that became a repeat problem after the initial injury. A lack of any advanced surgical techniques meant that it would have been impossible to properly repair the damage. At some point his shoulder had become permanently dislocated, leaving him with a serious disability for the balance of his life.[60]

Written slightly later than the account of Count Robert at Rocamadour was the Northern French *chantefable*, or sung verse, entitled *Aucassin and Nicolette*, in which the young knight called Aucassin dislocated his shoulder when he fell from his horse onto a rock.[61] It explains in simple terms just how these injuries were treated and here again is an example of a medieval woman with the skill and knowledge to treat such casualties. Aucassin was clearly in a great deal of pain and unable to use his arm after the fall, but turning to his lover Nicolette she used a combination of manipulation to return the shoulder to its proper position with a poultice to aid in healing:

She felt about, and found that he had his shoulder out of place.
She plied it so with her white hands, and achieved (as God willed,
who loveth lovers) that it came again into place. And then she took
flowers and fresh grass and green leaves, and bound them on with the
lappet of her smock, and he was quite healed.[62]

When Raimon of Avignon translated Roger Frugard's surgery into the Occitan language in the early part of the thirteenth century he included a note that explained just how often this injury occurred to knights who fell from their horses.[63] Bruno da Longoburgo was another surgeon who commented on treating soldiers with dislocations, cautioning practitioners to be wary of other injuries that might be associated with the warrior's profession, things such as lacerations, abscesses and ulcers.[64] Consulting Roland of Parma's thirteenth-century text for the repair of a dislocated shoulder, he followed Roger Frugard's instructions closely, as might be expected.[65] He suggested that the treatment begin by making a pear-shaped ball from stone or a piece of wood wrapped in cloth. While the patient was lying flat the doctor was to wedge the ball into the armpit using the force of his heel, while at the same time working the head of the humerus back into the shoulder joint. Once the arm had been returned to its proper position the area could be covered with a cloth pad that had been soaked in egg white. The ball was then to be removed from the armpit and replaced with a cushion and the whole area wrapped up to keep it in place. The arm could be bent at the elbow with the forearm placed against the chest and another cushion nestled underneath. If after three days, the shoulder joint did not remain in place Roland recommended that the procedure be repeated.[66]

Teeth

> He raised his fist and hit me in the teeth
> So fiercely that the blood ran down my beard
> *The Knights of Narbonne*[67]

Understandably, the teeth of those who fought on the battlefields of the early and high Middle Ages were easily loosened, broken or removed altogether by closed and mailed fists or by any number of weapons. Combing through the sources, even the most basic things like rocks were used to bash teeth, as an entry from the *Fragmentary Annals of Ireland* recalls from the year 860: 'One of the men of Munster came towards him and gave him a blow of a large stone on the mouth, and knocked all the teeth out of his head.'[68]

Waltharius includes the loss of teeth to a short sword when Waltharius took out an eye and six teeth of his former friend Hagano.[69] Within the sagas of the Vikings there is no shortage of, '… we who have sometimes got the toothache in our conflicts …', as Sturluson expressed it so vividly.[70] In *The Story of Burnt Njal*, for instance, the teeth of the helmet-less Thrain were spilled onto the ice by an axe called 'the ogress of war', wielded by Skarphedinn.[71] In the fantasy known as *Thorstein Mansion-Might*, Thorstein used the floor to smash four of Earl Agdi's teeth when he threw himself underneath him during a boisterous round of wrestling causing Agdi to land face first.[72]

References to those who specialized in treating sore, rattled and damaged teeth are really quite rare during this 500-year period. Occasionally though, a name or a find turns up that might just point to this occupation, like the teeth found in two Anglo-Saxon graves excavated at Dunstable in Bedfordshire. Both burials contained the bodies of adult males along with pouches of human teeth, which were not their own. In life, the teeth may have been carried by these men as evidence of their work as tooth-drawers or rudimentary dentists.[73] Within *Bald's Leechbook* there are remedies for sore teeth, including one made from cinnamon, honey and pepper that was to be placed over the area of discomfort.[74] *Leechbook III* contains a pain reliever made using '… henbane roots in strong vinegar or in wine …', which was to be held in the mouth.[75]

Henbane continued to be suggested for pain in the teeth during the eleventh and early twelfth centuries, as evidenced by the herbal of *Macer Floridus*. It was recommended that the roots of the henbane plant be soaked in vinegar, warmed and then kept in the mouth, just as *Leechbook III* had advocated previously.[76] The twelfth-century herbal of Henry of Huntingdon called *Anglicanus ortus* endorsed the use of oregano as a remedy, placed inside the mouth for a long period of time.[77]

Moving forward, this idea of vicious fighting and damaged teeth appears in most of the works of Chrétien de Troyes, including *Erec and Enide*. Erec ended up in single combat against a mysterious and much larger knight arrayed in arms the colour of vermilion:

> Such havoc did they inflict upon each other's teeth,
> cheeks, nose, hands, arms, and the rest, upon the temples,
> neck, and throat that their bones all ache.[78]

Similarly, during their final battle in *The Knight of the Cart*, Lancelot broke three teeth of the notorious Meleagant by striking the nasal protection of his helmet so hard that it was knocked into his mouth.[79]

It is possible that in the twelfth century there were those who specialized in treating teeth. In his seminal work on medicine in Anglo-Norman England, Edward Kealey indicated the existence of a couple of men of medicine who may have treated medieval mouths as part of their work. Practising in the first half of the century was a man called Hugh, while the other, a man from Essex called John, worked in the second half. Words like *dubbedent*, *adubedent* and *cum dentibus* attached to the names of these men may have represented the fact that they also looked after teeth.[80]

At the same time as de Troyes was writing his epic poems and John of Essex was practising medicine the miracle collection at Rocamadour was being gathered. One account offers an intriguing story of an aging knight who had four of his front teeth knocked out in battle.[81] This warrior, in his 60s by this time, was struck in the mouth by the hilt of a sword.[82] Quite naturally he was concerned with his appearance, but also with how he would sound when he spoke with four teeth missing. He was recounted as being quite worried about joining the many who sounded like incoherent fools because of their poor dental situation.[83] Not wishing to count himself among the masses, the record from Rocamadour indicated that the aging knight prayed vehemently that his teeth might be restored. According to the entry his teeth did come back, although it says that they were the colour of ivory, noticeably different from the rest of his teeth.[84] This does seem to have been a very unlikely scenario, but what does seem more credible is that this knight simply had ivory or bone replacements fashioned, which he then inserted into his mouth, perhaps binding them to his natural teeth by means of fine wire or silk, as suggested by Theodoric below. This account does raise the question of the use of false teeth during this time. One of the earliest mentions can be found in the mid-fourteenth-century surgery of Guy de Chauliac, who suggested:

> Et s'ils tombent, qu'on y mette des dents d'un autre, ou qu'on en forge d'os de vache, et soient liez finement et on s'en sert long-temps.[85]

> If they should fall out, put in their place the teeth of another or fashion new ones from cow bones. These should line up and last for a long time.

While the entry at Rocamadour is 200 years earlier than de Chauliac's work, the use of carved ivory or bone teeth or even the teeth of others makes far more sense than a knight in his 60s suddenly sprouting four new teeth, the colour of ivory.[86] Finally, this knight had four silver teeth made to offer as thanksgiving, which he brought to the church at Rocamadour when he went to show off the miracle that had happened.[87] It is perhaps no coincidence that within contemporary texts perfect teeth were frequently described as resembling ivory or silver such as those belonging to the beautiful Soredamors, in de Troyes' poem *Cligés*.[88]

Doctors such as Roger Frugard presented only limited material pertaining to teeth within their surgical texts. Roger offered a treatment for the pain associated with a dental cavity, which included the use of a hot cautery placed at the hollow behind the earlobe. Following that an equal mixture of garlic and henbane were to be heated over charcoal, while the patient breathed in the fumes of the concoction. Roger described the remedy as a good and reliable painkiller, but it seems likely that the second part was far more effective than the first.[89] The pain of teeth damaged and broken as a result of battle would certainly have stood to benefit from such a treatment. One of the few mentions of teeth in Theodoric's surgery relates to his ingenious method for realigning them when the jaw had been fractured in more than one place. He proposed the use of silver or gold wire or even silk thread to bind the teeth back together in their proper alignment while the bones healed.[90]

William of Saliceto offered a much more powerful medication for tooth pain, although to his credit he did note that it was not for simple dental discomfort, but for what he described as violent pain. It involved a mixture of opium and henbane made into a pill to be placed on the tooth or dissolved into wine. The pain was said to have ceased within an hour, which it no doubt did. Finally, he also offered a mixture to help steady teeth that had been loosened. It included a combination of red and white corals, putty, gum arabic and a sap called tragacanth. Once mixed and placed on the teeth it was said to help keep them firmly in place.[91] The benefits of such a sticky substance would appear to have been temporary and quite messy as it began to break down in the mouth.

Fractured Skulls

> The sword even reaches the skull and cuts a
> bone of his head, but without penetrating the brain
> *Erec and Enide*[92]

Of the many treatments performed on medieval skeletal injuries the one that surely sends a shiver down the spine like no other is surgery to repair a serious head injury, an idea made even more chilling by Theodoric in his mid-thirteenth-century surgical text. He recommended that a patient's ears be stopped up with cotton during such a procedure in order that '... he should not be bothered by the sound of scraping or perforation or by the hammer blow ...' caused by the surgeon's tools.[93] A practical example from York, which may predate the work of Theodoric by a few decades, manages to amplify the notion of these sounds even further. Discovered in a cemetery just outside the walls of the city, the skull shows a large sword cut through the top with the telltale marks of attempts to remove bone splinters that had broken away. The scalp had been peeled back in order to facilitate the surgery, which included widening the opening along the centre of the wound made by the sword. This was likely done to provide the surgeon with a larger entry point, making it easier to retrieve pieces of bone and other debris from the brain or dura. Scratch marks on the skull, around the area of the opening, look to have recorded where the surgeon slipped with his or her tools during the procedure.[94]

It is precisely these kinds of wounds to the head that are the focus of this section, not the sort with brains spilling out from skulls or staining the weapons of knights and warriors, so common in Viking sagas and epic poems, troubadour's songs and chronicles.[95] While that may make it sound like most other types of head injuries were quite treatable, the truth was of course very different. A fall or a blow from a weapon created the potential for serious concussion, a depressed skull fracture or, as the example above shows, dangerous bone fragments reaching the brain, which could lead to death. Extraordinarily, until the time of the First World War it is estimated the latter would continue to be lethal about 80 per cent of time, helping to provide some idea of the severity of these sorts of head injuries during the Middle Ages.[96]

Protection for the head at this time, in the form of a hood of mail or a metal helmet, was generally worn only by affluent professional warriors, an important distinction as it meant this type of personal defence was well beyond the means of the common soldier.[97] Master Wace even made the case for a wooden helmet within his chronicle *Roman de Rou*. The description is that of a warrior on the side of the English at the Battle of Hastings in 1066: 'He had a helmet made of wood, which he fastened down to his coat and laced round his neck.'[98]

The ordinary fighter would have had few options, but head protection made from hardened leather or even equipment looted from the battlefield may have been worn, with just about anything being preferable to facing axes and arrows with a head completely bare.[99]

The elite soldier usually wore a lightly padded cloth covering under the mail or helmet. Called a coif cap or an arming cap, it provided a buffer between the metal and the wearer's head, while adding a little extra protection. It is referenced less often than the helmet, but in his epic poem *The Song of Girart of Vienne* Bertran de Bar-sur-Aube credited the good coif cap worn by Roland as having saved his life when his helmet was crushed:

> And had the coif-cap on his white coat been frail,
> This blow would have sent Roland into his grave;[100]

A more lengthy and accurate discussion around medieval helmets and head protection is much better served by the more comprehensive and interesting studies that exist on medieval armour. The importance of helmets here lies simply in the protection that they may or may not have provided to the heads of soldiers in the Middle Ages. That was certainly the case in the ninth century for Charles the Child, the son of the Carolingian ruler Charles the Bald.[101] Just a teenager in the year 864, he survived a grim head injury, but only for a short time. The *Annals of St Bertin* recorded some horseplay, which resulted in a sword blow to the head and face of Charles caused by another young man named Albuin. The injury was large and deep spreading from his left temple, down and across his face to his right cheekbone and jaw. It certainly brings into question whether he was wearing protection on his head at the time. The chronicle indicated that the wound did not reach his brain, perhaps underestimating the gravity of the harm that had been done, as the injury hindered him greatly for what remained of his short life.[102] In spite of the best care available to the young Charles he struggled with serious epileptic fits as he lingered for the next two years before finally expiring on 29 September 866.[103]

In the stories and chronicles that describe the early centuries in Northern Europe, such as the sagas of the Vikings, helmets were constantly being split by swords and axes. In *The Story of Burnt Njal*, the title character's son-in-law had a sword he called 'Helmet-Hewer'.[104] Saxo Grammaticus included several helmet-smashing passages in his *Gesta Danorum*, like the rambunctious pre-wedding celebration of Rute and Agnar, the son of Ignell. One of the rowdy guests called Bjarke ended up being challenged to a duel by Agnar, after his bad behaviour had interrupted the party. Agnar struck the first blow, slicing through the front of Bjarke's helmet and scalp before the sword got caught in the vizor holes of his head protection.[105]

What is strange about these stories of helmeted Vikings thumping the heads of others is the fact that almost no Viking helmets have ever been discovered. Across the whole of Scandinavia just one complete metal helmet has ever been recovered, the Gjermundbu Helmet found in Norway in 1943.[106] One other of similar construction and date, called the Yarm Helmet, was found in North Yorkshire in the 1950s, but it has only recently begun to be understood.[107] Juxtaposed with this reality are studies like those completed by Caroline Arcini, noted earlier in this chapter.[108] In her appraisal of the cranial injuries she found that there were fewer damaged skulls in the late Viking Age examples from 990–1100 than from the group in the 1100–1300 date range, despite the nearly 3 : 1 ratio of skeletons in the earlier group compared with those from the second lot.[109] There are reasons of violence and politics that help to explain the cranial injuries in the 1100–1300 group, but with so few Viking Age helmets having been discovered the large number of earlier skeletons showing scarcely any skull damage seems counterintuitive.[110] Even at other Viking Age burials in Sweden, such as at Kopparsvik, Slite and Birka, very few skulls show any signs of injuries caused by weapons.[111] It would seem that there should either be a much larger number of excavated skeletons from the Viking Age displaying wounds to the head or a considerably larger quantity of Viking helmets. Therefore, the question must be asked, where are they? Did these warriors have a different means of protection, not made from iron or steel, which have long since degraded? Were they just superior fighters or are there more dead that yet lay undiscovered that will tell a different story?[112] A likely conclusion may be a combination of many things, but for now it remains an enigma.

Stopping to explore some of the medical advice for head injuries available in the Anglo-Saxon texts the options range widely, with *Bald's Leechbook* offering remedies to treat both simple and more serious types of a 'broken head'.[113] One involved the often-used betony plant, the leaves of which were to be bruised and then placed on the head of the injured person to reunite the wounded tissues. Another, meant for more serious wounds where the skull was exposed, could be made using a combination of honey, goutweed, maythe (camomile) and butter to produce a useful salve.[114]

In *Leechbook III* skull fractures were managed in a far more violent and controversial manner: 'If a man's, head-pan, or skull, be seemingly ironbound lay the man with face upward, drive two stakes into the ground at the armpits, then lay a plank across over his feet, then strike on it thrice with a sledge beetle, the skull will come right soon.'[115] It is difficult to understand just how this process would have been of assistance in treating such a serious injury. The fact that the force of a sledge beetle (a mallet or sledgehammer) was required seems only ever likely to have created more trauma.[116] Additionally, a large hammer like this would have been an unusual and valuable tool, likely the domain of a blacksmith. While it is only speculation to be sure, the use of such an instrument raises the possibility of a metalsmith's involvement in such an operation.

The abbey of St Foy recorded the details of a knight called William, from the now destroyed castle of Carlat in Southern France, who received a head wound.[117] Although it allows us to identify a particular individual, not much can be gleaned about the nature of his injury or the treatment received, however the details and unintended humour of the entry are worth recounting here. The injury to his head caused him to lose his sight, but after prayers to St Foy and the use of salves on his eyes he was able to see again. Shortly after his sight had returned William attempted to break up a fight between two men of his household, but as he did so he was accidentally struck in the eye by one of them. The bloody wound was so painful that he could hardly bear to open his eyes or even lift his head.[118] Returning to his intercessions to the good saint, he took rather a different approach the second time:

> O illustre sainte Foy, vous qui surpassez dans l'art de guérir les médecins les plus renommés, pourquoi avez-vous permis qu'il m'arrivât un accident si cruel? Ne deviez-vous pas protéger d'un tel malheur cet oeil auquel vous aviez rendu la lumière? Que m'a servi de recevoir de vous un bienfait si cruellement ravi? Puisque vous l'avez ainsi permis, rendez-moi ce que vous m'aviez donné.[119]

> O illustrious St Foy, you who surpasses even the most renowned of physicians, why have you allowed such a cruel and terrible thing to happen to me? Should you not have protected my eye against such an outcome? What was the point of receiving such a wonderful blessing from you? Since you have allowed it before, give me back what you gave me.

Grievances aired and faith in the saint restored, he decided to stop taking any food or drink until his eyes could be moistened with water that had been blessed at the abbey.[120] A member of William's household quickly made the journey to the abbey at St Foy and secured the holy water. While it worked to reduce the pain his eyesight hardly improved, so William made his own pilgrimage to the abbey, where he stayed for many days until he could once again see properly.[121]

The chronicles and epic poems of the twelfth and thirteenth centuries contain more of the same helmet- and skull-crushing blows so common in earlier works with stories of everything from survival to demise.[122] The famous Welsh historian Gerald of Wales (Gerald de Barri) wrote about his older brother, Robert de Barri, who was a member of the army that invaded Ireland in May 1169. Just a young soldier at the time, de Barri received a head injury while attempting to besiege the town of Wexford:

Among the wounded was Robert de Barri, a young soldier, who, inflamed with ardent valour, and dauntless in the face of death, was among the first who scaled the walls; but being struck upon his helmet by a great stone, and falling headlong into the ditch below, narrowly escaped with his life, his comrades with some difficulty drawing him out.[123]

It appears that his helmet was of some use in protecting his head as he escaped more or less unscathed, thanks to the work of his fellow soldiers. Strangely, Gerald did attribute the loss of Robert's teeth in later life to this earlier incident.[124]

The Knight of the Two Swords shows the prevalence and serious nature of head injuries suffered by warriors in battle. In this specific passage a number of knights, under the command of King Ris, turn up on King Arthur's doorstep. Among them were nine serious casualties, with head injuries ranking as the worst of the wounds. Arthur eventually had the men taken to two quiet rooms where their injuries were examined, cleansed, bandaged and cared for by his doctors. After some time had passed seven of the nine men managed to survive their wounds, but the other two did not make it.[125]

Looking to later surgical texts for evidence of the treatment of head injuries, Roger Frugard devoted several pages to the subject in his influential work, although it is worth noting that much of what he wrote was already available in earlier texts like the *Bamberg Surgery*.[126] Roger included different poultices for use on head injuries that did not involve fractures, again differentiating them by seasons, with one type for winter use and another for wounds occurring in the summer.[127] The matter of more serious head injuries was regularly managed using trepanation, a process of cutting or enlarging a hole or holes into the skull to relieve pressure on the brain or to allow for the removal of weapon or bone fragments. The skull found at York, noted at the beginning of this section, shows evidence of this procedure that has been in use for millennia. As outlined in Roger's surgery, it began with a cruciform-shaped incision being made into the scalp so that the skin could be peeled away from the skull with the use of a scraper.[128] Then a drill-like tool, called a trephine, was used to create a hole in the skull, although it is clear from the York example that some other instrument was used to enlarge the existing gap caused by the weapon.[129]

This was obviously a dangerous operation with the potential for life-threatening damage to the brain, but some surgeons may have had a way of trying to prevent fatal injuries. The skull of a male between the ages of 36 and 45 years with a date range of about 1200–1250 and showing evidence of trepanation was excavated at St Mary Spital in London. What makes it noteworthy is the faint evidence of a semi-circular mark just beyond the edges of the hole in the skull. It seems that it may have been made by some sort of guard that prevented the drill from going too deep and penetrating the outer membrane around the brain.[130] Another male from the same excavation, about the same age range and dating between 1250 and 1400, also shows evidence of trepanation. This individual suffered many serious injuries during his lifetime. Whether they all occurred at once or at different times in his life is difficult to ascertain, because he did survive his wounds including the trepanation procedure.[131] It is clear from excavated skulls like the York example and the two from London that patients could survive these drastic operations, some even going on to fight again.

Theodoric and William of Saliceto wrote extensively on head wounds. Theodoric, as always, relied heavily on his father's experiences throughout his chapters on these types of injuries, endorsing the fact that they must have been quite common on the battlefield.[132] The text of William of Saliceto provides the final example of a head injury, with its importance being in the details that confirm the surgeon's patience and care as he treated an injured man called Lazarino who came from Cremona in what is now Northern Italy. He had received a terrible blow to his head from a sword or perhaps a club, creating a wound that covered the length of his skull from his forehead right to the back and through to his brain. William began by shaving Lazarino's head and cleansing the wound of blood and debris to enable him to gain a proper view of the damage so he could remove the splinters of bone.[133] His initial investigation of the wound left William of the opinion that there was no hope for the young Cremonan:

> ... j'ai annoncé à ses parents et à ses amis que le cas était sans espoir et la mort du malade et, pour le moment, je l'ai laissé.[134]

> ... I explained to his parents and friends that it was a hopeless case that would certainly result in his death. I then left him for the time being.

Despite the severity of the damage and his proclamation to the patient's loved ones, William continued to care for the young man. He dressed the wound and kept watch over him, but by the third day Lazarino had become completely paralysed. He was unable to eat for a week, just sipping mixtures of sugar or honey with crushed rose petals and water. William looked in on him daily, cleaning and dressing his wounds. After about ten days the paralysis began to show signs of improvement and he was soon able to take some food, even requesting broth and wine. He was provided with a light chicken soup, but he was not allowed the wine. Incredibly Lazarino survived, recovering from his near fatal head wound and going on to live for another twenty years.[135]

Chapter 6

Disfigured and Disabled

> Half of your nose has been cut from your face
> *The Coronation of Louis*[1]

Warfare can maim and twist the human form in so many pitiable ways. Throughout history, weapons and devices of torture have continually been devised to cause mutilations, burn injuries and impairments of all kinds, bringing misery to so many soldiers and civilians alike and leaving lives forever changed. Tens of thousands were left with bodies and minds torn apart by the American Civil War of the nineteenth century, but after the fighting was over most disabled soldiers were unable to find work and the families of those who had been disfigured frequently hid them away out of sight so as not to cause embarrassment.[2] The horrors of the First World War left large numbers of men and women with the most dreadful injuries. Among British servicemen alone, there were more than 41,000 who lost one or more limbs, to say nothing of those from the many other countries that participated.[3] Conflict in the Middle Ages presented many similar situations and it certainly would not have been uncommon to see those missing an eye or using a wooden crutch and prosthesis to replace a missing leg.[4] Adam of Bremen reported one such group of men who barely survived an incident that occurred in 994 when Vikings from Sweden and Denmark met and defeated their smaller Saxon force, along the Elbe River near Stade in what is now Germany. Several high-ranking Saxon hostages were taken, but after one escaped the Vikings sliced away the noses, hands and feet of the remaining captives in retribution, before dumping them onto the shore: 'Among them were some noble men who lived a long time after ... a pitiful spectacle for all the people'.[5] *The History of Fulk Fitz Warine, an Outlawed Baron in the Reign of King John* described how ten knights '... lost their noses, others their chins ...' after being soundly beaten in battle by Fulk and his companions.[6] While this tale is a strange mix of fact and fantasy it represents the truth about many who were left disfigured by their wounds of battle or mistreatment as captured soldiers.[7]

Names also provided lasting representations of the damage done to individuals through violence, leaving little doubt about how they looked. Across the sagas and poetry of the Vikings descriptive names can be found at every turn with monikers like Ari the One-Eyed, Haki the Cheek-Cut One and Kettle Flatnose.[8] Injuries like these continued to make up some family names in the centuries that followed the Viking Age. Although some designations described unfortunate physical appearances that were the result of disease or punishment, in the form of mutilation, many other names would have denoted the terrible scars received in battle. The name *Denasez* is one that comes from the French meaning 'without a nose', a surname that might have been pinned to soldiers like those from *Fulk Fitz Warine* above. In 1086, at the time of the Domesday survey in England, a man called Reynaldus Stanceberd Denasez was among those recorded.[9] Another designation from the Old French word *borgne*, meaning 'one-eyed', can be found in the twelfth-century name le Borne, while the Old English word *hamal*, describing scarred or mutilated, is recorded in names like Hamill or Hammel.[10]

As seen above, some soldiers with scars and disfigurements were naturally looked upon with great pity, but then there were a whole range of reactions and emotions that covered these reminders of war during this period of time. Perhaps unsurprisingly Saxo Grammaticus explained that a Viking's injuries were viewed as marks of bravery because '… a man whose body was seamed with so many traces of wounds had no weakling soul'.[11] In some less expected places similar thoughts can also be found, including a mid-eleventh-century entry from the collection of miracles at St Foy where the scribe went into some detail about a warrior's bravery being shown through his scars of battle:

La plus belle gloire d'un héros c'est d'offrir sur son corps de larges cicatrices.[12]

The greatest glory of a hero is to end up with large scars on his body.

Outside of Europe, more of the same was set down by the twelfth-century Muslim chronicler Usāmah ibn Munqidh. He related the story of his father whom he said was addicted to war. He noted the many scars that covered his father's body resulting from the 'terrible wounds' he had received in battle.[13] There were several that decorated his physique, a pike wound on his chest, a spear injury to his arm that had required surgery, unidentified damage from a lance and possibly a scar on his nose from a javelin.[14] As terrible as these marks on his father may have been, they too seem to have been looked upon with great pride.

Within the written works of this time scars were regularly used as a means of identifying an individual. Take as an example Guibert of Nogent who included the story of a warrior bishop whose badly damaged body could only be identified by the wound on his neck, which he had received in a tournament.[15] Returning quickly to Saxo, in the sixth book of his *Gesta Danorum* the Danish king Fridleif was able to uncover a potential assassin by the marks he had on his body.[16] In de Troyes' *The Knight with the Lion (Yvain)*, the scar on the face of the knight called Yvain is what allowed him to be recognized when his unconscious and naked body was discovered in the forest where he had spent time in grief and madness.[17]

The mid-twelfth-century epic *The Coronation of Louis* is slightly different in this regard. The situation has a note of modern-day media spin to it, with the victim getting out ahead of his disfigurement to give himself a self-deprecating name before he could be labelled by others. In this epic the nobleman Count William (Guillaume) loses a portion of his nose while battling the giant Saracen called Corsolt.[18] When William was warned of the jeers and insults that he would have to endure as a result he soon took control of the situation by renaming himself after his mutilation, as if to take its away its power: 'The count baptized himself there again. "Henceforth, by all who love and would praise, by Franks and Lombards, I shall be named Count William Short Nose, the warrior brave."'[19] The damage to his nose became a badge of honour and a method of distinguishing himself elsewhere in the epic cycle of *Guillaume d'Orange*. In the poem entitled *Aliscans*, for instance, William had to show what was left of his nose to Lady Guiborc to prove that it was he, before she would allow his army to enter a fortress.[20]

As we have seen in examples from the miracle collections many warriors were quite happy to show off their scars to the scribes and witnesses scrutinizing their claims, evidence of the supposed divine intervention that had brought them back to good health.[21] The collection from Rocamadour offers several of these, including the young warrior called Gerald Hugh who received multiple wounds as he defended a castle from Basque attackers. He managed to survive his injuries, later showing his scars at the abbey.[22] During the first half of the eleventh century a warrior called Bernard, from the castle at Valeilles, was stabbed through the eye with a lance, but even after a serious infection he was left with just a '… slight scar that was visible to all eyes …'.[23] This is another example from the St Foy collection that uses a word like 'slight' or 'thin' when describing the cicatrice that was left by a wound, seeming to downplay the fact that they even existed at all, perhaps to make the healing seem all the more heaven sent. The young English knight from the Lascelles family who survived the injury to his intestines managed to impact other soldiers when he took himself to the palace of the English king to show off the scar on his stomach and credit his survival to St Godric. The visit of Lascelles prompted many of the soldiers present at the palace to make their own vow to visit the shrine of St Godric in the north of England.[24]

There were clearly those who were repulsed by the disfigurements of those close to them, but others who were just as disgusted by such shallow opinions. The twelfth-century Frenchman Andreas Capellanus, writing about love in the latter part of that century, included the compassionate and forthright thoughts of the lady of Narbonne. She reflected on those who rejected their lovers when they returned to them from the battlefield with disfiguring wounds:

> Opposed to this woman is the opinion of the lady of Narbonne, who said on the subject: 'We think that a woman is unworthy of any honour if she has decided that her lover ought to be deprived of her love because of some deformity resulting from the common chance of war, which is apt to happen to those who fight bravely.'[25]

She went on to say that if it was his courage that drew a woman to admire and love such a soldier in the first place then she should almost expect her lover to suffer an injury at some time. Equally, a warrior who had shown such valour should anticipate that his lady would continue to love and admire him for his bravery, even with a disfiguring injury.[26]

In the world of medieval medicine there were at least some attempts made to improve the appearance of some scars and disfigurements. While not related to battle or violence there is confirmation in *Bald's* that leeches attempted to provide a surgical repair for a cleft lip:

> For hair lip, pound mastic very small, add the white of an egg and mingle as thou dost vermillion, cut with a knife the false edges of the lip, sew fast with silk, then smear without and within with the salve ere the silk rot. If it draw together, arrange it with the hand; anoint again soon.[27]

This early procedure is one that is often quoted and with good reason. It represents fairly advanced medicine with the recognition that both edges required cutting and joining in order to knit together properly, plus the use of silk sutures, which would disappear or 'rot' naturally. The antibacterial properties of the salve, particularly the mastic, would have aided in healing, although the science would not have been understood. It is evidence that societies in the early centuries of the Middle Ages naturally recognized a disfigurement, but, more importantly, at times sought a viable treatment to repair it. Taking it further, principles such as these could quite easily have been applied to other disfigurements, such as poorly executed wound repairs.

The chronicler Matthew Paris noted, '... rub the wound where the steel has entered with superficial fomentations, and ... cause an ugly scar, not a cure'.[28] In his surgical text Theodoric wrote of his displeasure for wounds that had not healed properly, especially those on the face, noting his '... wont to destroy ugly scars ...'.[29] His section on wounds occurring from swords and other weapons warned that removing the dressing too quickly could result in a hideous cicatrice. In cases such as these he instructed that a gold cautery, which had first been boiled, be used to remove the scar tissue. After that, pieces of goose's fat and blood were to be used on the injured area. Once the inflammation had been reduced an ointment of chicken fat and mastic was to be applied to the scar. Theodoric also suggested ground-up pigeon dung and water as a useful cleanser for scars in order to promote proper healing.[30]

Burn Injuries

> ... a stooping shield-giant which breathes forth flame and fire.
> *The King's Mirror*[31]

The monk Peter of les Vaux-de-Cernay recorded many terrifying events in his chronicle of the Albigensian Crusade, including an episode that came during the siege of Moissac when Simon de Montfort, his brother Guy and others were nearly burned alive. They became trapped inside a siege weapon, known as a cat, as they attempted to attack the walls of Moissac. Under the cover of darkness, the defenders of Moissac began retaliating in earnest, perhaps aware of the high value targets that were inside the cat. They came out from behind their fortifications to try and burn the cat and those inside by using a weapon known as a petrary to hurl anything flammable at it, including dry wood, straw, meat, fat and oil. The crusaders used water, wine and earth in an attempt to extinguish the stubborn flames, but the fire continued to intensify around the cat. Under crossbow fire from the men of Moissac the crusaders continued to try and quench the fire, using iron hooks to keep themselves from the fierce heat as they tried to pull the lumps of meat and vessels full of oil out of the flames. In the end, the cat was pulled free and Simon and Guy were both saved, but it was at some cost to the others who did not fare so well: 'The anguish caused to them by the heat and their exertions was beyond belief and could scarcely be witnessed without tears ...'.[32] Perhaps feared above all other sorts of injuries, this horrifying scene highlights how fire and heat, when used as weapons of war, can cause panic and terror of the most primal sort. During these medieval centuries fire, boiling liquids, hot sand and chemicals were employed as weapons of terror to both attack and defend, spreading devastation and fear among soldiers and civilians alike.[33] The account of Abbo of Saint-German-des-Prés provides a hideous example of the kind of physical damage that boiling liquids could cause. As the Vikings attacked Paris in 885 a mix of wax, pitch and oil was heated in a furnace by the Frankish defenders who then spilled it from the top of their fortifications onto the assailing Danes. The damage caused to those who took a direct hit from the heated mixture was terrible as it '... made their skulls split open' and mercifully many did not survive.[34]

The sagas contain many cruel tales of men and women trapped inside buildings, which were then intentionally set alight. A stark illustration can be found in *The Story of Burnt Njal* when eleven members of Njal's family were killed by his enemies after they set fire to his house, with everyone inside. The only one to escape was Njal's son-in-law, Kari Solmund: '... by that time all Kari's upper clothing and his hair were a-blaze, then he threw himself down from the roof ... Kari ran till he came to a stream, and then he threw himself down into it, and so quenched the fire on him.'[35] Kari survived the flames and in a brief appearance in *The Saga of Grettir the Strong*, or *Grettis' Saga*, he is referred to as Scorched Kari, giving us an indication of the burn scars that were left on his head and body.[36] Within the original saga the author did not neglect the psychological impact of such an incident. We are told that Kari could no longer sleep at night, speaking of his grief on more than one occasion.[37]

The mid-thirteenth-century Norwegian educational text known as *The King's Mirror*, or *Konungs skuggsjá*, provided plans for a defence against siege weapons that included '... pitch, sulphur or boiling tar' thrown onto the assailants.[38] *La chanson de la croisade contre les Albigeois* describes a mix of water and quicklime dumped from the ramparts of Beaucaire.[39] This would have caused chemical burns to those who came into contact with the mixture. It would have quickly blinded those soldiers who were looking up and been very uncomfortable for those encased in mail or some other type of armour, as it slipped between gaps in their protection. A similar tactic was used by the English navy, under the command of Philip de Albiney, in 1217 against the French fleet off the coast of England. The English threw quicklime dust into the wind toward the French, which 'blinded the eyes' of many of them.[40]

It was Greek fire that came to be one of the most extreme weapons of the medieval era. It was a weapon that has taken on a near mythical status over the centuries. It could be thrown in clay pots and grenades or pumped through siphons to direct a larger stream of flame. Just the threat of its use managed to terrorize and frighten soldiers throughout the age. It is a weapon that seems likely to have originated in the Byzantine Empire, but the formula or formulae, as there was probably more than one type, are shrouded in some mystery. Sulphur, lime, tar, olive oil, naphtha and saltpetre are just some of the possible ingredients.[41] A partial clue is found in the mid-twelfth-century epic *The Conquest of Orange* that refers to a pungent smell associated with Greek fire.[42] *The Chronicle of the Third Crusade* also notes a very strong smell and goes a step further to describe flames that burned blue-grey in colour.[43]

At times Greek fire could be just as dangerous to the user as to those for whom it was intended. Its volatility was exposed in an incident in 1190, during the Third Crusade, when a man called Bellegemin and his men attacked a group of crusaders. Bellegemin was carrying a container of Greek fire, but when he was knocked off his horse it broke open, setting Bellegemin on fire and killing him.[44] It was also known to blow back against its attackers, as Matthew Paris highlighted in the year 1249: 'They [Saracens] threw against us the Greek fire in great quantity and force, which was very dangerous and destructive to us, because there was a strong wind blowing from the city towards us. But, behold, the wind suddenly shifting, carried the fire back upon the city, and burnt several of their men.'[45]

Water did little to extinguish the flames, which led to vinegar being one of the preferred methods used to put the fire out, as described by Roger of Wendover, '... by means of vinegar, gravel, and other extinguishing matter, the fire was subdued'. [46]

In 941, as Rūs Vikings made a raid on Byzantium they were repelled by the full shock of Greek fire when it was employed against their ships. An entry from *The Russian Primary Chronicle* for the same year described a naval battle between the Rūs and Byzantine sailors: 'Theophanes pursued them in boats with Greek fire, and dropped it through pipes upon the Russian ships.'[47] It goes on to explain how the Rūs were forced overboard to try and escape the devastation. There were those who survived, with some among them certainly requiring treatment for burns, later recalling the incredible weapon that was like lightning from heaven.[48]

This weapon of terror continued to be used extensively against European crusaders from the time of the First Crusade at the end of the eleventh century.[49] While it did find its way north to Europe, examples are a little more unusual, perhaps due to a lack of reporting, knowledge of its use or just fear of such a terrible weapon.[50] The French used it in 1195 against the port town of Dieppe, which was in English hands. They incinerated the English ships that sat in the harbour, along with parts of Dieppe that had only recently been constructed by Richard I of England.[51] Around the same time an entry in the Pipe Rolls of Richard I indicated that Greek fire was in England. The record from 1194–5 shows a shipment of weapons of war, such as shields, crossbows and *igne greco* (Greek fire), going north from London to Nottingham, specifically to an engineer called Urrico.[52]

A final reference to Greek fire that is of interest comes from the first Scottish War of Independence. A couple of records relate to its use against Stirling castle by the English in 1304. A writ of 31 March 1304, from Edward I of England at St Andrews to his treasurer and barons of the exchequer, ordered them to provide materials for Greek fire for the siege of Stirling castle. They included saltpetre and 'quick sulphur', which were sourced and shipped from York.[53] A second entry for expenses from July of the same year shows a payment of 47*s*. 8*d*. to a man called John de la Mullier for the use of Greek fire against Stirling castle. It was to cover the cost of things such as the employment of five men for eighteen days, a boy for forty days and the materials themselves. John de la Mullier received a significant payment of 36*s*. 8*d*. for his own involvement, supporting the idea that it was a highly specialized weapon requiring some mastery.[54]

One suspects that the tissue damage and infection related to severe burn injuries would have been difficult to survive. The chronicler of the Third Crusade notes of those attacked by Greek fire while at sea that only one of three fates awaited them, being burned to death, drowning or succumbing to their injuries.[55] References to those with burn scars, like Scorched Kari noted above, are uncommon. Still, there are others, such as Hugh de Lacy, a supporter of Henry II of England. Gerald of Wales described the burn on de Lacy's face, '… which much disfigured him, the scar reaching down his right cheek to his chin'.[56]

Remedies and pain-relieving procedures were developed and improved upon to try and treat those who had been injured by weapons of heat and fire. The first book of *Bald's Leechbook* included many treatments for burns like one incorporating the unusual component of goat's turd and another, 'Again, take lilly and yarrow, boil them in butter, smear therewith.'[57] Similarly, within the *Old Icelandic Medical Miscellany* there are a couple of treatments for burns that also involve the use of the lily, one of which was meant for areas of the body where hair grows.[58] The great twelfth-century German Abbess Hildegard of Bingen suggested something altogether different in a remedy that required flax seeds to be boiled in water. A linen cloth was then to be dipped into the resulting liquid and placed over the burned tissue of the body.[59]

As the twelfth century moved into its last two decades Roger Frugard noted the importance of first cleaning the burned area using olive oil that was mixed with cold water. The cold water was no doubt intended to cleanse, but just as importantly act to soothe the pain, even if only temporarily.[60] In the next century, a small, but significant refinement was made by Roland of Parma. He suggested that cold water be continually added to the mixture, which would have kept its analgesic properties working while the wound was being cleaned.[61] Roger also recommended three separate and different treatments, one of which involved pomegranate bark simmered in a wine of quality. The mixture was then to be boiled and the bark removed, ground up and mixed with egg white to make an ointment, which could then be spread over the burn.[62]

Relying on the Islamic physician Avicenna, in his chapter on burns, Theodoric too was concerned with the pain and discomfort that these wounds caused. However, he was just as interested in the growth of new tissue and the prevention of blistering. Acknowledging how delicate the damaged tissue could be the burned area was to be continually placed in a bath of strong vinegar. If soaking the burned area in a basin was not practical, then bandages drenched in the coldest vinegar were to be applied and changed frequently. Soothing medications like rosewater and snow were also suggested and so too were those containing the topical pain-relieving benefits of opium.[63] One such salve could be made in the following fashion using three parts of a red clay called Armenian bole mixed with one-part ceruse and a half-part of opium. These were to be mixed with vinegar and egg white and applied to the damaged area.[64]

Also writing on the subject, William of Saliceto recommended the application of a compress of snow or cold water to the burned area, again acting as an important analgesic. Cool mud is an alternative suggestion, because as he noted snow and cold water were not always readily available. The process was meant to be a continuous one in order to keep the area cool. A series of ointments were then to be applied to encourage the healing process.[65]

Torture and Cruelty

> They inflicted similar tortures on knights and others of every condition, some of them they hung up by the middle, some by the feet and legs, some by the hands, and some by the thumbs and arms, and then threw salt mixed with vinegar in the eyes of the wretches.
>
> Roger of Wendover[66]

The term *medieval torture* is one that often triggers in our minds terrible images of unspeakable deeds done to provoke fear and terror, to punish or cause a ransom to be paid. The above epigraph from *The Chronicle of Roger of Wendover* is the sort of ghastly picture that comes to mind, with the bodies of helpless soldiers and civilians strung up by their thumbs, hands and feet. This savagery took place in 1216 as King John laid waste to parts of England. The description becomes even more barbaric as the chronicler relates how some were grilled alive over coals until they expired.[67] At other times acts of extreme cruelty seem to have been performed just for the sake of it. Orderic Vitalis related details of an especially vicious count called Robert de Belesme, who in the late eleventh century ran riot with his armed men, mutilating and blinding many. He enjoyed devising new and diabolical methods for torturing his victims, preferring their pain to any ransom that he might receive for their release.[68] In the Middle Ages dreadful deeds of torture and cruelty like these were the cause of some of the most horrific injuries to the body and mind, regularly leaving victims disfigured and disabled. This section seeks not only to uncover more of these terrible acts, but to explore the few medical texts that sought to treat them.

In pre-Viking Ireland the *Annals of Ulster* recalled how six prisoners were tortured in the year 745, some of which may even have been crucified.[69] After the arrival of the Vikings the brutality continued, according to an entry for the year 830 in the *The Annals of Clonmacnoise*, which speaks of all sorts of cruelties used by the Northmen.[70] The same chronicle recorded more Viking brutality in the year 980 when others were tortured before being killed.[71]

Snorri Sturluson included an episode of the infamous Viking cruelty known as the blood-eagle within his *Heimskringla*: 'Thereafter Earl Einar went up to Halfdan, and cut a spread eagle upon his back, by striking his sword through his back into his belly, dividing his ribs from the backbone down to his loins, and tearing out his lungs; and so Halfdan was killed.'[72] This practice of opening the victim up from the back, separating the ribs and pulling out the lungs to look like wings has divided opinion among historians, being disbelieved by some. However, it seems to fit within a larger pattern of brutality that included things such as human and animal sacrifices performed at Uppsala in Sweden, as described to Adam of Bremen by an eyewitness.[73] As well, Ibn Fadlān and Ibn Rusta both recorded the Rūs burial practice involving the sacrifice of female slaves.[74]

The miracle collection at St Foy contains several records that piece together a larger picture of what it was like to be held captive and tortured in France and Spain in the first half of the eleventh century. A warrior called Robert from Auvergne was held prisoner by a man called Adalhelm, lord of the castle of Roche d'Agoux. He was kept with very heavy chains placed around his legs, forced to sleep uncovered on the bare ground and starved for two days only being fed on the third evening with mouldy crusts of bread. This was just the beginning of his torment as Robert was then forced into extremely tight shackles and placed inside a small, wooden cage.[75] Another called Oliba was captured and held for ransom in Calonge, Spain. He was treated despicably:

> Puis ce monster ... enferma l'infortuné dans une étroite niche et plaça autour de sa tête des pièces de bois armées de pointes de fer, de sorte que

le captif ne pouvait ni prendre sa nourriture, ni s'appuyer un seul instant pour dormir, ni reposer ses membres accablés de lassitude.[76]

Then the monster ... locked the unfortunate Oliba in a very cramped space and placed around his head pieces of wood that were bristling with iron spikes, so that he could neither eat, sleep nor rest his weary body in any manner.

The twelfth-century miracle collection from St William of Norwich in England shows similar traits to those employed on the Continent. A knight called William de Witewelle held his nephew, named Gerard, in iron chains, exposing him to the cold and depriving him of food for long periods. The knight also '... exercised a tyrannous violence against him'.[77]

Peter of les Vaux-de-Cernay related the torture of two crusaders, Walter Langton, the brother of the Archbishop of Canterbury Stephen Langton, and Lambert de Thury.[78] In the summer of 1211 they were captured by the Count of Foix. Both men were placed in deplorable conditions inside a tiny, stinking dungeon that did not allow them enough space to stand or lie down properly. They were kept in heavy chains with no light, except a candle that was provided when they were eating. According to Peter they were kept there for a long time until they were finally ransomed.[79]

Within the penultimate chapter of his book on wounds William of Saliceto included a remarkable piece on the treatment of injuries caused by torture. It is a very unconventional set of medical instructions for those who would read and practise the procedures he set out. It deals with all kinds of injuries resulting from torture, including bastinado, that is the whipping of the soles of the feet.[80] His efforts to help victims who had been treated so appallingly involved their diet, starting light and working them back up to their regular consumption of food over many days.[81] Bloodletting and the use of laxatives were also to be prescribed along with his regular treatments for contusions, wounds and fractures, taken from other chapters of his surgery.[82] A special ointment could be applied on the wounds and twice daily an immersion in a tub of water containing restorative and relaxing herbs and flowers such as camomile and cumin was recommended. Once the individual came out of the bath the ointment was then to be reapplied.[83]

In a final note on the subject William spoke about older doctors who had suggested that those suffering from the wounds of torture be wrapped in the skin of a newly flayed horse or sheep, while the hides were still warm. He had been told that this was a successful method of treatment, but it was not one that he himself had ever used.[84]

Perhaps the only other surgery or treatise from around this time containing anything to do with the injuries caused by torture can be found in the text of the French surgeon Henri de Mondeville.[85] These victims of torture, he noted, were often in severe pain, unable to move, comatose or suffering badly after being thrown from a wall. Others had endured dislocated and fractured bones, alongside many open wounds that resulted from their mistreatment.[86] While his work was compiled at the very end of this study, between 1306 and 1320, part of its value lies in de Mondeville's record of what he referred to as 'old-fashioned treatments', those methods used prior to de Mondeville's time.[87] Mirroring William of Saliceto in many ways, Henri noted that the recommended diet for victims of torture had consisted of small amounts of easily digestible food taken for three or four days before being returned to their regular meals. The second consideration had been bloodletting, which had been practised using the opposite part of the body. If the damage was to the upper body, then the patient was bled from the feet and if there were injuries to the lower body, the hands were used. In cases where the damage was severe and widespread over the body then the location used for the bloodletting was at the discretion of the doctor. The bowels of the victim were also commonly evacuated using laxatives prescribed by the doctor.[88]

Topical ointments and lotions were applied to the injuries, the first medicine being an oil made from myrtle or roses mixed with powdered myrtle rubbed into the bruised and damaged areas of the body. These were applied for the first few days, until the danger of infection had passed and the bruising had settled. Next came a remedy that was rubbed into the skin each day before the patient's morning and evening meals. It was a mixture of resin, wax, terebinth, frankincense and fenugreek combined with oil. Once every four days the victim was bathed using herbs to help them relax and after each of these baths the above salve was to be rubbed into the skin once again. This process was used until the victim had recovered.[89]

Henri de Mondeville then went on to describe some of the *modern* methods of treatment for torture that were being practised during the first two decades of the fourteenth century. He disapproved of many of them, including covering in horse manure those who had recently been released from abuse, a practice done for three or four days. Interestingly, de Mondeville also noted the method that William described, whereby the victim was wrapped in the freshly flayed skin of a horse. While William had never tried it, de Mondeville rejected it outright.[90] For the most part de Mondeville referred his students and readers back to his standard methods for looking after contusions, wounds and the like, although his treatise on fractures and dislocations was never written.[91]

Like mutilations, scars and burn injuries, torture takes a tremendous toll on the human mind, along with the damage that it causes to the body.[92] While the focus of both of these medieval surgeons was on the physical injuries associated with torture, both appear to have given the occasional nod to the psychological side of such abuse. William, for instance, acknowledged that some patients would fear being immersed in a restorative bath, in which case a sponge bath would suffice.[93] This was a small, but important note to his students as William must have witnessed such reactions among victims who had perhaps been forcibly held under water until they nearly drowned, were confined in small spaces or who suffered any number of gruesome mistreatments. Henri de Mondeville's rejection of burying victims in manure or wrapping them in fresh animal skins recognized the negative impact this would have had on those who had been tortured by being kept tightly bound in heavy chains or placed in small spaces and cages such as Walter Langton and Robert from Auvergne noted above.[94]

Prostheses and Devices

> Onund recovered and went about for the rest of his life with a wooden leg, wherefore he was called Onund Treefoot as long as he lived.
>
> *The Saga of Grettir the Strong*[95]

In the late thirteenth century the surgeon Lanfranchi of Milan noted that there were '... many tall-tales in circulation about persons who recovered parts of their sliced off noses and had them successfully remounted on their faces'.[96] He would go on to report that this was absolute nonsense, as once they were off there was no way to reattach them to the face. This passage from his surgery does raise other questions around what could be done for those who had lost a part of their body such as the nose or a limb. While prostheses constructed of wood and iron used to replace arms and legs are mentioned from time to time, sources suggesting facial appliances or masks are exceedingly rare. Infamously, the Byzantine emperor Justinian II, who reigned near the end of the seventh century and again at the beginning of the eighth, is one who is said to have received such a replacement. When he was overthrown at the end of his first reign his nose was apparently mutilated, but he would have one made from gold to take its place.[97] A second such appliance appears in Guibert of Nogent's *The Deeds of God through the Franks*, which relates much about the First Crusade. He recalled a delegate of the Byzantine emperor, an older man named Tetigus, whose nose had been sliced off and he too had a replacement made of gold.[98] Clearly, a nose formed from precious metal would have been beyond the means and practicality of almost everyone during this period. There must have been other, less costly attempts made to cover or hide such disfigurements. It seems likely that things such as cloth, leather or even wood, long since deteriorated, could have been used to cover facial mutilations and secured with a cord around the head or ears. Certainly, in later centuries simple and affordable methods were developed. During the sixteenth century, for instance, replacements were made from papier mâché.[99] Still, evidence from the last century shows that cloth was often the preferred option for many who had been damaged in this way. An entire industry arose out of the First World War to help conceal the facial disfigurements of the innumerable soldiers who no longer recognized the faces staring back at them in the mirror. However, there were a lot who chose not to wear such devices and simply tied a cloth around the mutilated portion of their faces.[100] No doubt this same solution sufficed to meet the needs of many in the Middle Ages.

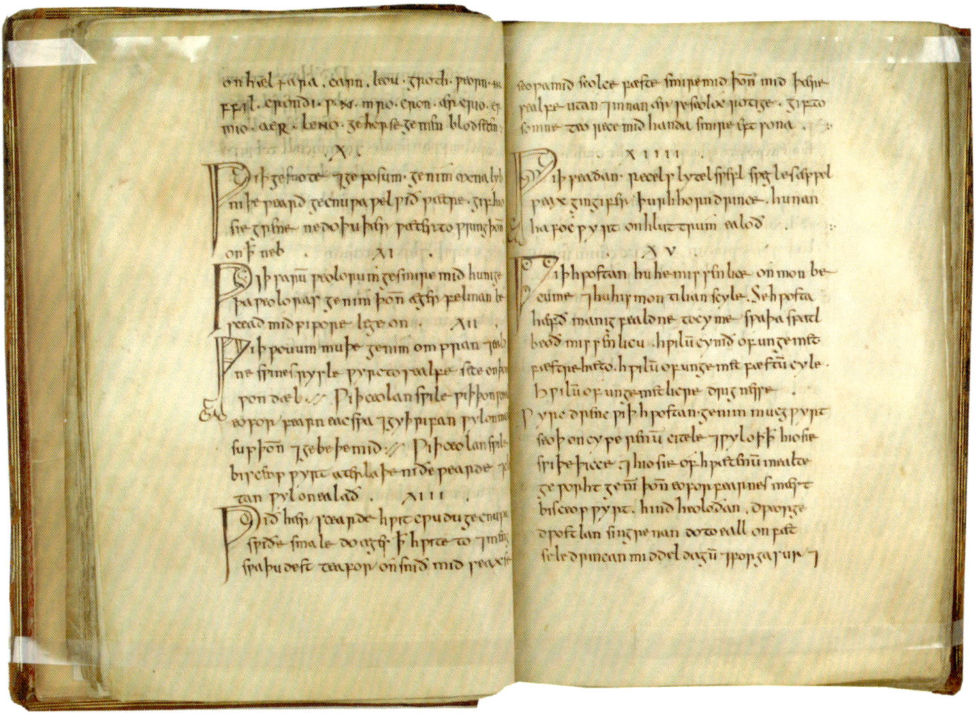

Bald's Leechbook, England (Winchester); second or third quarter of the tenth century, Book I, entry XIII being the instructions for the repair of a cleft lip in Old English. (*With the kind permission* © *The British Library Board, Royal MS 12 D XVII ff. 20v-21*)

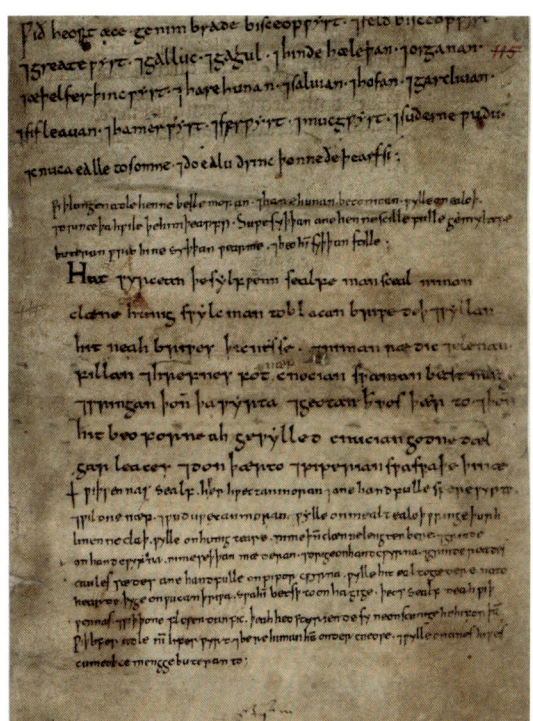

Anglo Saxon medical manuscript, featuring a collection of five recipes for heartache, lung disease, 'wenns' and tumours and liver disease; written in Old English by three different and contemporary hands. (*With the kind permission, Wellcome Collection, London. Attribution 4.0 International* (CC BY 4.0))

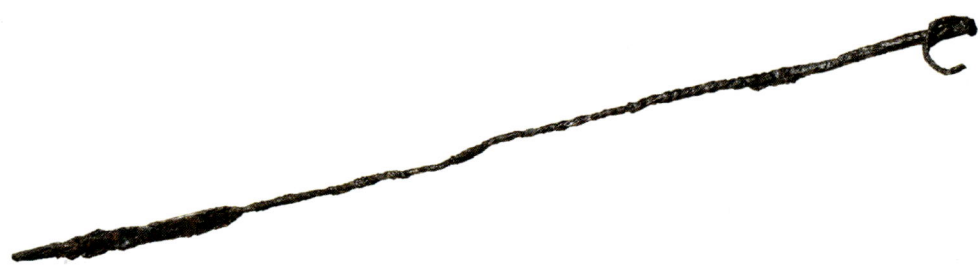

A cooking spit from the Viking Age grave of a seeress. The burial also included a metal wand, a purse containing Henbane seeds and other assorted items. The spit is made of a long iron bar with a square cross section. Found at Fyrkat outside Hobro in Jutland. (*Photo: CC-BY-SA, Arnold Mikkelsen, with the kind permission of the National Museum of Denmark*)

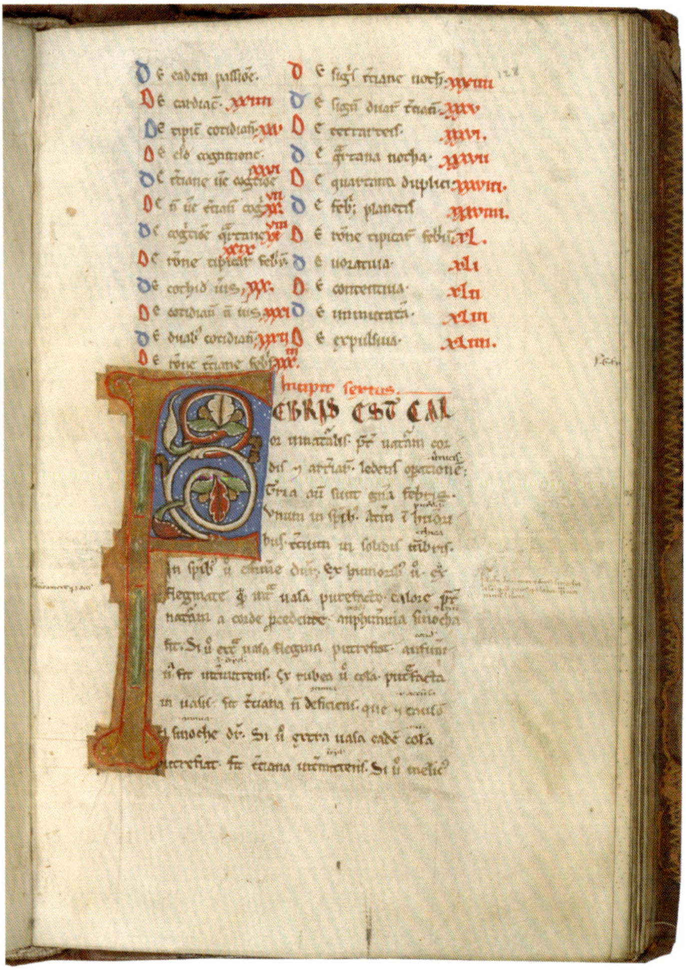

Initial page from the Passionarius of Gariopontus, book vi on Fevers. Gariopontus was one of the early teachers from the School of Salerno (died c. 1050). From a twelfth-century copy of a manual of special pathology and therapeutics of Byzantine origin, translated and edited by Gariopontus. (*With the kind permission of the Wellcome Collection, London, MS.MSL.133, 128r*)

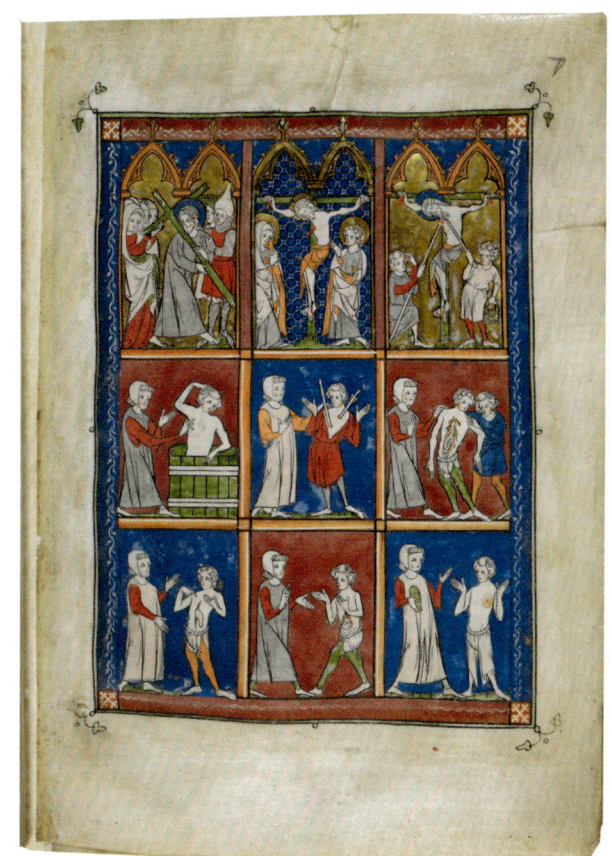

From a medical anthology including Roger Frugard's *Chirurgia* showing images of surgical procedures set alongside scenes from the life of Christ, fourth quarter of the thirteenth century–first quarter of the fourteenth century. (*With the kind permission, © The British Library Board, Sloane, MS 1977 f. 7r*)

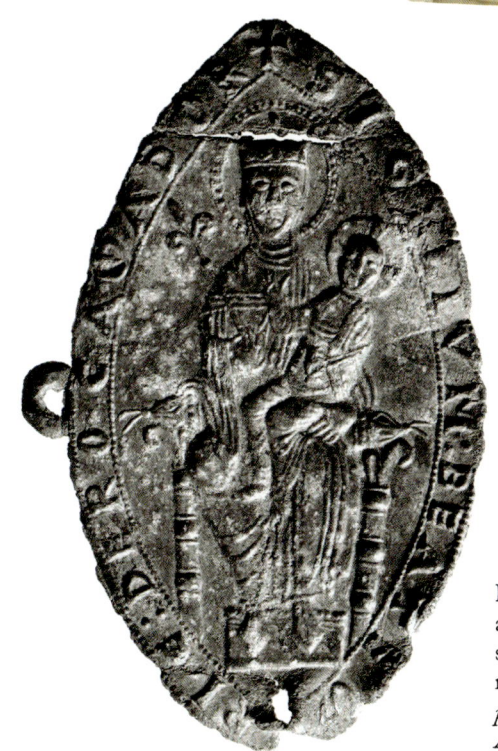

Pilgrim badge, a medieval souvenir from the Abbey at Rocamadour, France. Lead alloy with figures showing the seated Virgin holding Child, whose right hand is raised in benediction. (*With the kind permission of © The Trustees of the British Museum. All rights reserved, Object Reference – OA.666*)

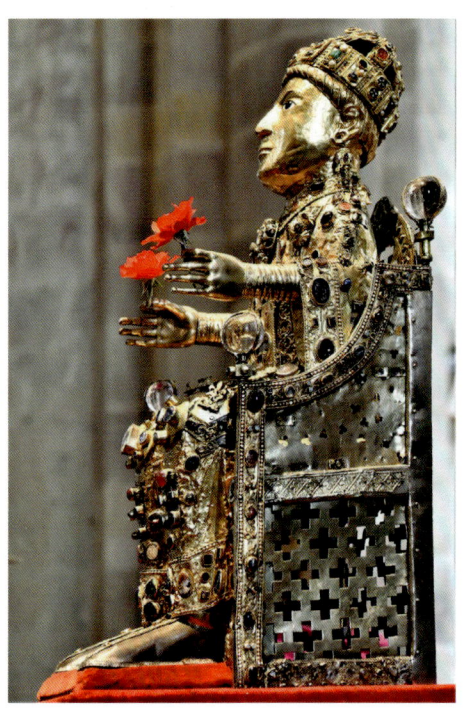

Reliquary statue from the Abbey of St Foy, Conques, France. Gemstones, given by pilgrims who visited the abbey, were added to the statue over the centuries of the Middle Ages. (*With the kind permission of G. Tordjeman2017GF-OTCM and www.tourisme-conques.fr*)

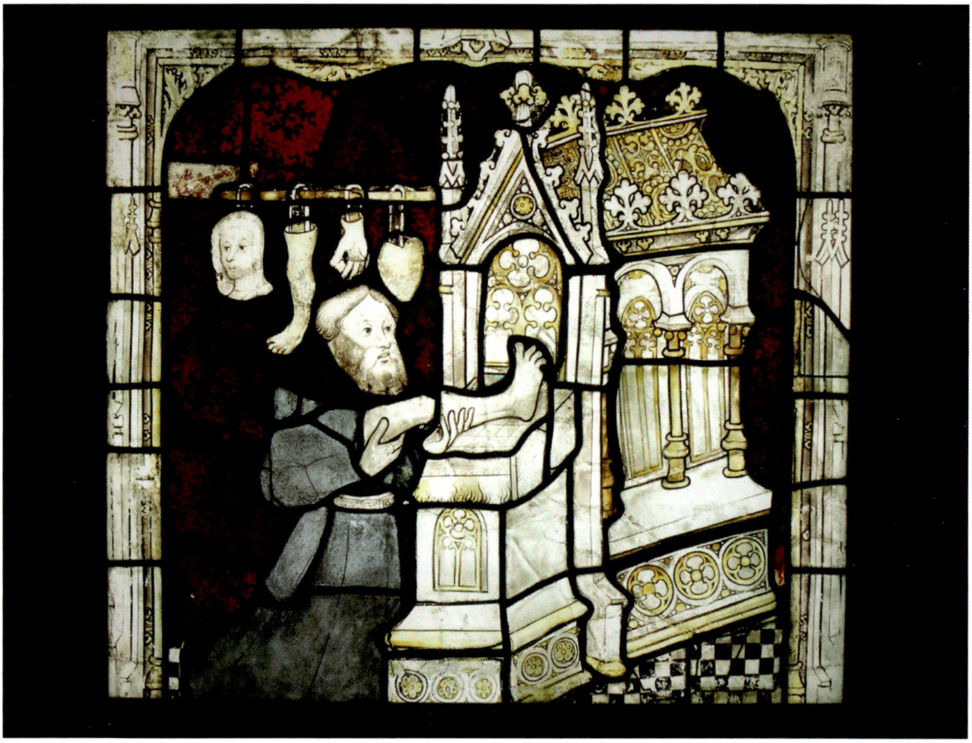

A pilgrim brings a life-sized wax leg as an offering to the shrine of St William in the York Minster. Other such offerings can be seen hanging in the background to the left, including a head and heart. From the St William Window, York Minster, early fifteenth century. (© *Chapter of York: Reproduced by kind permission*)

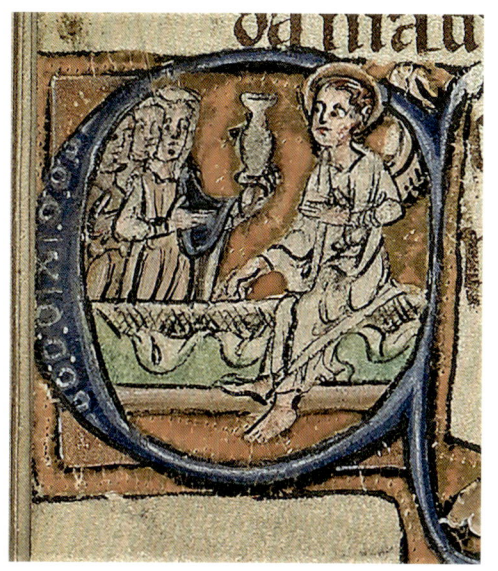

Illuminated letter containing an image of the three Marys bringing ointment to the tomb of Christ. To the right, an angel explains that Christ is no longer there, but has been resurrected. From a thirteenth-century English Book of Hours, possibly from Oxford. (*With the kind permission of Beinecke Rare Book and Manuscript Library, Yale University, Marston MS 22, page 81v*)

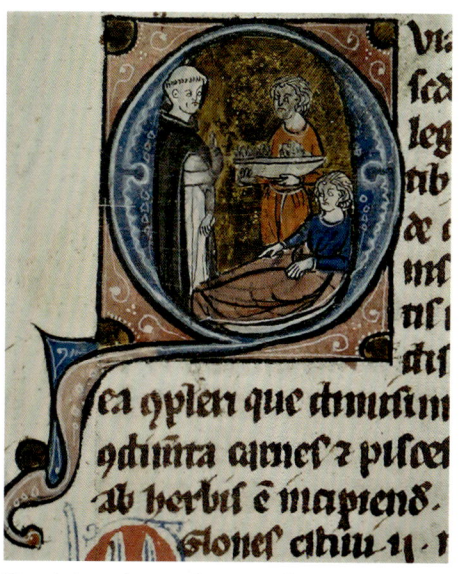

Dominican doctor shown with an assistant and patient. From a medical miscellany, mid-thirteenth century, Paris. (*With the kind permission of Kislak Center for Special Collections, Rare Books and Manuscripts, University of Pennsylvania, LJS 24, f. 65r*)

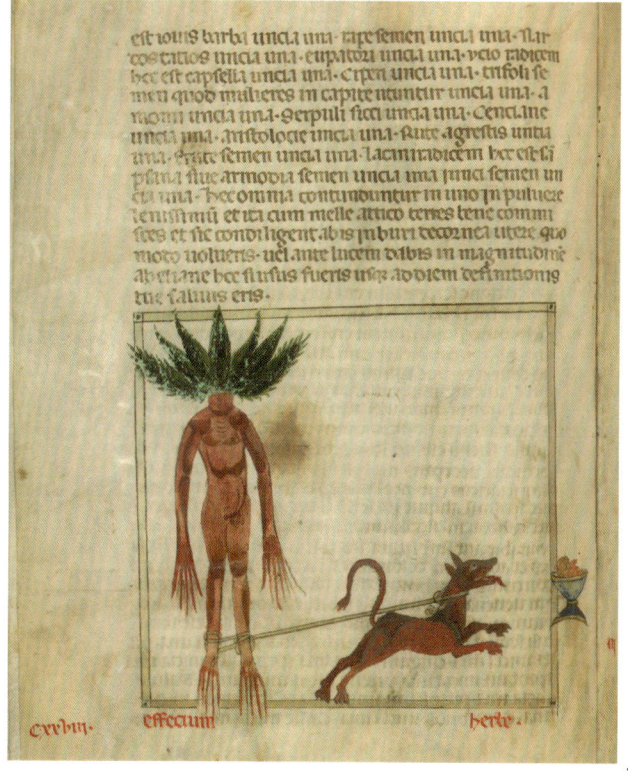

An illustration of mandrake from a mid-thirteenth century herbal. Often used for its narcotic properties in the Middle Ages, a legend grew around the harvesting of the plant with the quasi-human form. As it was pulled from the ground it was thought that its piercing scream would kill any who could hear it, so a dog was employed to do the job, often being enticed to pull toward a food item. (*With the kind permission of the Wellcome Collection, London, MS573, f. 35v*)

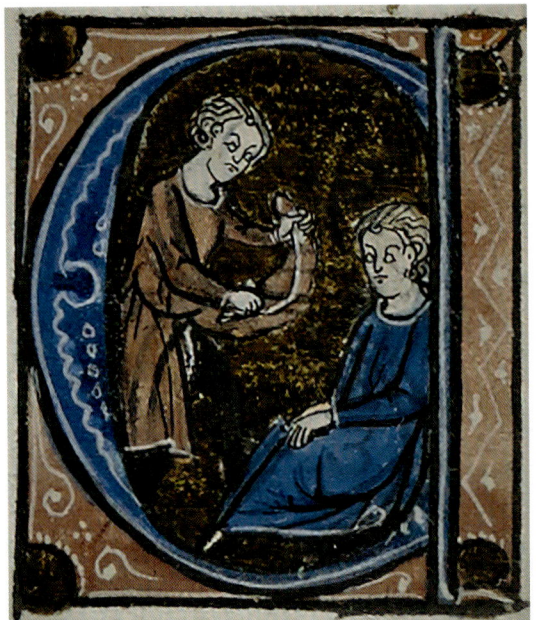

A doctor's assistant applying a poultice to a patient. From a medical miscellany, mid-thirteenth century, Paris. (*With the kind permission of Kislak Center for Special Collections, Rare Books and Manuscripts, University of Pennsylvania, LJS 24, f. 103v*)

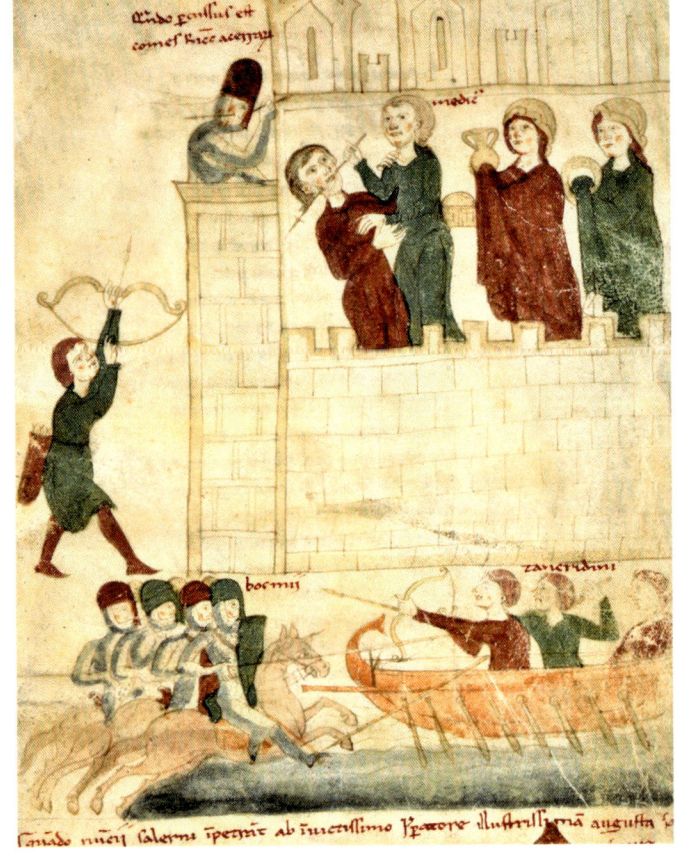

Treatment of an arrow wound to the face of Count Richard of Acerra at the Siege of Naples, 1191. Note the 'Medic' and his two female assistants carrying dressings and medicines. From a twelfth-century manuscript, Peter of Eboli's *Liber ad Honorem Augusti*. (*With the kind permission of Burgerbibliothek Bern, Cod. 120.II, f. 110r, Photograph: Codices Electronici AG, www.e-codices.ch*)

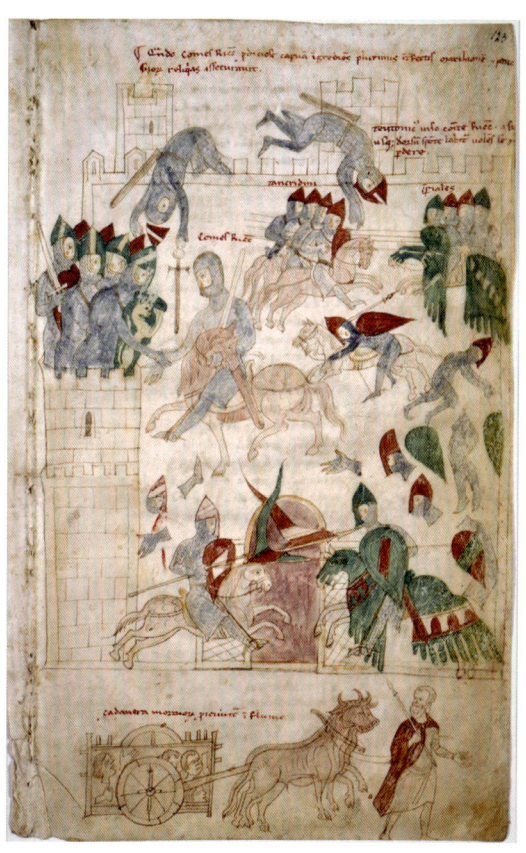

Assault on Capua by Richard of Acerra. The middle section shows many body parts cut away from unfortunate soldiers during the fighting. At the bottom, a cart is shown being used to remove the corpses, limbs and heads afterwards. From a twelfth-century manuscript, Peter of Eboli's *Liber ad Honorem Augusti*. (*With the kind permission of Burgerbibliothek Bern, Cod. 120.II, f. 123r, Photograph: Codices Electronici AG, www.e-codices.ch*)

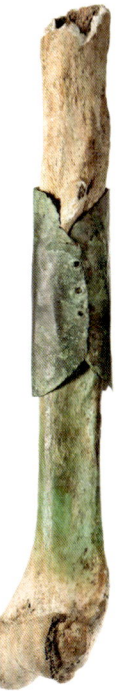

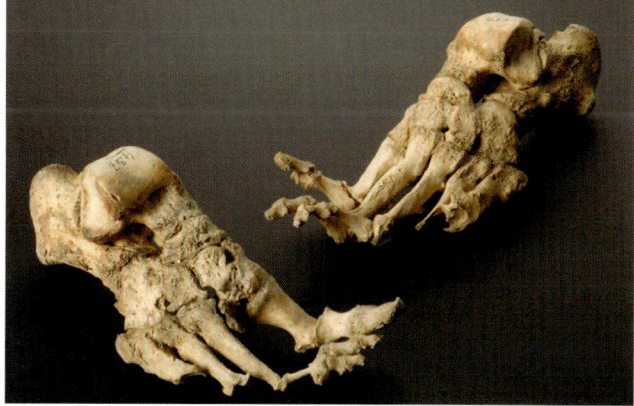

Feet from the skeleton of a mature female, showing the damaging effects of leprosy. From a medieval Danish leper's cemetery, reputedly *c.* 1350. (*Credit: With the kind permission of the Science Museum, London. Attribution 4.0 International (CC BY 4.0)*)

Successful repair of a humerus bone damaged by a sword or axe, done using a copper sheet wrapped around the bone and secured in place. From Varnhem, Sweden, as early as the twelfth century. (*Photo: Ola Myrin, with the kind permission of The Swedish History Museum/SHM (CC BY)*)

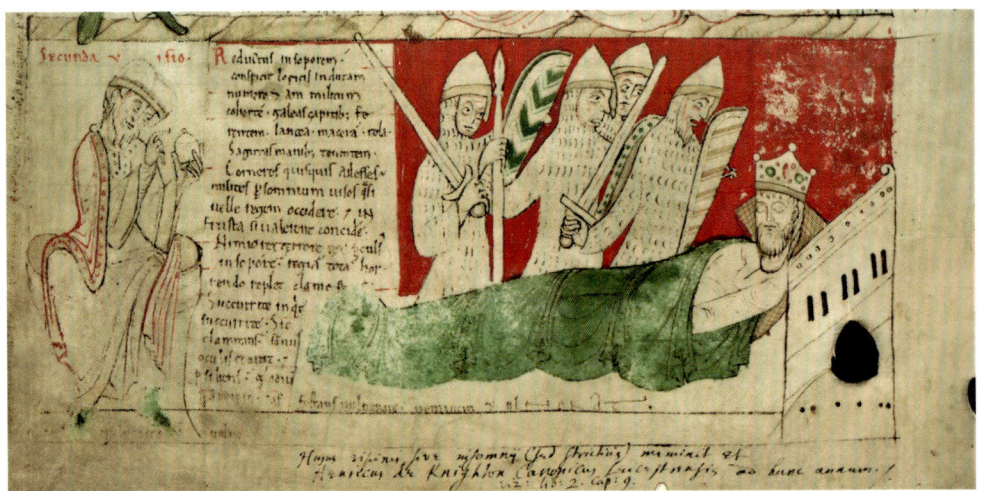

Dream (Nightmare) of Henry I, while on the left Grimbald, his physician, watches on recording what he witnessed. From the *Chronicle of John of Worcester*, twelfth century. (*By kind permission of the President and Fellows of Corpus Christi College, Oxford, CCC MS 157, p.382*)

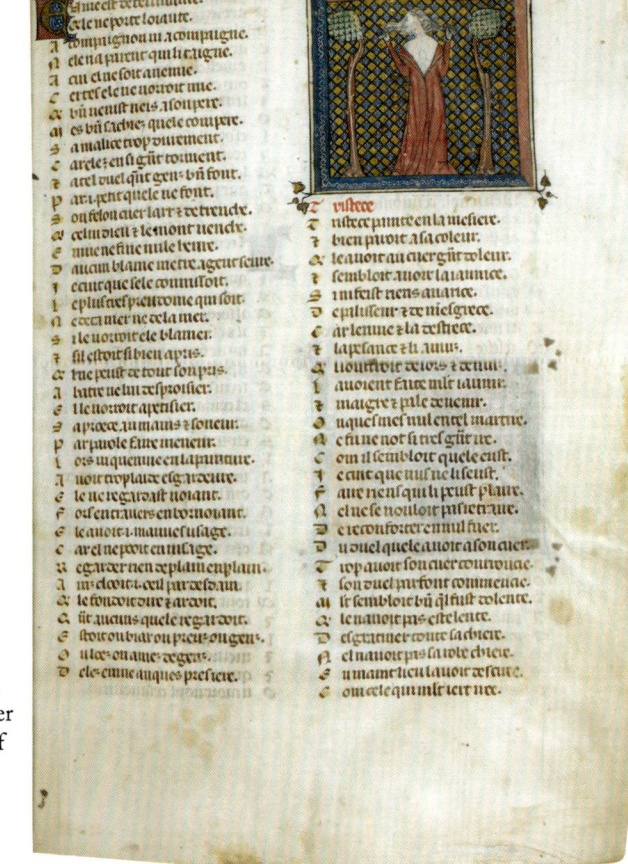

Tristece (Sorrow) from *Le Roman de la Rose*, France (Paris) c. 1320–c. 1340, text based on the thirteenth-century original. The image of a woman tearing her hair, scratching her face and exposing her breasts was a popular illustration of Sorrow during the Middle Ages. (*With the kind permission © The British Library Board, Royal MS 19 B XIII, f. 7r*)

When it comes to artificial limbs there are indications that the technology could at times be fairly advanced. In the story *Egil and Asmund* one of the title characters, known as Egil One-Hand, overcame his disability and could do more with the arm that was absent of its hand than with the other one. This was due to a sword, which had been created by dwarfs and attached to his arm just above his wrist. The story says that there was not a warrior alive who could handle his lethal sword strokes.[101] While this is a story of fantasy, a warrior like Egil, with a sword replacing a missing appendage, may not be so far-fetched. A grave with a body and equipment not unlike the character of Egil One-Hand was excavated near Verona in north-eastern Italy. This individual was a male between the ages of 40 and 50 discovered among 164 Longobard (also called Lombard) tombs dating between the sixth and eighth centuries. He was found with a well-healed right forearm at the site of an amputation that had taken his hand and part of the arm.[102] The critical point is that he survived the loss of a limb and lived for some years with quite a useful prosthesis. The evidence within the tomb showed a knife attached to a cap that had been placed over the end of his arm. His teeth showed considerable wear and flattening on the right side, compared to that of the left. His right incisor tooth is particularly worn down.[103] All of this indicates that this man wore a leather prosthesis with a knife on the end of it, adjusted and tightened with the assistance of his teeth, which he used to grip and secure the leather strap that attached it to his arm.[104]

Returning to the centuries of concern here, one of the earliest references to a prosthesis can be found in the year 886. In his description of the Viking attacks on Paris, Abbo of Saint-German-des-Prés made note of one of the defenders of the city called Oddo who had lost his right hand in battle. In its place was a hand made of iron, which according to Abbo was just as strong and useful as the real thing.[105] In an entry for 1125 Orderic Vitalis mentions the case of a Norwegian clerk who had been punished for killing a priest. The clerk had his eyes put out and his hands and feet were amputated before he was sent to live in England. While this account does not involve a battlefield injury, it is noteworthy because it refers to 'iron fingers which he used because he was maimed'.[106]

Prostheses used to replace damaged feet or legs have been discovered, but unfortunately these tend come from the centuries just before ours. A male skeleton excavated at Bonaduz, Switzerland and dating from between the fifth and seventh centuries had a replacement left foot made from leather and wood.[107] Another male, found at Griesheim, Germany, this time from the seventh or eighth centuries, had the lower portion of his left leg amputated. An artificial foot made from bronze was found in the grave, however just how it was attached and its practicality are certainly open to question.[108]

The sources within our timeline indicate a much more common type of replacement for a leg, the sort made from wood that was strapped to the base of the amputation and supported with the use of a crutch. The Viking sagas are filled with names such as Onund Treefoot and Thorir Wood-Leg, which suggest this kind of set up.[109] Found in the *Eyrbyggja Saga*, Thorir lost a portion of his lower leg when it was cut off by another called Thorarin.[110] He was treated and eventually given a limb made of wood, plus a new name to match, Thorir Wood-Leg.[111] The twelfth-century French poem *La Chanson de Guillaume* includes a similar reference after Guillaume took the leg of a Saracen called Alderufe, '… just worry about healing your thigh, making a wooden leg to help you walk, and getting a ferule on the end of the stump'.[112] Chrétien de Troyes provided a small clue about the type of wood that might have been used to make such artificial limbs for the common person, in late twelfth-century France at least. Near the end of de Troyes' unfinished work *The Story of the Grail (Perceval)* Gawain comes across a one-legged man of some wealth wearing a prosthesis made of gilt silver and encrusted with jewels. What is significant is the comment made by Gawain as he noted that the leg was not made from aspen wood, the usual material.[113] While it is important not to give too much weight to a single reference, the characteristics of aspen, being light and strong and not prone to splintering, would have made it an ideal choice for this sort of application.

The twelfth-century miracles of St William of Norwich contain a wide range of assistive devices used by the disabled. While the examples do not feature soldiers, they are still useful in offering an insight into the lives of those who had lost the use of their legs and yet still managed to get around using various appliances and means of transport. Seeking a cure for her deformed legs, a girl called Huelina was taken by her father to Norwich '… in a wheeled vehicle of the kind called a litter'.[114] Another lad, called Baldwin, who came from the area around Lincoln, had no use of his legs below the knees, not unlike many of those mentioned above. He was taken to Norwich by his father in one of these wheeled litters. When he arrived and wanted to move about on his own, '… he crept along on his knees leaning on hand trestles'.[115] Another disabled boy was taken to Norwich by his father in a 'handbarrow', while a woman named Matildis was unceremoniously laid across a horse '… like a sack …' by Peter the priest who looked after her.[116]

Disability

> The enemy pursued him in his flight and either killed, or in various ways disabled all of his men whom they could catch.
>
> Simeon of Durham[117]

What became of the survivors of mutilations, burn injuries, torture, the loss of limbs and other serious injuries in the long term? The answers are unfortunately few and far between, especially as it relates to the earlier centuries of this 500-year period. Families must have taken care of some of the disabled when they could, but the more general rule appears to have been true, as it has throughout history, which is those with power and money were usually provided with much better opportunities than those without.

There were some warriors who just seem to have carried on being soldiers, even if they had suffered wounds in previous battles and wars. The mass tenth-century grave discovered at Budeč in the Czech Republic contained several soldiers who showed evidence of injuries from previous battles, some of them being quite serious head and leg wounds. Many of these men appear to have been mercenaries in the employ of the Duke of Bohemia, some perhaps of Scandinavian origin, continuing to fight despite the damage that had been done to them previously.[118] Less than a century beyond our timeline, at least a quarter of those serving in the Provençal army were soldiers with severely scarred faces and hands from prior battles.[119] It is difficult to imagine that the most disabled among them would have been expected to fight. There were, of course, other roles that might have been more conducive to their impairments and would have kept them involved without actually having to carry a weapon, things such as supplying and feeding the other soldiers.[120] Still, there were those warriors whose afflictions were so severe that they could do little else but beg with the rest of medieval society's poor and forgotten.[121] Looking again to the period just beyond this study we find the example of English soldiers who were so terribly injured fighting against the French that the only opportunity left open to them was to seek charity.[122]

Contrast those requiring the mercy and assistance of strangers to those of privilege like the eleventh-century former soldier and senior London city official Godfrey de Magnaville, a man paralysed by the wounds he had suffered in battle. The *Carmen Widonis* recalled that his position in society meant that he was well looked after, despite his disability, being transported all over by litter.[123] Count Baldwin of Flanders was a nobleman who received a serious head injury during the siege of Arques in Northern France in September 1118. The account of William of Malmesbury underscores the disparity in treatment that was available to those with means and power, '… for the king sent a most skilful physician to the patient …'.[124] However, despite the expert help Baldwin improved little, lingering for several months before finally expiring in June 1119.[125] There were others who could afford to pay the fees of skilful doctors like William of Saliceto.[126] William's surgery included the case of a soldier who had been wounded by an arrow. While not named, he was from Cremona and described as the brother of a man called Henry Cinzarius. The wound was to his neck and it caused him to lose the use of his limbs from the neck down. With the passage of time and the care provided by William the man was able to make a partial recovery, going on to live for another ten years, gaining some mobility with the use of two canes.[127] The short entry gives the sense that William must have done some considerable work with the man to give him back some movement in his limbs. It is unfortunate that he did not go into further detail to describe the types of treatments and therapies he employed to get the man back on his feet again, even if it was with the aid of assistive devices.

There are a small number of records that show that there were some who were compensated for their injuries, being provided with charitable support for their needs, such as a severely wounded knight of the Hospitallers, returning from Crusade in 1177. The serious nature of his wounds meant that the soldier was no longer fit to fight or work. He benefited from a letter he carried with him from the grandmaster of his order, which allowed him to receive food and lodging wherever he presented the note.[128] Elsewhere, there are examples of towns and crowns looking after the casualties of war. Orderic Vitalis provided some insight into the state of things in England in the years following the Norman Conquest. In an entry for 1074 he stated that William I had given English lands to some of his seriously injured warriors, to begin with at least: 'To his (William's) victorious soldiers, covered with wounds, were allotted barren farms and domains depopulated by the ravages of war.'[129] There are a few things that are of interest here, the obvious fact concerns the physical state of some of these men who had fought on the Norman side, having been quite badly harmed during William I's conquest of England. However, that was not the end of the story as the record is book-ended by details of William's later mistreatment of some of these men. If Vitalis is to be believed here, it seems that in some cases William ended up taking back a portion of the land that he had given to some of his disabled soldiers and with others he took all of it back, leading to a general hatred and mistrust of the man now known as William the Conqueror.[130] We can find quite a different set of circumstances in an example of some Genoese archers who had their eyes put out by Emperor Fredrick II after he took Milan in 1245. In a far more sincere gesture to that of William I of England, these men were compensated for their injuries with a pension once they were able to return home.[131]

A few rare examples exist of those who were involved during the first Scottish War of Independence being looked after with a one-time payment or a benefit that continued for the balance of their lives. Some of these are listed below with the available details for each man:

- David Gough, a Welsh foot soldier, fighting against Scotland in Edward I's forces, was wounded during the assault on Brechin castle in August of 1303. Expenses of 6s. 8d. were allowed for his return home in August of that year.[132]
- A request from 13 April 1311 was made for payment to an unnamed English sailor. He was injured while fighting the Scottish at Dundee. The amount given to him was 50s.[133]
- In an entry for 12 August 1314 at York, a few weeks after the famous Battle of Bannockburn, Edward II of England agreed to pay for the maintenance of William, son of Thomas le Charetter of Grove, 'Scotch rebels having inhumanly cut off his hand whilst engaged in the king's service.' Unable to work, the request was to the hospital of St John, Brackele to look after him for the balance of his life, including the provision of food, clothing and any other necessities.[134]

- The entry that follows is for a second man called Henry le Lounge Fletewyk, with a similar request to the hospital of St John Ospringe that he would be looked after for the rest of his life.[135]
- A third entry, named John de Sheperton, was also to be looked after in this manner by the master and brethren at the hospital of St John, Oxford, here again for what remained of his life.[136]

These allowances and benefits are something of a mystery. The unanswered question is why any of them were looked after in this fashion. They all appear to have been quite ordinary men and this was certainly not something that was done for the average person, so just why it occurred in a few cases is extremely intriguing.[137]

The hospitals, such as those mentioned in the above examples, were not facilities in the modern sense of the word, but instead set up as part of a monastic complex. There were some that offered just short-term relief for the poor or sick, but it is clear there were others that must have acted in a more long-term or palliative capacity. The Grey Friars' monastery, on the banks of the Gipping River near Ipswich, England has recently become better understood through excavation and study. It was founded by Sir Robert Tiptoth (also spelled Tiptoft or Tibetot) who was himself a warrior, having been involved in the Ninth Crusade from 1270 to 1271, fighting alongside Prince Edward, the future Edward I of England. Sir Robert and his wife Una paid for the creation of the monastery some time between the 1270s and 1290s. There have been 150 medieval skeletons recovered from this site in Ipswich, with many of them showing signs of severe injury or disease that would have left them in need of constant care. It appears that they spent the last part of their lives being cared for by the Grey Friars until they died and were buried near the monastery.[138]

Occasionally, facilities were created especially for soldiers such as the one constructed in the village of Eagle in Lincolnshire, England between 1136 and 1148. Its name has been lost to time, but it was built on land granted by King Stephen to house Knights Templar who were either aged or sick.[139] In Winchester, St John's Hospital was built around the year 1275. It was specifically intended to help those soldiers who were lame or sick, along with others who were poor or in need of assistance. Meant for the short term, it provided food and lodging for one night, but at times allowed for longer stays, depending upon the individual's ability to travel.[140]

In Poland, there is the example of the high-ranking warrior named Kwiecik. He held a large area of land in his home country, a settlement called Kwiecikowice, which contained a monastery that had been founded within its boundaries. Being a violent man, he accumulated several serious sword wounds over the years. By 1228 his injuries were such that he had become completely disabled, forcing him to live within the monastery under the care of the monks who looked after his daily needs.[141]

We are given a rare glimpse and whiff of the reality of these facilities that housed the sick and injured, soldiers and civilians alike, in France and England.

In around 1220 the Bishop of Acre in Palestine, Jacobus de Vitry, wrote his *Historia Occidentalism* in which he spoke about these hospitals and those who served the sick and wounded: 'These servants of Christ, sober and sparing towards themselves and rigid towards their own bodies, abound in compassion towards the poor and sick, and at once minister to them all necessaries to the best of their ability. For Christ's sake they bear the filth and impurities of the patients and the annoyance of almost unbearable smells.'[142]

The centuries can make it difficult for us to understand and appreciate the thoughts and emotions of those whose lives were turned upside down by the kinds of injuries outlined in this chapter, disfiguring scars, terrible burns, amputations and those caused by torture. Sources and stories certainly help, but time has made the lives of these warriors distant and impersonal. In the wheelchair bound former footballer from Wilfred Owen's poem of the First World War *Disabled* we may just catch a glimpse of what some of these medieval soldiers felt and thought as they lived out their days in the 'Institutes' of the period, the monasteries with their schedules and rules. The young man of Owen's poem sat each evening waiting for night to come, while he:

> … shivered in his ghastly suit of grey,
> Legless, sewn short at elbow.[143]

Once admired and cheered by the crowds, he had lied about his age and dreamt of glory when he joined up, only to find himself a maimed old man before he was 20:

> Now, he will spend a few sick years in Institutes,
> And do what things the rules consider wise,
> And take whatever pity they may dole.
> Tonight he noticed how the women's eyes
> Passed from him to the strong men that were whole.
> How cold and late it is! Why don't they come
> And put him into bed? Why don't they come?[144]

Chapter 7

Illness and Infection

To heal the sick the leech's art sometimes will fail, and, spite of remedies, disease weigh down the scale.

Matthew Paris[1]

Disease and illness were commonplace among Europeans of the Middle Ages. Most people played host to some sort of parasite-like roundworm, maw-worm or tapeworm, that caused complaints such as chronic abdominal pain and diarrhoea.[2] As irritating as these illnesses must have been they would have seemed fairly insignificant compared with some of the more serious outbreaks of plague and disease that were to come along like leprosy and ergotism (St Anthony's fire), which caused panic, sickness, brutish disfigurements and death among so many. A lack of detail provided in the sources make many more of these afflictions difficult to identify, but apparently no less dangerous or lethal as evidenced by the *Annals of Ulster* for the year 813. It relates the terrible suffering caused by 'heavy diseases', but with few other words of description for posterity.[3] The chronicles written by Herman and Berthold of Reichenau list a catalogue of mystery plagues and afflictions that occurred during the eleventh century.[4] The monk Orderic Vitalis was a witness to several such illnesses that spread across France and England during the latter part of the eleventh century and the early decades of the twelfth. He wrote about the situation in France during 1105, identifying and recording some of the problems, while others he was only able to speak of in more general terms: 'In the month of May a contagious influenza spread through all the West ... Burning fever and other febrile diseases with a variety of disorders grievously afflicted mankind and prostrated numbers who took to their beds.'[5]

Efforts to quell the impact of these diseases varied widely. In the world of the Vikings, the Arab traveller Ibn Fadlān recorded the common-sense approach taken by the Rūs traders he met in the tenth century. When one of them became ill they were placed in a tent away from the others with bread and water being left outside until they recovered. He discovered that if the individual died then the body would be burnt, unless they had been a slave in which case they were left to the dogs and wildlife.[6] Adam of Bremen provided some detail about the role of the gods in the pre-Christian world of the Vikings. He spoke about the important temple complex that existed at Uppsala where the statues of Odin, Thor and Freyr could be found. Priests were appointed to look after the statues and offer sacrifices for the people during certain times and events. In the case of war, a libation would be poured out to Odin and when plague or famine struck then the liquid offering went to Thor's statue to put an end to the sickness or hunger.[7]

In Christian Europe disease and illness were frequently deemed to be punishments sent by God for sins that had been committed, especially sexual sins.[8] Pilgrimage was one way of obtaining God's forgiveness and healing, although it was not always free from superstition as an eleventh-century example from the south of England highlights. Interested to know which saint's shrine would be best to cure his leprosy, a high-ranking noble carried out a race with a trio of identical candles, each representing one of the three most popular saints in England at that time, St Edmund at Bury, St Æthelfrith at Ely and St Cuthbert at Durham. He deemed the saint whose candle burned down the quickest to be the most powerful and hence best to cure his leprosy. St Cuthbert at Durham ended up as the eventual winner.[9]

When it came to soldiers and illness the great Roman writer of the late fourth century called Flavius Vegetius Renatus, or just simply Vegetius, included the subject in his seminal treatise *De Re Militari*, or *Concerning Military Affairs*. In this military manual Vegetius underscored his great concern for the damage that disease could do to an army, 'For little can be expected from men who have both the enemy and disease to struggle with.'[10]

He stressed a suitable location for encampment, a good water supply, the right time of year, plus exercise and medicine as cornerstones of proper health and disease avoidance for any army. This treatise was still being followed by several military leaders of the Middle Ages some centuries later. Popular at the time of Charlemagne, it was also a favourite of Henry II of England and his son Richard the Lionheart, both of whom carried copies of *De Re Militari*.[11] However, there were many armies that lived in close quarters, regularly without proper hygiene and sanitation, clean water and fresh food, making them susceptible to things like dysentery and fevers. The Viking army that attacked St Denis in 865 'became ill with various ailments', including sores and diarrhoea.[12] Exploring the annals compiled by Herman of Reichenau, he described a plague that ran rampant among the army of Holy Roman Emperor Henry II in 1022 killing large numbers of soldiers.[13] In July 1038, while on the coast of the Adriatic Sea, something similar occurred when a plague attacked the army of Emperor Henry III killing a great many of his warriors.[14]

The impact of disease and infection has long been more dangerous to armies and their soldiers than the arrows and swords of the enemy and this was certainly the case during this period.[15] Four different kinds of illnesses or groups of them, as most involved more than one type or strain, are under review within this chapter, dysentery, St Anthony's fire, sexually transmitted infections (STIs) and leprosy. These were not only quite common, but most were greatly feared because of their potential to do such terrible damage to their human victims. The focus here is of course on how each of them affected the armies and individual soldiers of the time, with a look at just a few of the potential treatments that were available. The lack of understanding of germs and contagion meant that these remedies and cures frequently treated just the symptoms, offering some temporary relief, but no real healing. Lastly, infections in wounds, at times caused by the malpractice of some doctors, are also considered at the end of this chapter.

Dysentery

> If God had not sent them a plague, as he did with dysentery, they would never have been taken.
>
> *La chanson de la croisade contre les Albigeois*[16]

Dysentery is a disease almost tailor made for warfare with soldiers living close together and human waste often so near to water and food supplies. During the Middle Ages a general misunderstanding of germs and proper sanitation, handling food with unwashed hands and the popular practice of using human faeces as fertilizer led to many soldiers becoming infected. Symptoms of the illness can include inflammation of the intestines, stomach pains, diarrhoea that frequently contains blood and mucus, vomiting, dehydration and fever. It is something that can quite easily be fatal if it is not properly controlled and treated.[17] Rampant during the American Civil War, it was estimated that about 70 per cent of soldiers had it at any one time, providing some idea of just how bad it could become when left unchecked.[18] Erich Maria Remarque's novel of the First World War, *All Quiet on the Western Front*, offers a depiction of the disease among soldiers, a picture that could hardly have changed much since the Middle Ages. In fact, without the knowledge that this is a reference to the First World War this scene is one that could almost be describing the Rūs in Azerbaijan or Danes in Canterbury noted below:

> … dysentery dissolves our bowels. The latrine poles are always densely crowded; the people at home ought to be shown these grey, yellow, miserable, wasted faces here, these bent figures from whose bodies the colic wrings out the blood, and who with lips trembling and distorted with pain, grin at one another and say: 'It is not much sense pulling up one's trousers again.'[19]

The *Royal Frankish Annals* include an outbreak of dysentery in 820. In January that year a council of Frankish leaders was assembled at Aachen to discuss the rebellion led by Ljudovit the First, Duke of Lower Pannonia, a part of the area now known as the Balkans. The Franks decided to send three separate armies in different directions to attack Ljudovit and his soldiers. Along the way one of the armies was stricken with a serious outbreak of dysentery. The entry records that much of the army died after contracting the sickness.[20]

The Persian historian Miskawayh recorded a detailed picture of a Swedish Viking raid on the city of Bardha'a (Barda) in Azerbaijan in 943, which he based on eyewitness reports.[21] In it he recalled a severe epidemic, long thought to have been dysentery, which claimed the lives of many of the Rūs forces that had taken the city. Miskawayh blamed the sickness on the different types of fruit that were grown in that region, noting that the Vikings overindulged on this produce, which was otherwise unavailable to them in their cold climate.[22] It is clear from the large numbers of Rūs who died and the fact that '... the epidemic became even more severe' that Miskawayh was in fact talking about a serious illness, rather than a bit of diarrhoea and stomach upset from eating unripened or unfamiliar fruit.[23]

Danish Vikings met with a serious outbreak of dysentery as they attacked Canterbury in 1011. Many chronicles, including that of Simeon of Durham and Florence of Worcester, relate the Danish attack on the city that involved plunder, destruction, torture, killing and the taking of slaves. However, it seems that the Danes did not escape without some divine retribution, as Simeon of Durham explained: 'In the mean while the anger of God being aroused against the murderous people, destroyed two thousand of them by pains of the intestines.'[24] Most of the chronicles that recall this incident remain with the figure of two-thousand dead, a number that is almost certainly embellished, as is usual. The *Chronicle of Florence of Worcester* is one that goes further suggesting that the surviving Danes were given an opportunity to make reparations to the archbishop, but when they did not repent, they continued to die off, ten and twenty at a time.[25]

Dysentery had no respect for position, rank or wealth, everyone from common foot soldiers to kings were susceptible to the illness. Louis VI of France and John of England were among the kings whose lives were taken by dysentery.[26] King Edward I of England was another who suffered, eventually losing his life to the illness. As the summer of 1306 approached the English army marched rapidly towards Scotland under the leadership of Edward I's son, while the king himself was carried slowly by horse litter, all the while making frequent stops. At times he could only manage a few miles at a time. By this point he was well into his 60s and struggling with other afflictions, including those which hindered his feet and legs. On 8 September 1306 Edward had to send his apothecary Richard de Montpellier back to London to collect more of the necessary spices and remedies required to treat his ailments. Richard rung up a hefty bill for items such as rose sugar with ground pearls, silver, gold and pomegranate wine. The total cost of the king's prescriptions was £134, an amount that was left unpaid by Edward I.[27] Working in conjunction with de Montpellier was the king's physician, Master Nicholas de Tyngewyke. Through winter and spring 1307, the king seemed to get better under their care as he convalesced at Carlisle. On 3 July 1307 Edward got back into the saddle of his charger to continue to Scotland, but his improvement lasted only a short time and he was again struck down by the dysentery that had slowed his journey so badly. Master de Tyngewyke tried to relieve his suffering, but this time the medicines did not aid the king and he died of dysentery on 7 July 1307, not far from Carlisle.[28]

Today the treatment for dysentery includes antibiotics and plenty of hydration, but in the Middle Ages most remedies that did exist only provided some mild and temporary relief. *Bald's Leechbook* contains a few remedies for dysentery and among them is one that was a mix of superstition, religion and medicine. It called for a new bramble root, from which nine chips were to be cut and placed into the left hand of the leech. The doctor was then to sing Psalm 51 three times, as it focuses on forgiveness from sins and then the Pater Noster nine times, '… then take mugwort and everlasting, boil these three, the worts and the chips, in milk till they get red'. The liquid was to be sipped at night and then the patient could be wrapped up warmly and given rest. According to *Bald's*, the patient could require a second or third dose before beginning to feel better.[29]

We need to turn to the herbals to find other cures, many of which contain elements of the rose. Still used today as a natural remedy to treat diarrhoea, rose-based concoctions were widely prescribed for dysentery throughout these medieval centuries, as the list of items for Edward I shows above. *Bald's Leechbook* suggested drinking rose water, as did the later herbal of *Macer Floridus*.[30] In the middle of the thirteenth century the English medical writer Gilbertus Anglicus made a whole host of suggestions for dysentery, including one that also made use of rose water.[31]

St Anthony's Fire

> This year many persons were attacked by the Holy Fire, which made their limbs as black as coal.
>
> *The Chronicles of Robert de Monte*[32]

Almost forgotten today, *ignis sacer*, or *holy fire*, was one of the most prominent illnesses of this period in history. Later referred to by the more familiar names *St Anthony's fire* or *St Martial's fire* and now known as ergotism this frightful sickness peaked during the eleventh and twelfth centuries, causing the mutilation and deaths of many.[33] It is caused by a very toxic type of fungus called *Claviceps purpurea* that grows on grains, especially rye, creating a potent poison when consumed. The fungus was prevalent in the cooler, moister climate of Northern Europe, which enabled huge outbreaks of the illness to occur in places like France, Germany and the Low Countries. The two principal forms of the sickness, convulsive and gangrenous, can bring with them a whole host of symptoms, some of which take hold within the first few hours of being ingested, things like headaches, nausea, vomiting, hallucinations and diarrhoea. These can last for long periods before giving way to the violent burning pain in the limbs that gives the illness its name.

Convulsions, the loss of appendages and limbs or even death can then follow the initial symptoms.[34]

Its very nature would have made this illness absolutely devastating to any army that carried or foraged grain products that contained the fungus. *La chanson de la croisade contre les Albigeois* provides a sense of the dread attached to the illness. During the siege of Beaucaire in summer 1216 the situation for the crusaders began to deteriorate rapidly. Having slept little and struggling in full armour for days on end in the sweltering August heat of Southern France, their supplies of food and drink began to dwindle quickly. One of the crusaders, Sir Hugh de Lacy, was meant to have noted that if their situation had continued in that fashion for much longer then they would have suffered a fate worse than the holy fire.[35] Whether or not this was something uttered by de Lacy is hard to know, but the chronicler's inclusion of the illness as a gauge of a situation as dire as this one provides an idea of the level of fear and suffering that was attached to the *ignis sacer*.

The winters of 856 and 857 were very destructive seasons for the sickness. *The Annals of St Bertin* noted a cold, dry winter in 856 along with a serious, but unidentified pestilence.[36] The *Annals of Xanten*, however, specifically described a large outbreak of the gangrenous variety of the illness in 857, one of the earliest accounts of ergotism: 'A great plague of swollen blisters consumed the people by a loathsome rot, so that their limbs were loosened and fell off before death.'[37] The Danish armies of the ninth century had been attacking North-Western Europe for a few decades by this point and must have come into contact with the illness and those who were afflicted by its terrible traits. In spring 856, for instance, they were assaulting places around Orleans and would continue to make further incursions into the areas around Paris, Tours and Saxony. Xanten too would be sacked just a few years later.[38] At the beginning of the tenth century, Rouen and the surrounding area was given over to the Norse leader Rollo by Charles the Simple, as he attempted to quell future Viking raids into West Francia.[39] This new settlement of Northmen, which was to become known as Normandy, would find itself dangerously close to the significant outbreak of the holy fire that occurred around Paris in 945.[40] A more northerly link to the illness can be found near the end of the Viking Age in eleventh-century Norway when the Norwegian king called Magnus II Haraldsson died from it in 1069, aged just 20.[41]

This sickness would carry on unabated for the next two or three centuries becoming more frequent and causing even more damage to the population.[42] The very wet summer of 1128 led to one of the worst recorded outbreaks. In Northern France and the Low Countries the illness was noted as having mutilated the faces of some of its victims.[43] Barger's text on the subject lists example after example of the sort of suffering it caused during its peak: 'Many were tortured and twisted by a contraction of the nerves; others died miserably, their limbs eaten up by the holy fire and blackened like charcoal.'[44]

Instances involving soldiers and ergotism do appear in the miracle collections, such as one found among a small group of records from the abbey of St Foy that dates from the first half of the twelfth century.⁴⁵ William, the son of a rich nobleman called Guy from Reims, was part of an army that made a long-distance expedition to fight against an unspecified enemy. Things did not go as planned and the soldiers were soon out of food and struggling in the cold weather. William gave in to his hunger and ate some rye bread poisoned by the toxic fungus.⁴⁶ It is not mentioned whether the bread had been transported by the army or if the poisoned loaf had been foraged by the soldiers. Satiated by the 'unhealthy foods', he fell into a deep sleep in the cold, but it would not be long before the illness began to take its course and William was soon in agony and burning up with fever. He became terribly thirsty and likely delirious, so to add insult to injury he drank from a nearby stagnant pond. Perspiring profusely, his stomach swelled and his limbs began to contract.⁴⁷ The story then jumps to William being back at home under the constant care of physicians who were able to restore function and movement to his upper body, but his lower half was completely paralysed. His parents, wealthy as they were, could do nothing further to help their son. The doctors had done everything in their power to help the young soldier.⁴⁸ No clues are offered about the sorts of therapies used by the physicians, although some possibilities are explored below.

About fifty years later the scribes at Rocamadour would record an excellent account of a knight who was left crippled by the holy fire. The story surrounds a warrior called Harduin from Indre-et-Loire in Central France. Harduin met a pilgrim who was on his way to the shrines at Rocamadour and Compostela in Spain. He liked the look of the pilgrim's cap and offered to buy it from him. The religious traveller said thanks, but no thanks, as he needed the cap to protect himself from the sun and rain. Used to getting what he wanted, the knight became angry at being turned down and so he attacked and injured the poor pilgrim.⁴⁹ At some point around this time the knight must have eaten something made with infected grain. The record says that as evening approached the knight began to feel the burning in his foot. As the pain went from Harduin's foot to his knee he thought that his whole body was going to be consumed by the internal fire, so he had his leg amputated at the knee. The procedure did not help matters, because soon enough his other foot was being consumed by the same painful burning. Harduin was left a maimed man, eventually losing both feet and at least one of his lower legs.⁵⁰ The coincidence of the knight's assault on a pilgrim and his attack of *ignis sacer* meant that this would become a morality tale among the collection at Rocamadour.

There are many accounts of limbs lost to ergotism, either amputated intentionally to try and halt the progress of the holy fire or that were taken by the illness itself.⁵¹ Shrines to St Mary became popular with sufferers flocking to them in hopes of a cure and the same was true of the hospitals dedicated to St Anthony. In 1093 a French nobleman called Gaston of Valloire established the Hospital Brothers of St Anthony, constructing such an infirmary beside the Church of St Anthony at La-Motte-Saint-Didier, near Vienne. Sufferers from all over began to make their way to the hospital for treatment.[52] Many more of these facilities dedicated to St Anthony began to spring up throughout Europe, such as the one established at Salerno, committed to the treatment of those who had fallen ill after consuming the poisoned grains.[53] Distressingly, the surgeons attached to these hospitals of St Anthony became very skilled at amputating limbs afflicted by the poison, leaving thousands in a similar condition to the knight from Indre-et-Loire.[54]

The influential herbal *Macer Floridus* was written at a time when significant outbreaks of ergotism would have been fresh in the memory. This work contains several recipes that were meant to cure the illness or help those suffering from its effects. Unfortunately, only some of them would have been of any use in providing temporary, but very welcome relief from its symptoms. Among the plants recommended was the opium poppy. The leaves were to be ground up and used as a plaster. This was said to have destroyed the sickness.[55] Hemlock was another plant mentioned, its leaves too were to be bruised and used as a plaster.[56]

While it never completely disappeared, outbreaks of ergotism did begin to dwindle or perhaps just fade into the background as the Middle Ages moved on to more frightening and devastating diseases that would soon dwarf even the largest of eruptions of the holy fire.

Sexually Transmitted Infections

> When some evidence of disease begins to show after coitus with an infected woman ...
>
> William of Saliceto[57]

It is a story as old as warfare itself; soldiers away from their loved ones, facing the uncertainty of combat, with money and spare time on their hands have regularly sought comfort and distraction either through prostitutes, casual partners or slaves. History is absolutely clear about what follows when there are soldiers and sex, sexually transmitted infections (STIs). Previous wars, rules, religious and personal morals have done little over the centuries to change attitudes or quell the urges of warriors, leaving a clear path for venereal disease to strike, quite often in huge numbers.

The world wars of the twentieth century would see the rates of infection absolutely skyrocket. The illustrations are many and at times quite shocking, such as the more than 1 million French soldiers who were admitted into hospitals for the treatment of STIs during the First World War.[58] While the armies of the Second World War were desperate to learn from the harsh lessons of the previous global conflict, efforts failed miserably. In North Africa alone, between 1943 and 1944, more men of the Allied forces were put out of action by gonorrhoea than were wounded by the bombs and bullets of their enemies.[59]

During the American Civil war hospitals had to set aside specific wards for those suffering from gonorrhoea and syphilis. Perhaps as many as one in twelve soldiers contracted these infections, with the reported cases of gonorrhoea in the Union army being 109,400, alongside 73,000 instances of syphilis.[60] Miserably, prostitution increased apace with these diseases as many women, without the support of their husbands, were forced to sell themselves to feed their families.[61] Elsewhere, in 1846 the British surgeon William Acton found that annually more than 18 per cent of British soldiers admitted to hospital had primary venereal sores.[62]

Soldiers with STIs are also found among the characters featured in the plays of the Elizabethan and Renaissance periods, such as the early seventeenth-century *The Knight of the Burning Pestle*. It included a knight called Sir Pockhole whose name and patch over his disfigured nose proclaimed the damage done by syphilis.[63] The Dutch writer Erasmus incorporated something similar in the syphilitic soldier from his sixteenth-century colloquy *The Soldier and the Carthusian*.[64]

While gonorrhoea, genital warts, lesions and other diseases and infections remained a constant throughout the medieval period, syphilis did not arrive on European shores until well after the period covered by this study.[65] It began its ugly reign in earnest in around 1494–5 with the invasion of Italy by the army of Charles VIII of France. The French army included large sections of mercenaries, many of whom took this unwanted souvenir back home with them to countries all across Europe once the fighting had ceased.[66] Today these afflictions are quite curable or at least treatable, but throughout the ages the various salves and cures, containing things like lead and mercury, tended to do just as much harm as the disease itself. Mercury would continue to be used as a cure, especially for syphilis, until the twentieth century.[67]

Specific examples of soldiers suffering from these STIs in the early and High Middle Ages are unusual. However, treatments for these diseases and references to warriors spending their idle time in brothels, bathhouses and taverns of cities and towns throughout Europe and while on crusade make it clear that things were no different at this time.[68] Some brothels were even set up by soldiers, like William of Poitou, who returned from fighting in the Holy Land, ironically having abandoned his faith.[69] In William of Malmesbury's account for the year 1119 he described how William of Poitou built a structure that resembled a monastery to house his brothel. He planned to fill it with prostitutes, using the common and sardonic naming practice of calling the manager of the establishment the Abbess.[70] She was responsible for looking after the day-to-day running of the brothel, choosing the women and ensuring they were single and disease free.[71]

In twelfth-century London, legalized brothels, or *stewes*, were located south of the River Thames at Southwark on the Bank-Side, beside the Bear Garden. These stewes were licensed establishments for the purpose of, 'The entertainment of lewd persons, in which were women prepared for all comers.'⁷² At Parliament in 1162, Henry II of England confirmed a number of laws and ordinances governing these stewes, including when they could be open, how much could be charged and the fact that they would be checked by the bailiffs and constables on a weekly basis.⁷³ Standing out among the regulations is the mention of the *burning* or venereal disease, which in this case was likely gonorrhoea: 'No Stew-holder to keep any woman that hath the perilous Infirmity of Burning, nor to sell bread, ale, flesh (meat), wood, coal, or any sort of victuals.'⁷⁴ These laws show the genuine concern that officials had about the spread of venereal disease, but with that said there was no shortage of unlicensed premises where prostitution could be found. Taverns were a popular place for solicitation, with alcohol and gambling among the other vices that were available inside these premises, unlike the certified stewes.⁷⁵ Twelfth-century London was a city that was full of taverns and their associated vices, as outlined by Richard of Devizes, a monk who provided a scathing report of the city. According to Richard, the city was a den of iniquity that was to be avoided at all costs. He described the houses full of 'flocks of prostitutes' and 'lewd singing girls' alongside the gambling establishments, taverns and every other vice imaginable.⁷⁶ While seemingly overexaggerated and clearly the view of a monk, this does show the kind of thing that was easily available to city dwellers and those passing through like soldiers, priests and traders.

Tournaments were another place where prostitution could be found in abundance. Like the fairs of the age, these gatherings of knights and spectators brought with them all sorts of vices to fill the evenings and nights, after the fighting of the day had ended. At Cambridge, the swords and sex of these tournaments finally caused their downfall when complaints by scholars and citizens to Henry III of England meant that they were made illegal anywhere within 5 miles of the town after the year 1245:

> Tournaments and tilting of the nobility and gentry were commonly kept at Cambridge, to the great annoyance of the scholars ... Much lewd people waited on these assemblies; *light housewives*, as well as, *light horsemen*, repaired thereunto. Yea, such the clashing of swords, the rattling of arms, the sounding of trumpets, the neighing of horses, the shouting of men, all day-time, with the roaring of riotous revellers all the night ...⁷⁷

The fighting and fun were just too much for some to ignore, such as the knight Ralph de Kamois who continued to hold '... a riotous tilting in the very town of Cambridge' despite the ban. He would later be sanctioned for his actions, but quickly forgiven.⁷⁸ With or without Cambridge there were tournaments to be found in all sorts of other places, both in England and on the Continent and each had a similar format of day and night entertainment to please participants and observers alike.⁷⁹ Of course, what all of this meant was the opportunity for STIs, such as the *burning*, to quickly spread far and wide by means of those knights, soldiers and prostitutes who went from tournament to tournament looking for fame, fortune and excitement.

In the absence of antibiotics, once again it was the symptoms being treated and not the disease. Beginning with *Bald's Leechbook*, it contains a few treatments for '… a mans instrumenta genitalia'. Swelling and soreness in afflicted genitals were to be bathed with a liquid made from ground betony, mixed with wine. In the case of '… mucous, or in eruption …' the liquid made by boiling sage in water was to be used to bathe the infected area. Another option was a salve made from burnt dill and honey that could also be applied in the same area.[80]

In the eleventh century, Constantine the African included treatments for gonorrhoea among the works he translated and wrote about while at Monte Cassino, not far from Salerno.[81] This was doubtless a common complaint among the large number of soldiers returning from crusade who made a stop at Salerno to be treated for wounds or disease on their way back to Europe. The twelfth-century *Trotula*, a work that primarily focuses on women's health, is another that was compiled at Salerno. It too contains a section on the treatment of STIs in males.[82]

Hugo de Lucca's role in treating soldiers of the Bolognese army must have included many who had contracted STIs and it seems that William of Saliceto may have encountered a few in his experience, as well. Hugo's son Theodoric recorded a frightening and invasive treatment for genital warts discovered on the penis. It would surely have required a steady hand on the part of the surgeon and a patient with a strong constitution: 'When they occur on the end of the prepuce and are soft, split them open with scissors and fill the whole cavity with well-ground salt and press it down with the finger for a long time.'[83]

In his surgery William of Saliceto spelled out the connection between sexual intercourse and venereal disease, specifically gonorrhoea. He understood the urgency of treatment, recommending a special ointment and powder to be used at the first sign of infection after sex. For those that had symptoms of a more advanced nature, William called for proper cleansing of the genitals and a diet that would aid in the healing process, but in the most extreme cases he used a cautery to remove the dead and diseased tissue.[84]

When faced with something sharp or hot near their genitals the cure must have seemed so much worse than the disease itself, but as always, it is unlikely that any of these treatments would have done much to stop warriors from pursuing what they desired.

Leprosy

> Just then there had come up a hundred lepers, deformed men with pitted and livid faces, limping on crutches to the clatter of hand-rattles.
>
> *The Romance of Tristan and Iseult*[85]

The Black Death of the mid-fourteenth century was undoubtedly the worst disaster of the Middle Ages and certainly one of the most dreadful plagues in the history of humankind. Before the mid-fourteenth century though there was another disease that was widely feared in Europe and beyond its borders, unnerving everyone from peasants and priests to knights and kings: leprosy. It caused damage to limbs and faces, blinding some of its victims and the 'loathsome disease' brought with it a whole host of other symptoms, forcing many to live outside of society.[86] One of the great tragedies of the disease, and there were many, came from the fact that it became a catch-all term for just about every type of skin disease. Psoriasis, alopecia, lymphedema and ringworm were among the many skin ailments that were mistaken for leprosy, because few people understood or were willing to take a chance that these other conditions were anything but the dreaded disease.[87]

Unlike many other diseases, leprosy *Mycobacterium leprae* is one that can be identified in skeletons excavated from medieval cemeteries and battlefields. One such early burial ground, found near modern day Molise in Eastern Italy, contained the bodies of ethnically varied origin. The area seems likely to have been an advanced military outpost of Lombards and Avars trying to protect themselves against a Byzantine invasion from the south. The body from tomb 144 comes from the second half of the seventh century and is that of a young male soldier between the ages of 20 and 25 who suffered from leprosy during his lifetime.[88] How he was looked upon when he was alive is impossible to know. The fact that he was buried alongside his comrades in the same manner as the rest of the bodies in the cemetery, which included two females that were also found to have evidence of the disease, is certainly of interest. One of the reasons that these burials are worth noting is the fact that five centuries later the Third Lateran Council of 1179 made this practice illegal, declaring that leprosy sufferers were to live away from the rest of society and be buried in separate cemeteries, as well.[89]

Fear of this disease can be found in the late ninth century thanks to the Welsh monk Asser who wrote a biography of the famous Anglo-Saxon warrior and ruler King Alfred. Within the pages he spoke about Alfred's long suffering with a painful illness, '… a severe disease, unknown to all physicians …'.[90] He had struggled with it for more than twenty years and at one point Asser found him lying prostrate and praying to God to relieve him. Alfred asked God to exchange whatever it was that he had for something lesser, as if he were at some sort of medieval disease customer service department. What he did not want in trade was leprosy, because, 'He had a great dread of leprosy …'.[91] He felt the disease would immediately make him an object of loathing and contempt among his people, a fact that was sadly all too true at this time.

Just how leprosy was treated in other parts of Northern Europe, in the centuries dominated by the Vikings, is a complex question. The disease had certainly become quite common in Scandinavia as the Viking Age ended. However, evidence of leprosy between the centuries 500 and 900 is more difficult to find, because many of the burials tended to be cremations, leaving little in the way of buried clues.[92] Later inhumation burials do show lepers mixed within common cemeteries, although at Lund, Sweden the earliest leper burials are found on the edge of the cemetery. It would be at Lund where the first Scandinavian leper hospital would be opened, but not until the mid-twelfth century.[93]

There are only a few references to outbreaks of leprosy elsewhere within the world of the Vikings, such as the *Annals of Ulster*, which mentions the disease being in Dublin in the year 950.[94] The earliest code of laws from Norway, the Gulathing code, excused lepers from war service.[95] Saga references are also very thin on the ground, with *The Saga of Thorstein, Viking's Son* being one of the very few exceptions. The tale involves a warrior called Viking who was stricken after drinking from the lower part of a magic horn that left him '... confined to his bed by the disease called leprosy'.[96] Near death, he was given a drop of liquid from the restorative upper portion of the same horn and was returned to health, with the disease dropping away from his body like fish scales.[97]

Three references from the eleventh and twelfth centuries that involve soldiers and leprosy help to provide an understanding of just how the disease was viewed on an individual level and by the wider population as time moved forward. The first comes from Orderic Vitalis who related details about the great soldier and brilliant physician called Ralph Mala-Corona. He spent the latter years of his life at the Abbey of St Evroult in Normandy.[98] He contracted leprosy, which he felt he deserved as a result of the sins he had committed during his life: 'This noble soldier having obtained from the Lord by earnest prayers the disease of leprosy to expiate the multitude of sins which burdened his conscience ...'.[99] A chapel was built for him and he had a monk called Goscelin who was assigned to look after him, as well. Despite his affliction, Vitalis noted that people still flocked to Ralph Mala-Corona for his advice and counsel.

In Ireland, the Leper Hospital of St Mary Magdalen, Maudlinstown was founded in around 1170 by the leader of the invading Anglo-Norman forces called Raymond Fitzgerald or Le Gros, as he is also known. It was endowed by Raymond's friend William Ferrand, a knight who himself had become a victim of the disease.[100] Gerald of Wales noted that Ferrand tried to get himself killed in battle, preferring that to the long and slow death of leprosy.[101]

The third illustration comes from Canterbury and highlights the shame and embarrassment involved with the disease. The twelfth-century Bishop of Clermont, speaking at a council in Bourges, France, described a knight called John the Scot who lived in Clermont: '... and who, having been seized with leprosy, had been cut off, in the ordinary way, by the decision of the clergy and laity, from public intercourse, being abandoned also by his wife'.[102] This knight went to Canterbury to seek a miracle cure and after spending six months there he was well again. The council summoned the knight to come before them to confirm the details of his return to good health, but he was so ashamed of the horrible disease that he simply refused to be seen by them as '… it was bad enough that any one knew he had been a leper'.[103]

Literature of this period contains far more tales involving leprosy than it does illnesses such as ergotism or STIs, possibly because it was so feared, making it the ideal ugly antagonist. One of the most famous examples is the late twelfth-century German poem *Der Arme Heinrich*, or *Poor Henry*. It tells the tale of a knight of high status called Heinrich who contracted leprosy in the prime of his life:

> He fell a prey to leprosy.
> Now when it easy grew to see
> The heavy scourge that God had sent
> Upon him as a punishment,
> That marred his limbs and body then
> He grew repugnant to all men[104]

The leprous knight desperately searched for a cure, finally settling upon a doctor at Salerno who explained that to become well he required the blood of a young virgin who would willingly give up her life for the knight. As expected, he found such a girl, a kindly peasant who was happy to agree. The two made their way back to Salerno and just as the doctor was about to kill the girl the knight had a change of heart, deeply regretting something so horrible and selfish just to save his own life.[105] He stopped the physician from killing her and the two made their way back home. On the way, the knight was miraculously cured of his leprosy and despite the gulf in class between the two they were married.

Despite tales like *Der Arme Heinrich*, knights who contracted leprosy were left in a quandary, because even with the disease they were still well-trained and high-status warriors. The question became what to do with them, a problem partially solved in the early twelfth century by the Order of St Lazarus where some of them found refuge and a new life.[106] While they were still forbidden from military service within Europe, they were a welcome part of the crusading armies in the Holy Land under their own banner of St Lazarus.[107] After all, Baldwin IV, or Baldwin the Leper, was the King of Jerusalem between 1174 and 1185. These leper knights were noted as having served in many battles in the thirteenth century, including the year 1250, during the Seventh Crusade in Egypt. The chronicler Matthew Paris counted the leper knights among the crusaders during a crushing defeat: 'The whole Christian army, consisting of the nobility of all France, the Templars, Hospitallers, the knights of the Teutonic order of St. Mary, and those of St. Lazarus, was cut to pieces in Egypt.'[108] To prevent the further spread of infection it is likely that some distance was required between the knights of the Order of St Lazarus and other parts of the crusading army. David Marcombe, who has traced their history, suggests that their role may have been more strategic than military, perhaps involving reconnaissance or foraging work.[109]

While St Lazarus was a possibility for the knightly classes the average soldier would have found himself ostracized by society, having to turn to begging or perhaps going on pilgrimage in search of healing.[110] A fortunate few would have ended up in one of the hospitals that were set up all over Europe to house lepers, as an act of mercy and a method of trying to control the disease. One such hospital from Dudston, near Gloucester, England, was founded in the twelfth century. The rare extant rules of the hospital, which come from the latter part of the century are of great interest. The twenty-three laws set out to govern the house included the separation of men and women and regular religious practices. Sexual intercourse meant instant expulsion from the hospital, as did persistent backchat to the master of the facility. Remarkably, patients were given some freedoms, such as the ability to take a break outside of the hospital, provided they were chaperoned.[111]

With the stakes being so high for those infected by the disease remedies varied widely and there were many of them. These cures extended across the centuries and varied widely, with everything from a salt and horse-fat mixture known from *Bald's*, which was meant to be spread over the body, and the use of the sperm of a rorqual whale set out in the Norwegian text *The King's Mirror* from the first half of the thirteenth century.[112]

Infection

> … and gangrene started in the intestines.
> *Les miracles de Notre-Dame de Roc-Amadour*[113]

Infections in wounds were also among this group of invisible enemies that were a persistent threat to the lives and limbs of medieval warriors and they would continue to endanger soldiers through to the twentieth century.[114] There are many examples of just how dangerous these contaminated injuries could be, with death a common outcome. The Viking sagas are certainly not without their stories of minor scrapes and cuts becoming a major problem, including Sturluson's *Heimskringla*, which relates the bizarre story of the lethal infection that took the life of Earl Sigurd. A battle arranged against a rival named Melbridge Tooth (also Máel Brigte the buck-toothed) was supposed to settle differences between the two men. It was agreed that the fight would be between forty men on each side, but Earl Sigurd brought eighty warriors who soon slaughtered their opponents. The heads of Melbridge and his smaller army were taken by Sigurd and his soldiers and tied to their saddle straps. Karma or at least the head of Melbridge Tooth soon bit the deceitful Earl Sigurd and the resulting infection killed him: 'Earl Sigurd killed Melbridge Tooth, a Scotch earl, and hung his head to his stirrup-leather; but the calf of his leg were [*sic*] scratched by the teeth, which were sticking out from the head, and the wound caused inflammation in his leg, of which the earl died …'.[115]

Medieval malpractice was often the cause of these infected wounds as the account of an unnamed soldier from the mid-eleventh-century miracles of St Foy can attest. Practioners of medicine who were less than skilled or just plain charlatans seem to have been quite easy to come by, very often causing infection or further injury. The French writer Rutebeuf highlighted these quacks in his thirteenth-century comic monologue called *Dit de l'herberie*, or *The Tale of the Herb Market*, which features a doctor of fake medicine and his bogus wares.[116]

Returning to the soldier from the St Foy account, while his name is not provided, he was a follower of a nobleman called Gerald. In a conflict against citizens from an area in South-Western France formerly called Quercy this soldier was struck in the side by a spear as he tried to help one of his comrades. The record notes that he received poor medical treatment at the hands of the unskilled doctors who looked after him.[117] They bandaged his injuries too quickly without cleansing the area, trapping clotted blood and other decaying matter inside of the wound, which of course caused the injury to become badly contaminated.[118] There is some inference that the original bandages were never changed, creating further problems and giving the injury no chance to heal properly.[119] Trying to unfetter the truth of this miracle account from St Foy can be a little troublesome. Nevertheless, it appears that the warrior was in some considerable danger from the infection that built up in the wound causing him a great deal of pain and discomfort. This contamination seems to have resulted in the soldier's delirium, seeing a saint when in fact he was being treated by a doctor:

> La sainte, tournant vers lui son visage toujours radieux, toucha légèrement de sa verge la plaie du blessé. Ce contact fut si efficace, que de la plaie, rouverte comme par un tranchant, il s'échappa une humeur fétide qui souilla le pavé. Le chevalier, saisi par cette odeur, témoignait du dégoût.[120]

> The saint turned her bright countenance toward him, gently touching the wound of the injured man with her rod. This contact worked to reopen the wound as if it had been a knife, causing fetid liquid to soil the pavement. The knight was repulsed by the smell and showed his disgust for it.

The release of the infection, probably by a doctor's knife, almost certainly worked to save him, as the account notes that in the end he did survive.[121]

Orderic Vitalis offers a twelfth-century record of an infected wound in William, Count of Flanders whose hand was injured by a foot soldier at the siege of Aalst in summer 1128. Whether it was the result of a lack of knowledge, improper treatment or malpractice on the part of those who looked after him the contamination took his life.[122] In his account, Vitalis believed that *ignis sacer* had played a part in William's death, along with the infection relating to the wound, something not included by other chroniclers.[123] In fairness to Vitalis, summer 1128 saw the beginning of a violent eruption of the illness, which may explain its inclusion, however, whether it contributed to the death of the young Count William is debatable.[124]

While doctors lacked a basic understanding of the bacteria that caused these infections there were some methods employed to try and treat the resulting contamination that were known to work. Things such as vinegar and alcohol, usually wine, were used with varying degrees of success. The leechbooks contain remedies with these ingredients, *Bald's*, for example, mentions vinegar as part of a solution to treat skin infections like erysipelas.[125] Usāmah ibn Munqidh provided an example of the use of vinegar by a Frankish physician in the 1130s. A knight called Bernard, the treasurer to Fulk of Anjou, King of Jerusalem, received a serious kick to his leg from a horse. It became badly infected and impossible to close, as soon as one opening was sutured another would appear. The ointments that were applied to his leg failed to work, so a Frankish doctor was summoned. He immediately washed away the salves from Bernard's leg, using only strong vinegar to cleanse the knight's lower limb. This led to its healing so that Bernard was soon 'up again like a devil', as ibn Munqidh noted in his memoir.[126]

About fifty years later at Rocamadour the collection of miracles contains a record of a serious wound treated in a similar manner. The injured warrior in this case was called Siger of Subrigien, likely Saarbrücken in Germany.[127] His chest had been run through by the spear of another called Count Theobald, causing life-threatening injuries to Siger. The wound, which was to Siger's lungs, became very badly infected, filling with pus and fetid matter that continued to ooze out of him. The contamination was treated daily with wine, poured onto the wound to cleanse it, in the same way that armour was cleaned with sulphur, as the scribe colourfully explained. Siger was in a bad way during this time, so much so that those close to him were sure that he was going to die, but to everyone's surprise the therapy was eventually successful and Siger survived.[128]

Nearly a century after Siger's pus-filled injury, Theodoric would insert into his surgery one of the most groundbreaking sections on the treatment of wounds that had been written in some time, suggesting that the formation of pus was not necessary for proper healing. It would put both him and his father completely at odds with the ancients, as well as surgeons like Roger Frugard and Roland of Parma who had believed that pus was a required part of the healing process.[129] At times Theodoric even called them out by name within his text, referring to them as 'stupid men' for believing in the old approach.[130] In terms of the formation of this discharge, white or 'laudable pus' had long been seen as a positive sign of a healing wound, while foul, watery contamination, like that found in the account of Siger above, meant that the injury had become infected and the victim was likely to die.[131] With this so-called 'dry healing' technique Theodoric wrote that suppuration of any type served only to hinder the proper healing of a wound. He and his father recommended that wine be used to cleanse the area around the wound before bandaging it without the aid of any ointments. It was then to be left for several days to allow the body to begin to heal the injury naturally.[132] Henri de Mondeville would continue to endorse this method of dry healing in the early part of the fourteenth century, especially after treating large numbers of battle-related wounds.[133]

Once again giving the casebook of William of Saliceto the last word, a record involving the healing of a man called Gabriel de Prolo shows the general lack of knowledge and understanding of bacteria and contamination in a wound.[134] The injured man came from Cremona and had been hit at the back of his knee by a crossbow bolt. The wound itself does not sound overly serious, the bolt having penetrated through to the bone, but causing it no harm. In de Prolo's case it appears to have been the subsequent contamination that became the real cause for concern as he lay at death's door for two months with a serious infection that caused him severe chills among other things. William mistakenly believed that the chills were an indication that the soldier's brain had been affected by damage to a major nerve, part of the original wound. He went on to say that this usually indicated that death would be the outcome, especially if the chills were accompanied by diarrhoea, fever or insomnia. William's recommendation in these cases began with a strong laxative to purge the body. If the symptoms started to subside then nature had a chance to heal the individual. Water and a light diet were suggested for the patient, although in some cases a little wine was acceptable. In the end William's treatment meant that Gabriel the soldier survived his injury and most importantly the infection that resulted from it.[135]

Men like Gabriel de Prolo and Siger of Subrigien were, of course, the exceptions, surviving their contamination and qualifying them for entry into the casebooks and miracle collections. The reality for most was quite different, with illness and infection killing untold numbers during this period of five centuries. It seems that soldiers were uniquely qualified to become afflicted by disease or hindered by infection. Living in cramped and dirty conditions often promoted illnesses like dysentery and of course exposure to the swords and arrows of their enemies meant that the chance of life-threatening infection was always high.

Chapter 8

Tormented Minds

> But now all his happiness has passed away!
> *The Wanderer*[1]

Combat has caused appalling damage to so many minds over the millennia, from those in the ancient world such as Achilles in Homer's *Iliad* to later examples such as Major George Wither (1588–1667), an officer and poet during the English Civil War of the seventeenth century who was haunted by terrible nightmares.[2] The twentieth century, with its two world wars and numerous other conflicts, left an untold number with minds wounded by the violence and savagery. The Middle Ages were no different for those such as the eleventh-century warrior Rigaud who was caught up in a fierce struggle between two lords in the region of the Albigeois in Southern France.[3] He was a soldier of great skill and experience whose arm became paralysed when he was struck by a sword in battle. He became severely depressed and so hopeless that he felt it would be better to be dead than to continue with what he considered to be a useless life. He stopped practising the fighting arts and completely gave up on riding horses, something that had brought him great joy before his injury.[4] The hopelessness, melancholy and loss of interest in what used to bring such pleasure seem instantly identifiable as symptoms of a mind tormented by the trauma of the battlefield. Compare the thoughts and feelings ascribed to Rigaud to those of the character of Paul Bäumer in the novel *All Quiet on the Western Front*, written by Erich Maria Remarque who was himself a soldier of the First World War: 'I was a soldier, and now I am nothing but an agony for myself, for my mother, for everything that is so comfortless and without end.'[5] Bäumer's words, so fraught with pain and anguish, seem as if they could have been spoken by almost any soldier throughout the ages, including Rigaud himself nearly 900 years before the First World War.

There will be those who question trying to examine the mental health of a soldier like Rigaud based on just a few lines written many centuries ago and there is no doubt that it can be a difficult task and one that is at times open to scrutiny and different interpretations of the evidence. However, for a moment reconsider Rigaud's situation had he been a modern soldier returning from some war-torn part of the world having lost the use of one arm. His depression and desperation would immediately be considered probable symptoms of Post Traumatic Stress Disorder (PTSD) or some other issue of mental health resulting from his experiences of war and worthy of further investigation. The same is true of these more ancient examples, they are at least a starting point. If we can accept the fact that Rigaud's paralysis was the outcome of his sword injury, then the connection between violence and his mental health should not be a great leap.

In any era, the terrible reality of war is not just the gruesome physical toll that it takes, but likewise the significant psychological cost in damage done to the minds of soldiers and civilians alike.[6] Those warriors who fought a thousand years ago faced fear, wounds, sickening smells, terrifying noises and the shocking scenes of war. It is trauma or stress like this, be it physical, mental or emotional, that can cause changes to the human brain altering the way in which it processes memories and new information, triggering things such as acute depression, fear and nightmares.[7] As examples throughout this chapter will show, physical wounds like Rigaud's are not necessary for this type of damage to occur to the mind. This is not to downplay the relationship between combat injuries and a damaged psyche because there is clear a link joining the two, as numerous studies have confirmed.[8] Oftentimes though it is the shock of violence, seeing comrades with limbs hacked away or surveying a battlefield filled with rotting corpses or being in fear for one's own life that impacts the mind. Indeed, as the First World War dragged on physicians such as the Englishman Dr Harold Wiltshire began to realize that there were other significant causes of psychological trauma beyond what was being blamed on shell shock. In the medical journal *The Lancet* Dr Wiltshire reported that the largest number of his patients who suffered severe emotional scars did so because of the terrible things that they had seen, rather than from any physical injuries.[9] Wiltshire was not alone, his contemporary the German psychiatrist Robert Gaupp was of a similar opinion. He too recognized that the main cause of harm to the minds of so many was the significant fear and anxiety brought about by things such as seeing 'maimed or dead comrades'.[10]

This chapter attempts to search for and analyse those soldiers and their families who were victims of war many centuries ago and who suffered with things such as depression, nightmares, strife in the home and suicide. The final section explores the methods and medicines used to try and assist in the recovery from such difficulties.

Vikings

> … some strange terror stole upon him …
> Saxo Grammaticus[11]

Thinking again about the evocative nature of the word *Viking* it can stir up images of an almost invincible character; a muscular, battle-hardened warrior who feared nothing. This stereotypical image can make it difficult to fathom that they could have been haunted by their experiences of battle, but the truth was much different. They bled, felt pain and fear like anyone else and importantly for this chapter there were those whose mental health suffered as a result of combat. Looking once more at the entry in the *Annals of St Bertin* for the year 865, it described several ailments and illnesses that struck the

Northmen who sacked St Denis, north of Paris late in that year. It noted that some Vikings were covered with sores, while others suffered with watery diarrhoea and there were those who 'went mad', which sadly is just about as broad and unhelpful a definition of mental health issues as is possible.[12] Quite the opposite is true of Viking sagas and poetry, because among the tales of heroes and bloodshed are rich and varied descriptions of identifiable problems pertaining to mental health. In fact, research into this subject has laid bare vivid and accurate accounts of a wide range of issues found within these chronicles and verses, with everything from depression and bipolar disorder to things such as autism.[13] It should not be surprising then that the intersection between this warrior culture and minds wounded by battle is found time and again in the sagas and poems of medieval Scandinavia.[14] It seems that more recorded examples may be found here than in just about any other culture within these five centuries.

While it is true that many of these oral traditions were not transcribed until the twelfth and thirteenth centuries and some even later, there are those, such as the poem *Sonatorrek*, or *The Loss of Sons*, which were recorded much earlier, in this case the middle of the tenth century.[15] Full of heavy and palpable sorrow, it was composed by the famous Viking, Egil Skallagrímsson, lamenting the loss of his two sons who died while still young. Within the poem Egil also expressed the continued sadness he felt at the loss of his older brother Thorolf who was killed in battle many years earlier.[16] *Sonatorrek* is significant because it does expose the inner thoughts and feelings of a Viking warrior like Egil. It shows that issues of mental health, such as depression, were just as possible in the tenth century as any other. Egil's relationships with the gods are also interesting in this poem, mainly with the tricky Odin whom he felt had let him down:

> I was friendly with the Lord of the Spear; I trusted him without misgiving until the Lord of ears, the awarder of victory, broke friendship with me.[17]

Within other stories and poems that describe the gods of the Norse pantheon there are acknowledgements and indications of minds tormented by violence. After all, these gods and the mythology associated with them were a product of the human mind and a way of explaining the world. Contemplating the poem *Hávamál*, or *The Lay of the High One*, it provided eighteen charms that were given to Odin after he was meant to have suffered for nine nights, hung from a tree. The first of them was directed at those suffering from melancholy and grief:

> I know incantations
> Which no king's wife knows,
> And no man's son.
> Help is the first one called,
> And it will help thee
> Against strife and sorrows,
> Against all kinds of grief.[18]

Unfortunately, none of the details of these spells were provided, just their general intent and outcome. The next couple of these are similar, with the second charm intended for those wishing to become physicians. The balance of them pertain to other issues, such as success in battle, so perhaps it is significant that these charms, directed at a warrior society, should begin with issues relating to health, especially mental health even before speaking of war. This must have been something that was required in some measure.

Another god of war and member of the Aesir, called Tyr, was detailed in the *Prose Edda* as wise, bold and incredibly brave, so much so that he was often invoked by warriors as they went into battle.[19] It was because of this fearlessness that Tyr ended up losing his right hand. He was the only one among the Aesir brave enough to feed the young wolf Fenrir, an offspring of Loki. As the wolf became larger the gods realized that it was too dangerous to be left unchained and so shackling it became a job that fell to Tyr.[20] As Tyr attempted to bring the beast under control it bit off his hand. The stirrings of Tyr's torment seemed immediate when the other gods laughed at the situation, but Tyr could find no humour in it whatsoever.[21] Later in the poem *Lokasenna*, Tyr and some of the other gods are found arguing with the troublesome Loki. The state of Tyr's psyche appeared to be getting worse when he said to Loki, 'I miss my hand, you miss famed wolf: both suffer bitter loss.'[22] Little else is ever said on the subject, but in the *Lokasenna* there is a fairly strong hint of the torment in Tyr's mind after suffering the loss of his hand so violently.

An earthly illustration from the sagas is laid out in some detail in *The Saga of Grettir the Strong* involving one of the early principal characters, Onund Treefoot, who was described as a great Viking who raided and fought throughout the British Isles and beyond. He lost his leg below the knee while fighting at sea and once his physical injuries had healed, he was fitted with the wooden limb that gave him his alias.[23] As the months passed the injuries to Onund's mind began to become apparent, something not uncommon in soldiers with both physical and psychological wounds.[24] He described to his friend the hopelessness and melancholy he felt because of the damage done to him by the war axe:

> No joy is mine since in battle I fought.
> Many the sorrows that o'er me lower.
> Men hold me for nought; this thought is the worst
> of all that oppresses my sorrowing heart.[25]

As time passed Onund Treefoot continued to struggle with his emotional scars, concerned that he was little more than a maimed, one-footed man.[26]

Of the different representations of a mind wounded by the trauma of combat there is one that can be found in several stories and poems of the Vikings. Known as battle-fetter, war-paralysis or any number of other similar expressions, it denotes the sudden immobility or seeming lack of common sense on the battlefield, which can cause a soldier to become temporarily disconnected from reality. It is a dissociative state, often caused by chronic trauma, becoming a third part of the body's 'fight or flight' response, which is to *freeze up*.[27] It can create extreme danger for that individual, along with those who are nearby or depending upon him or her for their safety. It has been depicted in many modern films and television programmes about warfare, including the 2001 television series *Band of Brothers* that brought to life the exploits of the US Army's 'Easy' Company, 506th Regiment of the 101st Airborne Division, during the Second World War.[28] Portrayed more than once within the series, in one disastrous scene a lieutenant was sent to lead his men on an attack against a German held position in the town of Foy in Belgium. As they began their assault the American officer soon froze up, becoming confused and unable to make decisions before directing his men into what was a dangerous situation.[29]

According to Norse mythology battle-fetter was something that came from Odin.[30] The *Ynglinga Saga*, which explains some of his accomplishments, mentions that he '… could make his enemies in battle blind, or deaf, or terror-struck …'.[31] In the same manner, within *Hávamál* Odin was said to be able to paralyse his foes whenever he wished.[32] These ideas around paralysing his enemies describe this notion of battle-fetter. Since Valkyries were believed to play a major role in deciding how a conflict and certainly how a warrior's life would play out on the battlefield it was thought that Odin used them to place this paralysis on combatants as they fought.[33] Each Valkyrie was given a name that reflected some facet of war and importantly one was called Herfjotur, a name that means battle-fetter.[34]

One of the most detailed examples of war paralysis comes from *The Saga of Hord*. Within the tale the story's namesake, an infamous outlaw and warrior, found himself surrounded by many of his enemies as they fought with one another. Three times during the fighting Hord was overcome by this paralysis and as the struggle carried on, he was mortally wounded eventually succumbing to his injuries.[35]

Specific spells and charms were thought to be useful in releasing a warrior from these fetters of their mind. The poem *Grógaldr*, or *Groa's Chant*, contained a charm that was instructed to be chanted over the thighs of the afflicted person. Here again, the details of this loosening spell are not explained.[36] There is, however, another such incantation found in other pagan Germanic culture from around the ninth century, which does provide the particulars for this kind of spell.[37] The *Merseburg Charms*, as they are known, are keys to two different spells. While the second one pertains to the treatment of the horse belonging to the northern god called Balder (Baldr), the first provides for the loosening of fetters related to battle. This initial incantation is called *Losesegan*, or *The Blessing of Release*. The last two lines are said to be the enchanted portion of the charm and by reciting it to the warrior it was meant to cause their mind to become clear:

> Once sat women,
> They sat here, then there.
> Some fastened bonds,
> Some impeded an army,
> Some unravelled fetters:
> Escape the bonds,
> flee the enemy![38]

There are more examples from the Viking world that are presented in the specific sections that follow dealing with things such as nightmares and suicide. These preceding cases represent just a few from their literature, which focus on depression and the intense confusion on the field of battle felt by so many Viking soldiers.[39] Those who had suffered injuries to the mind and body would seem to have had no trouble in identifying themselves or their state of mind within these tales, as they were told again and again within this warrior society.

Beyond the Viking World

> I myself too, in my misery and distress, have constantly had to bind my feelings in fetters
>
> *The Wanderer*[40]

Like the French warrior called Rigaud, who appeared at the beginning of this chapter, there are examples of others from these centuries whose minds were wounded by the violence of combat. They too suffered from things such as depression and battlefield paralysis. These examples represent a cross-section of some of them:

- In the most well-known Anglo-Saxon epic poem *Beowulf* is the character of Hrothgar, the King of the Danes who fell into a deep depression for a time. According to the story Hrothgar had once been a great warrior and leader.[41] However, as the monster Grendal began to attack those he cared for Hrothgar found himself faced with the melancholy that would soon grip him much harder.[42] Perhaps because of his wartime experiences, but certainly the result of the carnage and fear created by the monster Grendel, Hrothgar became very depressed. The terrible sorrow and grief that were triggered within him nearly crushed the leader of the Danes.[43]
- Another Anglo-Saxon poem known as *The Wanderer* may provide the most complete and engrossing picture of a soldier whose mind had been tormented by his experiences of war.[44] Found within the tenth-century *Exeter Book*, this anonymous work explores the crushing loneliness and vulnerability of a homeless warrior whose lord and comrades had been killed in battle, as some of the opening words of the poem convey:

> These are the words of a wanderer whose memory
> was full of troubles and cruel carnage, wherein his
> dear kinsmen had fallen:[45]

The poem is thick with melancholy and examines the loneliness and distress of a soldier who, as a result of war, appears to have lost everyone and everything that was dear to him, making his thoughts '... full of homeless wanderings'.[46]

- During the second half of the twelfth century the area around Toulouse was ravaged by war. The miracle collection from Rocamadour, which was assembled around this time, recorded a knight called Raymond who was himself from Toulouse. He was taken by his parents to the abbey at Rocamadour for care and comfort. He had become incoherent and struggled to respond to those who spoke to him, only managing to repeat what was said to him by others and swearing against God.[47] The entry is a short one with only a few details, but his distorted speech patterns strongly resemble others suffering from a wounded mind.[48]
- Seemingly written before 1197, one of the most detailed descriptions of battlefield terror comes from the Middle Irish tale *Buile Suibhne*, or *The Frenzy of Suibhne (Sweeney)*.[49] Within the story, as the Battle of Magh Rath began, Suibhne froze completely, being overcome by the paralysis referred to as battle-fetter by the Vikings:[50]

> he looked up, whereupon turbulence, and darkness,
> and fury, and giddiness, and frenzy, and flight, unsteadiness,
> restlessness, and unquiet filled him, likewise disgust with
> every place in which he used to be and desire for every place
> which he had not reached. His fingers were palsied, his feet
> trembled, his heart beat quick, his senses were overcome, his
> sight was distorted.[51]

- There is a great deal of evidence that shows that civilians too can be impacted by warfare, just as the thirteenth-century example of John of Ancaster shows.[52] He had fallen victim to war, likely the terrible destruction caused by the fighting between the English and French after the death of King John of England in 1216. The conflict was fierce in the area around Lincoln, where John of Ancaster resided. During 1217 pillaging and violence was done on an almost industrial scale.[53] The record notes that John of Ancaster lost so much that was good in him. He was taken by his father to the tomb of St Hugh of Lincoln in the hope that the saint might assist in the healing of his son's madness, which had been brought on by the violence.[54]

Nightmares

> Hard have been my dreams ...
> *The Story of Burnt Njal*[55]

Wilfred Owen, the great poet of the First World War, was heavily influenced by his experiences of violence in the trenches of the Western Front. Killed just a week before the guns of the First World War fell silent, his most famous work *Dulce et Decorum Est* details a recurring nightmare in which he saw one of his men choke to death, unable to get his gas mask on in time.[56] Nightmares like these, sleep disturbance and insomnia are all hallmarks of a mind haunted by the terror of warfare.[57] Psychiatrists who have treated veterans of conflict have repeatedly heard how their patients become so fearful of their nightmares that they are afraid of falling asleep. Difficult to treat and repeated night after night, these dreams can replay the scenes of horror that the sufferer has witnessed in incredibly graphic detail.[58]

Unfortunately, these bad dreams do not tend to diminish with time. In a survey of Second World War veterans completed in 1983, the majority were found to be suffering from PTSD and among the symptoms uncovered were continued nightmares, more than four decades after the war that damaged their young minds had ended.[59] These same sorts of bad dreams troubled warriors of the Middle Ages in a similar way.

The homeless soldier in *The Wanderer* suffered routinely with the same nightmare or what might be described as a reverse nightmare in which he dreamt that his lord and comrades were very much alive and all was right with his world, only to be tortured when he awoke to find:

> The grievous wounds, which the loss of his lord has made in
> his heart, are all the harder to bear, and his sorrow comes back
> to him when the memory of his kinsmen passes through his mind.[60]

Almost worse than a bad dream and served up nightly this would have only brought into sharp focus the misery that was this poor warrior's life.

The title character in the Viking tale *Gisli Sursson's Saga* became so frightened of his nightmares that he too could no longer sleep. Written around the end of the thirteenth or the beginning of the fourteenth century, this saga portrays a brutal picture of Viking life. The story's namesake was a warrior who had experienced a great deal of brutality in the form of combat, killing, maiming and perhaps worst of all he had witnessed the horror of people being burned alive.[61] These experiences left Gisli so damaged that he hid himself away in an underground hideout to feel safe.[62] He experienced frequent nightmares, which became progressively worse making Gisli afraid of the dark, fearful of being alone and eventually unable to sleep.[63] Whatever the truth of this tale might be, the presence of these dreams is indicative of the author's understanding of the genuine connection between trauma and these nightmares.[64]

Returning to Kari Solmund, the son-in-law of Njal from *The Story of Burnt Njal*, mentioned in the section on Burn Injuries in Chapter 6, he too had witnessed scenes of horror when he narrowly escaped the intentional burning of his father-in-law's home and all who were inside. The event and the physical injuries that he received impacted him greatly, as the song he would later sing portrays:

> Bender of the bow of battle,
> Sleep will not my eyelids seal,
> Still my murdered messmates' bidding
> Haunts my mind the livelong night ...[65]

In the early 1130s the regular nightmares experienced by the English king Henry I were witnessed and recorded by a physician called Grimbald. He noted that during these nightmares the king would leap naked from his bed, grab his sword and begin yelling and thrashing violently at the imaginary visions from his dreams before chasing away his guards.[66] Henry was an experienced soldier, which may in part explain some of these dreams and the jumping from bed to take his sword. A similar case from the fourteenth century involved a knight called Sir Peter Béarn. Although outside our timeline it is worth reporting here because of its details, which are nearly identical to those of Henry I. Sir Peter's mental health had also been badly impaired, becoming so acute that his wife and children were no longer able to live with the knight. He too suffered from frightening nightmares and would arm himself while asleep and thrash about. His servants were charged with trying to wake him from his bad dreams to keep him from harm.[67]

Interesting to note is the fact that Roger Frugard included the sort of behaviour shown by men like Henry I and Peter Béarn in his surgery, but under a section on depressed skull fractures where the scalp was not broken. Nightmares are common in sufferers of PTSD, as well as those with mild brain injuries, but the coincidence between Roger's findings and the other two is remarkable.[68] In any case, it seems clear that Roger had witnessed or had knowledge of soldiers exhibiting such behaviours: '... the patient has nightmares of himself in combat with an enemy and he awakens from sleep and seizes his own weapons and acts as if he is wide-awake'.[69]

Unless they occur nightly or regularly, nightmares are not something that can be predicted or require a preventative treatment. The fact that remedies for these bad dreams existed at all is perhaps one of the best indicators that there were those who were seriously afflicted by these horrors of sleep. A cure for nightmares is contained in the *Old English Herbarium*, which names the plant *betonica* (wood betony or bishopswort) as a powerful preparation. It was said that '... it shields him against monstrous nocturnal visitors and against frightful visions and dreams ...'.[70] Picked in August, without the use of iron tools, betony was to be shaken until the mould was off its leaves. It was then to be dried in the shade and ground into a powder, roots and all. The instructions go on to note, '... then use it, and taste of it when thou needest'.⁷¹ The Rhineland Abbess and healer Hildegard of Bingen also suggested betony for nightmares, although her prescription is somewhat less complicated. The sufferer was simply meant to take betony leaves to bed with them and this would help to reduce the bad dreams.⁷²

Suicide

> ... he intended to kill himself at once ...
> *The Knight of the Cart (Lancelot)*⁷³

The writers of this period were not shy about using suicide as a romantic device to pull at the heartstrings of their readers. Warriors and their lovers, betrayed or broken-hearted, often took their own lives or at least attempted to do so within these tales. Saxo Grammaticus included the suicide of Gunnhild, the wife of Asmund, in the first book of his *Gesta Danorum*. Gunnhild chose to stab herself with a sword, rather than carry on without her beloved husband who had been killed by Hadding, one of Odin's heroes.⁷⁴ Perhaps the most famous of these stories is the tangled plotline of two near suicides in Chrétien de Troyes' tale of Lancelot in the *The Knight of the Cart*. Certain that the flawed reports were true that the other was dead, Lancelot and his lover Guinevere each tried to take their own lives, but both managed to survive, remaining very much alive within the tale.⁷⁵

Away from the fantasy of works like these there is nothing romantic about the trauma of warfare that has far too often led to the suicide of soldiers, catastrophically eliminating all hope of something better and leaving behind devasted friends and loved ones. The incidents of soldiers and former soldiers taking their own lives are sadly all too easy to find throughout the history of warfare. In the middle of the nineteenth century dire examples of self harm and suicide can be found throughout the American Civil War.⁷⁶ In his poem *Suicide in the Trenches*, Siegfried Sassoon wrote about a young soldier who, amid the mud and lice of the trenches, blew his brains out.⁷⁷ Recent data on military veterans has shown that as many as 6,000 US ex-service personnel took their own lives in 2018, while in Scotland in 2019 a former soldier committed suicide every 6 days.⁷⁸

There are no figures or percentages to help us to judge whether suicide among those who fought during the Middle Ages was more or less common than it is now or at any other point in history. Neither do we have such figures for those who took their own lives after the fighting had stopped. What does exist is a handful of accounts of soldiers who took their own lives or attempted to do so, most of which were recorded by eyewitnesses or contemporaries:

- Reported by the philosopher and historian Miskawayh, he described the suicide of a young, fresh-faced Swedish Viking, the son of a chieftain. In Azerbaijan, in 943, days of disease, fighting and exhaustion between

Rūs and Muslim forces left hundreds dead on both sides. According to eyewitness reports a skirmish took place between a group of five Rūs warriors and a much larger Muslim force. As the fighting began it was said that the Vikings, who had taken refuge in a garden, slew great numbers of their enemies, but eventually four of the Rūs were killed, leaving just the chieftain's son. When it became evident that the battle was lost, he climbed a tree and stabbed himself through the stomach until he died.[79]

- A king with a Scandinavian name about whom little is known forms a part of this small group. The reason he took his own life is also a mystery, as the entry in the *Anglo-Saxon Chronicle* for the year 962 noted only that, 'King Sigferth killed himself and his body lies at Wimborne.'[80]
- The early eleventh-century miracles from St Foy present a detailed case of the attempted suicide of a young knight of high rank named Gerbert. The circumstances began with a violent and ruthless man called Guy who ruled a castle at what is today known as Le Monastier-sur-Gazeille in South-Central France.[81] Guy had taken three men hostage, holding them prisoner in his castle. Gerbert made arrangements to help them escape, but when Guy the Castilian discovered the plot he was furious, employing his henchmen to find and mutilate Gerbert by gouging his eyes out. They soon tracked Gerbert down and though he fought back fiercely he was left blind and disfigured. The violence and grave nature of his injuries drove him to try and take his own life. It was Gerbert's understanding that those who had recently been injured and then drank goat's milk would drop dead on the spot.[82] He wandered the countryside with two of his servants trying to find someone who would give him the goat's milk he so desired, but no one was willing to provide him with the drink. Gerbert then decided that he would starve himself to death, but after eight days and nights of eating nothing he began hallucinating before collapsing. The vision caused him to have a change of heart and he soon began eating again.[83]
- A little more than a century later, in 1124, a knight and troubadour called Luke de la Barre fought against Henry I of England. He was captured and then released by Henry, only to rejoin the English king's enemies and once again be captured. He was due to be punished by having his eyes put out, but he chose instead to take his own life by smashing his head against a stone wall.[84]
- In his surgery William of Saliceto included a couple of thirteenth-century examples of attempted suicide. The first being that of a prisoner held in jail at Cremona who managed to retain his knife while in his prison cell. William explained that it was an act of despair that caused him to try and take his own life by cutting his throat and lung with the weapon.[85] He noted that he was able to save the man, who recovered after a month.[86]

- The second involved a soldier named Jean de Bredella, mentioned previously, '… who wounded himself in the stomach with a knife …'.[87] He caused considerable damage to his intestines. Initially, another physician from Pavia was called out, but he felt that de Bredella had no chance of surviving such terrible damage. However, the friends of the soldier along with the physician requested that William provide a second opinion. He agreed and was able to assist in saving the soldier's life.

There is another group of warriors, including, for example, Bernard from Auvergne, who seemed to have reached a point in their depressed state when they desired death over life:

Tant de peines aigrirent son esprit et le jetèrent dans un tel trouble que sa raison commençait à en être ébranlée: la mort lui semblait moins dure qu'une telle vie.[88]

His mind was in so much pain and threw him into such turmoil that he began to question his existence: death seemed to him a better option than life.

However, like Rigaud, noted at the beginning of this chapter, their accounts do not indicate that they took the next step. Nonetheless, since this is an examination of the mental health of medieval soldiers, their thoughts and emotions are still of value here and worthy of inclusion at face value.

The men noted in this section represent a wide span of time, geography, social standing and personal details. The chance to learn more about their lives, to ask questions of those who knew and cared about them is of course long gone, making it impossible to better understand their lives and reasons for taking such drastic actions or even desiring to do so. The one man from whom we might have hoped to gain some insight was the surgeon William of Saliceto who treated two of the men. Unfortunately, their mental health issues are barely discussed, beyond the unnamed prisoner whom he noted acted out of desperation.[89] Perhaps it is too easy to draw a connection between war and suicide among these men of the Middle Age, but on the other side of the same coin it is difficult to ignore the findings of mental health professionals who continue to understand and define the clear and significant link between trauma and suicide.[90]

Family Matters

> With pity and with grief for us they'll mourn.
> *The Song of Roland*[91]

The devastation of a loved one lost to violence in the Middle Ages is reflected by the medieval German poet Heinrich von Morungen (d. 1222), in the poem *On the Heath on a Morning*:

> Alone in her bower
> I found her weeping tears like rain;
> For only that hour
> Word had reached her that I was slain.[92]

True today as it was a millennium ago, the loss of a soldier to war is indescribably tragic for those left behind. Perhaps the only thing worse than losing a family member or loved one to war is having more than one taken, like many families did during the world wars of the last century.[93] A recent discovery made among the bones of the Viking warriors of the Great Army that invaded England in the ninth century has offered up a parallel scenario. DNA testing has shown that two of the men who were buried near St Wystan's Church at Repton were father and son, originating from the southern portion of Scandinavia, perhaps Denmark. The older of the two men was about 35–45 years of age and the second was 17–20 years of age. Both men suffered serious battle trauma, likely dying from their wounds within a short time of each other.[94] Two-and-half centuries later the chronicler Orderic Vitalis provided a glimpse into the miserable end for two French knights, brothers who died in the year 1119 as Louis VI of France was at war with Henry I of England. The two belonged to the de Trie family, Wallon being the eldest and his younger sibling Enguerrand. Vitalis first described the death of Wallon de Trie, who was involved in an exchange of prisoners with the English. Shortly after being traded back to the French side he died of his injuries and the poor treatment he had received at the hands of Henry I.[95] Enguerrand de Trie died his own grim death not long after his elder brother, being wounded in the face above his eye as Louis VI's forces abandoned their siege of the castle Chateau-Neuf held by Henry's men. He lingered for several days before succumbing to his wounds.[96]

Strangely, the same sympathy felt for those who lost family during more recent wars is so often hard to find for individuals who lived centuries ago. However, it is fair to say that during the ninth century and later in the twelfth century there were likely parents, spouses, siblings and others who were crushed by the news that they had lost two of their loved ones, killed as a result of war. Families related to soldiers, particularly parents, do suffer in ways that others can never fully appreciate. Studies have shown that the mothers and fathers of children serving in armed forces across the world regularly struggle with the symptoms of a troubled mind themselves. An eye-opening investigation of the parents of soldiers in the Israeli army, published in 2017, uncovered high rates of depression, anxiety and other PTSD-like symptoms among them.[97] There are a few examples of the pain and anguish suffered by medieval parents that mirror the lives of modern mothers and fathers of soldiers, one of which can be found in *The Saga of Gunnlaug Serpent-Tongue*. Illugi the Black, the father of the warrior Gunnlaug, endured some of the same symptoms, such as depression and vivid nightmares. Illugi had witnessed the violence of single combat involving his son while he was alive. Much later, his son Gunnlaug would die a brutal death in battle.⁹⁸ After the loss of his son Illugi became severely depressed, even turning to extreme violence murdering one man and maiming another.⁹⁹

Mothers of those defending Paris against the attacks of the Vikings in 886 were said to have endured a great deal of mental anguish, manifested in thinning hair, self-harm and even exposing their breasts.¹⁰⁰ Across the Middle Ages, this was a common illustration of women who suffered the grief of a loved one gone off to war. The very figure of *Sorrow* from the thirteenth-century poem *Le Roman de la Rose*, or *The Romance of the Rose*, is described as a woman who '… had not been slow to scratch her whole face …', tear her dress until it was worthless and pull out her hair.¹⁰¹ These details also form part of an emotive illustration of a mother that comes from the final account in the miracle collection of St Foy and dates to the first half of the twelfth century. It recalls a mother who was in a very bad way after her son, Bernard Gerald, was mortally wounded when he was struck in the back of the head by a bolt fired from a powerful crossbow weapon.¹⁰² His mother's mental and physical health declined rapidly once she found out that her son was unlikely to survive such a serious wound:

> … sa mère éclata en sanglots sur le malheur de son fils et ne sut à quel parti se résoudre. Alors dans sa douleur, elle se meurtrit le visage, laisse tomber se cheveux épars, déchire le vêtement qui couvre son sein et, dans l'anxiété de son âme, ne sait où porter ses pas.¹⁰³

> … his mother burst into tears over her son's condition and did not know what to do. In her worry and pain she bruised her face, pulled out her hair and tore the garment that covered her breast and, in the anxiety of her soul, did not know where to go.

Bernard remained alive for some three months, which continued to take an enormous toll on his mother's health. We are told that she was barely alive as her son finally passed away.¹⁰⁴

Parents are not the only ones who feel the anxiety and misery involved with having someone they love in military service. Those spouses and partners living alongside soldiers suffering from a mind tormented by the trauma of combat can sadly end up dealing with their own serious issues of mental health. There are many modern, comprehensive studies of the subject that have uncovered the significant mental health problems, such as stress and depression, which exist among those living with men and women in the armed forces. The statistics involving the abuse and deaths of children have also brought to light a similarly shocking number of cases within military families. In her 2015 book *Homefront 911 – How Families of Veterans are Wounded by Our Wars*, Stacy Bannerman noted that in the USA the instances of soldiers' children who had been killed by that parent or their partner had more than doubled since 2001.¹⁰⁵ In 2012 there were nearly 13,000 reported cases of children who had been abused, assaulted, neglected or murdered among the combined branches of the American armed forces, a figure that had increased by 40 per cent over 2009.[106] This bleak family situation exists across the globe and has done so throughout history.[107] There is evidence that shows that the Middle Ages were no different:

- In the later medieval period the Dominican cleric Johannes Herolt recalled a story with a scenario that will no doubt seem quite familiar. Originally recorded in the first quarter of the thirteenth century, it involved a Frisian soldier who regularly abused his wife, both verbally and physically. The soldier, who is not named, routinely came home drunk and beat his wife. Desperate for any way to stop the violence, even just once, the soldier's wife feigned illness so that a local monk could come out to visit and provide her with the Holy Communion. According to the story, the monk and the woman's husband met each other as they made their way to the house where the soldier and his wife lived. The soldier, who was carrying a pot of beer with him, attempted to offer the monk a drink. When the monk declined, the quick-tempered soldier used the pot of beer to smash the pyx containing the host, which the monk carried.[108] The alcohol abuse, the quick temper and the violence shown by the soldier are all characteristics of a scenario that has played out among so many military families throughout history.[109]
- A different sort of case involving the wife of an injured fighter comes from the second half of the eleventh century. The account involved the spouse of a soldier called Mathfred who can be found elsewhere in this volume.[110] It is valuable because it shows a wife who was affected by her husband's '… darkest of all emotions …' as it is related by the record.[111] While the entry mentions Mathfred's deteriorating mental health, it also notes the psychological pain and anguish that his wife suffered alongside him. It was the spouse of another soldier who recognized what Mathfred's wife was going through and intervened to bring her comfort and assistance.[112]
- An entry from the twelfth-century miracle collection at Rocamadour involved the story of a knight's wife who tried to take her own life along with that of her unborn baby.[113] The woman and her husband were together when some good-natured joking quickly turned into a fit of jealousy and rage by his wife. After threatening to do so she took a large knife and stabbed herself through her stomach.[114] Here again, it is not the miracle portion of the story that is important, but instead the distraught and heavily pregnant wife of a knight who tried to kill both herself and their unborn child. It is only supposition, but since the child never again features after she had stabbed herself it may well be that the child did not survive. This shocking situation may at first appear strange and even unrealistic, but the anger, suspicion and drastic action taken are all too common among the spouses and partners of

soldiers.[115] Modern and tragic echoes of the past are unfortunately very easy to find, such as the situation involving the pregnant wife of a soldier in Fayetteville, North Carolina, who after threatening to do so shot and killed herself. Another instance from Fort Hood in Texas concerned the husband of a private first class who had just come back from Afghanistan. Shortly after her return he took the lives of their two young children before taking his own.[116]

Healing

> Straightway he sought medicine for his grief ...
> Saxo Grammaticus[117]

The examples presented in this chapter underline the terrible damage that war has done to the minds of so many throughout the centuries. Despite the 1,000 years between them the figure in *The Wanderer* could just as easily be a hunched and weather worn silhouette in a modern shop doorway with a piece of wrinkled cardboard that reads 'Ex-Serviceman – Please Help'.[118] As has happened after modern conflicts, the wars and major campaigns of the Middle Ages would have produced an influx of soldiers like the character in *The Wanderer*, as well as others outlined throughout this chapter. The Third Crusade of the late twelfth century provides evidence of this sort of inundation. According to the chronicle, which recalls so much of this campaign, there were many veterans who were left physically uninjured, but suffering mentally because, 'Their hearts were pierced by swords of sorrows from different sorts of suffering.'[119] They had seen so many scenes of horror, comrades and civilians killed and wounded in the most horrific manner, hacked to pieces, crushed to death, burned alive or killed by infection and disease and indeed had been in danger of losing their own lives.[120] These soldiers returned home to Europe with their minds already suffering from what they had gone through only to find themselves being taunted by some who perceived them as having accomplished little in the Holy Land.[121] Examples from other more recent wars spring to mind here, like soldiers returning home to America from the Vietnam War in the 1960s and 1970s who were treated so poorly by some members of the public.[122] Fortunately, the chronicler of the Third Crusade, who may well have been a crusader himself, was quick to come to the defence of his companions in arms who had been so unfairly taunted and mistreated.[123] He rebuked their detractors stating quite strongly '... they were criticising things which they had not experienced and knew nothing about'.[124]

Soldiers, like those returning from the Third Crusade, used a wide range of medications, remedies and therapies in a desperate attempt to find ways to heal their troubled minds. Some cures and treatments seem ahead of their time, while others appear to us rather odd and misplaced as perhaps some current drugs and treatments will seem to those in the future. Saxo described the grief of the famous Viking hero Ragnar Lothbrok after he lost his wife Swanloga to disease. His depression was not related to battle, but Ragnar turned to some sort of medicine to treat himself, while he kept himself hidden away indoors.[125] What is unfortunate is that Saxo did not divulge the nature of the remedy for melancholy, although St John's wort *Hypericum perforatum* must be a possibility. Widely used for many centuries as a natural antidepressant, St John's wort continues to be employed today for the same purpose.[126] It is worth noting that caches of St John's wort, mixed with the seeds of common valerian and stinging nettle, have been discovered at the medieval monastic complex at Soutra Aisle in Scotland, among the other combinations of healing and anaesthetic plants and seeds.[127]

The world of the Anglo-Saxons contained some cures for mental illness such as that found in the *Lacnunga* for '… heaviness of the mind …', which recommended radish with salt and vinegar.[128] While gas seems the only likely outcome of this radish cure, the placebo effect of such a treatment perhaps associated with magic cannot be underestimated. It would have been far less damaging than the cruel remedy found in *Leechbook III*: 'If a man be lunatic; take the skin of a mereswine *or porpoise*, work it into a whip, swinge the man therewith, soon he will be well. Amen'.[129]

Within the Islamic world of the tenth century a far different approach was being taken by those such as the Iraqi physician Ishaq Ibn Imran. He wrote what may be the oldest known treatise on mental health.[130] His work was significant, in part because it was translated into Latin by Constantine the African while at Monte Cassino in the latter part of the eleventh century, bringing these thoughts and ideas into Europe.[131] Ibn Imran devoted more than half of this work to the treatment of melancholy. He understood that it was more than just depression and could encompass elements such as fear and panic in the individual. Many of the treatments offered up within his treatise feature ingredients such as opium poppy, plants and nut oils.[132] A sense of something similar, called an 'elixir of grief', is offered against depression in the late twelfth-century Georgian poem *The Man in the Panther's Skin*.[133] It is noted as a medicine made from opium or hashish and was said to have worked remarkably well.[134] Ibn Imran also included things such as music as a part of the therapy, which would later be included by other practitioners in medieval Europe.[135] This idea that music has a therapeutic effect was something that Gerald of Wales thoroughly endorsed. In his twelfth-century *Topography of Ireland* he devoted a great deal of ink to validating the benefits of music in the healing of both mental and physical pain.[136]

The surgeon Roger Frugard included a much more invasive approach to healing the mind. Patients were to be restrained first before a cross-shaped incision was cut into the scalp to enable the skin to be peeled back. The skull was then trepanned to allow the perceived harmful vapours in the head to be released.[137] Usāmah ibn Munqidh explained a similar treatment for mental illness, performed by an unnamed Frankish doctor, decades earlier than

Roger's text. The doctor examined a woman whom he claimed was possessed by a devil. He too shaved her head before cutting a deep, cross-shaped incision into the top of her head. Something obviously went terribly wrong during the operation as Usāmah ibn Munqidh stated that she was killed almost instantly.[138]

About seventy years beyond the work of Roger Frugad the Franciscan monk and scholar Bartholomew Anglicus discussed the subject of 'madness' in his encyclopedic work *De proprietatibus rerum*, or *On the Properties of Things*. Within it he wrote about specific types of mental health issues, along with potential treatments for healing them, some of which had been noted by others before him:

> Other men darken and hide themselves in privy and secret places. The medicine of them is, that they be bound, that they hurt not themselves and other men. And namely, such shall be refreshed, and comforted, and withdrawn from cause and matter of dread and busy thoughts. And they must be gladded with instruments of music, and some deal be occupied.[139]

There were others too, such as Guglielmo da Brescia, who was physician to three popes and had helped to develop the medical curriculum at Montpellier.[140] Guglielmo recommended and applied very modern sounding techniques to the treatment of mental illness that included things such as exercise, music and nature.[141] These more benign treatments, including musical therapy and distractions that otherwise occupy the mind of the sufferer very often form a part of many modern therapies. In Britain there are now programmes for veterans who have been wounded in mind and body, involving them in archaeological investigations to aid their recovery. Forming part of their overall therapy, programmes like this can work to focus and occupy the mind away from the damage caused by the wounds of war.[142]

The recognition of the serious psychological harm that warfare can cause has never been more prevalent than it is now. Doctors and therapists have gained more understanding around the fact that without proper treatment the impact of these psychological wounds just continues to pile up, becoming a much larger issue.[143] However, even with a better understanding of the connection between the trauma of combat and damaged minds treatments have lagged well behind the advancements in medicine used to repair the physical body.[144] Today the numbers of those soldiers and their families who suffer problems of mental health, family break-up and suicide remain much higher than those who have not been impacted by war, so the fact that these same problems plagued medieval society should not be surprising. What may be unanticipated are some of the ideas of those such as Ibn Imran and Bartholomew Anglicus that would not be terribly out of place in the modern treatment of soldiers struggling with a psyche wounded by war. Sadly, the advances made during these medieval centuries would be displaced by hysteria and superstition in the later Middle Ages. In fact, those suffering mental health issues, including so many soldiers, would continue to be treated very poorly right up to the modern day.[145]

Conclusion

A hard-fought battle ensued, in which there was great effusion of blood on both sides, vast numbers being slain with brutal rage. At last the furious attacks of the English secured them the victory, and the king of Norway as well as Tostig, with their whole army, were slain. The field of battle may be easily discovered by travellers, as great heaps of the bones of the slain lie there to this day, memorials of the prodigious numbers which fell on both sides.

Orderic Vitalis[1]

This study began with a passage from *La chanson de la croisade contre les Albigeois* listing many of the battlefield injuries that were all too common during this 500-year period. It also included the efforts made by some soldiers to extricate their wounded comrades from the fighting, providing at least some sense of hope to the few grim lines.

Allowing Orderic Vitalis the concluding epigraph, it evokes something altogether different in terms of the bleak reality of warfare in the medieval era and the many who did not survive the brutal fighting. This site was the location of the Battle of Stamford Bridge, fought on 25 September 1066 not far from York, pitting Harold Godwinson's Anglo-Saxon army against a large contingent of Vikings led by Harold's brother Tostig and Harald Hardrada of Norway. Harold Godwinson won the battle, but large numbers on both sides were killed. Writing several decades later the words of Vitalis acknowledge the level of slaughter that must have gone on that day. The 'heaps' of bones, twisted skeletons with arms and legs detached, ribs crushed and skulls missing must have presented the most surreal scene to those who passed close to the site of the battle many years later.

The *Anglo-Saxon Chronicle* added that Godwinson's men continued to attack the rear of the surviving Viking army as they attempted to return to their ships following the battle, noting that some were drowned and others burned alive.[2] At times it must have seemed like the horror would never end. The same could also be said of the centuries that would follow those highlighted by this book. The Late Middle Ages would bring with them new and ferocious gunpowder weapons that had the potential to kill even larger numbers of unfortunate warriors and leave others with hideous injuries. Long drawn-out campaigns such as the Hundred Years War would be fought over many decades. One of the worst disasters in human history was also on the horizon following devastating crop failures and famine, the Black Death of the mid-fourteenth century with its gruesome curtain calls made every ten years or so afterwards. Still, the battles would be fought and millions would lose their lives to the fighting, famine and disease creating many more 'great heaps of the bones of the slain'.

Glossary of Chroniclers, Surgeons and Miracle Collections

Abbot Suger: The Abbot of St Denis (near Paris) was born some time around the year 1081. He wrote an account of his friend King Louis VI of France. It provides a great deal of insight into the first few decades of the twelfth century, especially as it relates to France. Abbot Suger died in 1151.

Abulcasis: Sometimes referred to as the 'father of modern surgery', Abulcasis was born after 936, near Córdoba, Spain. The works of this influential physician were relied upon by medieval surgeons like Theodoric and Bruno da Longoburgo. He was one of the first to provide illustrations of medical and surgical instruments. Abulcasis died in 1013.

Adam of Bremen: Living and writing during the second half of the eleventh century, Adam of Bremen was a German chronicler who detailed much of what happened in and around Northern and Western Europe, including many of the exploits of the Vikings.

Ahmad ibn Fadlān: A tenth-century Muslim traveller and writer from Baghdad, ibn Fadlān encountered Swedish Vikings called Rūs as he made his way along the Volga River. He described their customs and practices in rich and graphic detail, including the funeral of a Rūs chieftain.

Annals of Fulda: This ninth-century chronicle relates much about Europe, particularly the eastern portion of the Frankish kingdom, from 838 to the year 901. It is full of information on everything from the weather and disease to kings and Viking attacks.

Annals of St Bertin: Chronicling the history of Europe, especially the west Frankish kingdom between 830 and 882, it contains details of daily life, as well as the world of kings and princes during this time. Many of the attacks of the Vikings are also recorded throughout these years.

Avicenna: Known as the 'Prince of Physicians' by his countrymen, this Persian doctor was born around the year 980 and would write his first book on medicine by the time he was 21. He would go on to pen more than forty works on a variety of subjects before he died in 1037. Many European doctors like Theodoric relied upon the work of Avicenna.

Bald's Leechbook: Owned by a physician called Bald and transcribed or compiled by an individual call Cild, this medical resource, written in Old

English, is actually two books, which are survivors from the tenth century and may reflect information from an even earlier date. Two otherwise unknown physicians, called Dun and Oxa, are also mentioned and relied upon within the books. These comprehensive texts include details on the healing of wounds, diseases and other ailments.

Bamberg Surgery: Written by an unknown author, the *Bamberg Surgery* is named after the Bamberg Royal Library where two copies of the manuscript were uncovered. It is a lesser known work, which is earlier than Roger Frugard's seminal surgery, although it is not as comprehensive as Roger's work. With that said, Roger almost certainly relied upon the *Bamberg Surgery* in the writing of his own text.

Bede: Frequently referred to as the Venerable Bede, this English Benedictine monk and historian was born in Northern England, where he spent much of his life. He wrote the important *Historia ecclesiastica gentis Anglorum*, or *History of the English Church and People*, providing a view of everyday Anglo-Saxon life from inside and outside of the Church. Bede died in 735.

Bruno da Longoburgo: Also known as Bruno the Arabist, the work of this mid-thirteenth-century surgeon, as his alias implies, was heavily influenced by earlier doctors like Avicenna and Abulcasis. Around 1252 Bruno produced a major work called *Chirurgia Magna* and later a shorter version of basically the same text known as *Chirurgia Parva*. He died in 1286.

Carmen Wido: Also known as the *Carmen Widonis*, this song contains some 835 lines that recall the Norman Conquest of England. Attributed to Guy of Ponthieu, bishop of Amiens, and written as early as 1067, just a few months after the Battle of Hastings, it is considered one of the most accurate accounts of the battle.

Constantine the African: Born originally at Carthage, in North Africa, Constantine was something of a mysterious figure before arriving at Salerno in around 1070. Once there he was sponsored by Alfanus who encouraged Constantine to move to the abbey at Monte Cassino where he became a monk. Constantine translated many works of medicine from Greek and Arabic into Latin making them usable to European practitioners of medicine, especially at Salerno. He was still living at Monte Cassino when he died in the late eleventh century.

Galen: Born in Greece around 129, Galen would begin studying medicine as a teenager. He moved to Rome in 162 where he climbed the ladder in the medical field becoming physician to Roman emperors Commodus and Septimius Severus. He wrote several medical texts that would continue to be influential for centuries to come. Galen died in around 216.

Gilbert Anglicus: Born sometime around the year 1180, Gilbertus was the first of the notable English medical writers and put together a compendium of

Glossary of Chroniclers, Surgeons and Miracle Collections 133

medicine. At times he, like so many others, relied heavily on the works of Roger Frugard. He recorded a large number of medicinal recipes for everything from headaches to stomach discomfort using more than 400 substances including things like mint juice, licorice and fennel. He died some time around the middle of the thirteenth century.

Guy de Chauliac: Born in France at the end of the thirteenth century, he wrote the valuable *Chirurgia Magna*, which included much about the state of medicine in the fourteenth century. Contained within is a history of medicine that covers many of the influential surgeons of the 500-year period explored in this volume. He survived the Black Death discovering that there were at least two types, pneumonic and bubonic. Guy de Chauliac died in July 1368.

Henri de Mondeville: Henri was born around the year 1260. He appears to have studied medicine at Montpellier and Paris, as well. Henri would later become the surgeon to French kings Philip the Fair and Louis X. Although written just outside the period covered by this study (between about 1310 and 1320), his work does at times reflect on pre-fourteenth-century medicine.

Henry of Huntingdon: The English writer and cleric Henry of Huntingdon was born in the mid-1080s and died in 1155. Influenced by those such as Constantine the African and Macer Floridus, Henry's work includes an important herbal, written in verse form, called *Anglicanus ortus*.

Hildegard of Bingen: A twelfth-century abbess of the Benedictine order in the Rhineland area of what is today Germany, this remarkable woman was a healer, poet and writer in addition to her many other talents and skills. A focus of the Benedictine order is healing and among her works are those that deal with the treatment of illnesses and injuries. She died in 1179.

Hugo de Lucca: Also referred to as Ugo de Lucca or Master Hugo, he was the town surgeon of Bologna in the early decades of the thirteenth century. A part of Hugo's commitment to the town was his attachment to the Bolognese army in the same role as surgeon. He went with them on the Fifth Crusade, between 1218 and 1221. He was the father of Theodoric, whose surgery is based in part on Hugo's knowledge and experiences.

Jordan Fantosme: An Anglo-Norman poet, chronicler and supporter of Henry II of England, Jordan Fantosme recorded the war between England and Scotland in 1173 and 1174 in the form of a verse. He died in about 1185.

***La Chanson de la croisade contre les Albigeois* or *The Song of the Crusade Against the Albigensians*:** This poem relates the history of the Albigensian Crusade that occurred during the first few decades of the thirteenth century, in what is today Southern France. Pope Innocent III declared a crusade, led by Simon de Montfort, to crush the Cathars of Languedoc and their perceived heresy. It was written by two authors, William of Tudela to begin with and a second anonymous writer who recorded the balance.

La Chanson de Guillaume or *The Song of William*: It is one of the oldest works of its type, along with *The Song of Roland*. At times quite grisly, the poem outlines the adventures of William of Orange. Only a single Anglo-Norman copy of this twelfth-century French epic poem still exists.

Lacnunga: A collection of about 200 herbal recipes, folk remedies and charms written in Old English, this less than scholarly work relied on sources from all over the Mediterranean and Northern Europe. For all its faults it has much that is of value including a couple of pagan charms, which are of interest.

Lanfranchi of Milan: Likely born in Milan during the first half of the thirteenth century, Lanfranchi was a student of William of Saliceto and likely had contact with Theodoric at some point. He became a Master Surgeon in Milan, before fleeing to Lyon in 1290. From there he would go to Paris and write his *Chirurgia Magna* in around 1295. It would become a source that would be widely used.

Leech: Derived from the Old English word *læce* or the Old Danish word *læke* meaning physician or healer.

Leechbook III: Found as part of the same manuscript as *Bald's Leechbook*, this Anglo-Saxon medical text is an otherwise separate text. It best represents the medicine of Northern Europe at the time, being the one furthest from the influences of the Mediterranean.

Macer Floridus: A highly influential French herbal, *Macer Floridus De Viribus Herbarum* contains seventy-seven plants and their uses for things such as the healing of wounds and the treatment of other ailments of the body. There are questions as to its author and original date, but Odo de Meung, a French physician, seems the most likely. It appears likely to have been created in the eleventh century, although an earlier date has now been suggested as possible. This herbal is mentioned many times by Theodoric in his surgery.

Master Wace: According to the chronicler himself, he was born in 1100 on the island of Jersey. Master Wace was brought up and educated at Caen in Normandy. A patron of Henry II, Master Wace chronicled much of Norman life, including the Conquest of England. He relied upon other chroniclers, tales from his father and witnesses of major events to help him with his work. He died as late as 1184.

Matthew Paris: Born some time in around 1200, Matthew became a monk at St Albans in 1217 where he would stay for the rest of his life, making several trips to the royal court and one significant voyage to Norway. He chronicled many of the events of the thirteenth century, which he also illustrated himself. Matthew died in around 1259.

Miskawayh: The Persian historian Miskawayh (932–1030) used eyewitness reports to detail quite an evocative description of the Swedish or Rūs Vikings as they attacked what is now modern Azerbaijan.

Old English Herbarium: This illustrated herbal is the only one that survives in Old English. It is a translation of a combination of much earlier works, which describe the uses for plants and animals.

Old Icelandic Medical Miscellany: Known also as MS Royal Irish Academy 23 D43 with supplement from MS Trinity College (Dublin), it is perhaps the most important of the existing medieval Icelandic documents on medicine. A copy was discovered in Ireland, during the last century, among a group of Celtic manuscripts that were being catalogued. While it was compiled in the latter part of the fifteenth century, some of the material can be attributed to earlier centuries. It combines a few Scandinavian texts, including Norwegian and Danish.

Orderic Vitalis: Orderic was born in around 1075 in England and began his early studies at Shrewsbury before being sent to a monastery in Normandy. He was still just a boy when he arrived in Normandy, where he spent most of his years as a monk at Saint-Évroult. Before he died in around 1142 Vitalis wrote a large volume of work that provides an interesting and useful look at the Anglo-Norman world during this time.

Raimon of Avignon: Before the year 1209 Raimon, a troubadour, produced one of the earliest translations of Roger Frugard's work. It was converted into the Occitan language in verse form.

Rocamadour – Miracle Collection: The miracles of Our Lady of Rocamadour come from an abbey and site of pilgrimage of the same name in south-west France. They are based upon accounts from the twelfth century, many of them from the 1160s and 1170s, having been transcribed during 1172 and 1173. Separated into three books, they contain miracles and morality tales involving knights, soldiers and many of the ordinary folk of the time.

Roger Frugard of Parma: Also called Roger of Parma or simply Roger Frugard, he is credited with one of the most seminal works of medieval medicine. Roger's surgical text was put together by his students, led by Guido II of Arezzo, between 1170 and 1180. It is arranged from head to toe, with much of the focus being on the treatment of wounds and ailments. It was instantly successful at Salerno and was soon being copied, translated and spread across Europe.

Roger de Hoveden: Also called Roger Howden, this twelfth-century chronicler was close to the courts of both Henry II and Richard I of England. He accompanied Richard I as a royal clerk to the Holy Land during the Third Crusade. Roger died *c.* 1202.

Roger of Wendover: Only a little is known of the chronicler Roger of Wendover who died in 1236. As the name suggests he seems to have been from Wendover in Buckinghamshire and like Matthew Paris he too became a monk at the abbey of St Albans. He was then prior at Belvoir, which belonged to

St Albans. His extravagances would lead to his downfall and he was eventually stripped of his office.

Roland of Parma: Roland of Parma produced his surgical text after 1240, being published in around 1250. Most of his work was taken directly from Roger Frugard's groundbreaking text, although he added a few of his own experiences and observations. Other surgeons, like Theodoric and his father, were extremely critical of Roland and his work, because it fell so close to Roger's surgery.

Royal Frankish Annals: Written in three main parts by more than one chronicler, these annals record the years between 741 and 829 taking in the time of Charlemagne, a man who was himself interested in history and wanted to be certain that this period was recorded for posterity.

St Thomas of Canterbury – Miracle Collection: Miracles attributed to the martyr Thomas, Archbishop of Canterbury (St Thomas à Becket) who was murdered on 29 December 1170. Within just a few days of his death miracles were being ascribed to him, the result of which meant that Canterbury became a famous pilgrim site, attracting the sick and wounded from all over Europe.

St William of Norwich – Miracle Collection: Based on the miracles attributed to St William, the son of a tanner and only a boy when he was killed in 1144, with the local Jewish community being wrongly blamed for his death. They were recorded in the second half of the twelfth century by Thomas of Monmouth, at Norwich.

Sainte Foy – Miracle Collection: The abbey of St Foy (St Faith) is located near the town of Conques in south-west France. The collection of miracles is made up of four books, with a few additional accounts. The miracles are attributed to the young female saint, Foy or Faith. Most of these records come from the first couple of decades of the eleventh century, many having been transcribed by Bernard of Angers, but there are later accounts as well, a few of which come from the twelfth century.

Saxo Grammaticus: Saxo was a Danish historian and writer who was born in the second half of the twelfth century. He wrote *Gesta Danorum*, or *Danish History*, a combination of both history and myths. Saxo died in around 1220.

Simeon of Durham: Born in the second half of the eleventh century, he would later become a monk at Durham Priory, as his name implies. Simeon chronicled the history of England, relying on the works of others for a significant portion, but latter parts were his own. He likely died during the 1130s.

Snorri Sturluson: An historian and writer, Sturluson was born at the end of the 1170s. So much of our modern understanding of Norse mythology comes from a collection he wrote known as *The Prose Edda*. Another of his works called the *Heimskringla* recalls the history of the Kings of Norway. Sturluson was killed in 1241.

The Song of Roland: Perhaps written by a Norman poet called Turold, this epic poem is one of the earliest of its type. Recorded in around 1100, *The Song of Roland* (*La Chanson de Roland*) is an exaggerated and embellished chronicle of the Battle of Roncevaux Pass in August 778 between Charlemagne's Frankish army and Basque forces. It recounts the exploits of Charlemagne's nephew called Roland.

Theodoric: The son of Hugo de Lucca, in around 1265 he produced his own surgery, which was a combination of ancient, Islamic and contemporary medical knowledge. Theodoric also relied heavily on his father's experiences as a surgeon, as well as his own. He and his father were proponents of 'dry' or pus-free healing.

Trotula: Likely written by a woman called Trota or Trocta, this volume is an assemblage of three works compiled at Salerno in the twelfth century. While it focuses on the health of women, it also contains some information on men's health, especially as it pertains to STIs.

Usāmah ibn Munqidh: An Islamic writer and poet, Usāmah ibn Munqidh (1095–1188) provided first-hand accounts of the Muslim world and European (Frankish) crusaders. He included several fascinating interactions between the two sides, Islamic and Christian, which could occasionally be quite friendly.

William (Guillaume) de Congenis: A teacher at Montpellier, William's work is known only through one of his students who copied some of his lessons. They were clearly based on Roger Frugard's surgery, with some of William's own additions. During the Albigensian Crusade, William acted as surgeon to Simon de Montfort.

William of Saliceto: Born in around 1210, William was widely regarded as one of the top surgeons of his time. His surgery would be written in around 1275 and would remain an important work long after it had been completed. Individual cases involving the wounded are catalogued throughout the text providing insight into the world of medicine in the late thirteenth century. William was also a teacher of those such as Lanfranchi of Milan and Henri de Mondeville.

Notes

Preface
1. Angel Flores (ed.), *An Anthology of Medieval Lyrics* (New York, Modern Library through Random House, 1962), p. 292.

Chapter 1 – Leechbooks and Surgeries
1. Paul Meyer, *La chanson de la croisade contre les Albigeois* (La Société de l'histoire de France, 1879), p. 328, 'Là vous eussiez vu tomber maint chevalier armé, fendre maint bon écu, ouvrir maint côté, et les jambes rompues, les bras tranchés, les poitrines ouvertes, les heaumes brisés, les chairs déchirées, les têtes fendues, le sang répandu, les fesses (?) coupées et les barons combattre ou occupés à emporter ceux qu'ils voient à terre.'
2. Joseph and Frances Gies, *Life in a Medieval Castle* (New York, Harper & Row Publishers, 1981), p. 179, See also, Thomas Leckie Jarman, *William Marshal First Earl Of Pembroke And Regent Of England (1216–1219)* (Oxford, Basil Blackwell, 1930), p. 12.
3. Jarman, *William Marshal*, pp. 11 and 12. See also Alice Horton and Edward Bell (trans), *The Lay of the Nibelungs* (London, George Bell & Sons, 1901), p. 7, 'From old knights and from young ones went thrust and parry there, Till crash of breaking lances re-echoed through the air'.
4. Laura A. Hibbard, *Three Middle English Romances* (London, David Nutt, 1911), p. 140. The early fourteenth-century story of *Sir Beves (Bevis) of Hampton* managed to describe the odd mix of violence and competition that was the medieval tournament: 'The trumpets blew and the knights rode out in a row. Madly they laid on with spear and mace, and no man knew another. Knights were hurled from their saddles and steeds were won and lost.' See also, Lady Doris Mary Stenton, *English Society in the Early Middle Ages (1066–1307)* (London, Penguin Books Ltd, 1986), pp. 83–5, for the names of some of the great and good who lost their lives at these tournaments, including Geoffrey, the son of Henry II of England in 1186.
5. Gies and Gies, *Life in a Medieval Castle*, p. 178.
6. C. Hedenstierna-Jonson, A. Kjellström, T. Zachrisson et al., 'A female Viking warrior confirmed by genomics', *Am J Phys Anthropol* (2017), pp. 854–5, the burial of a high-status female Viking warrior found at Birka in Sweden, grave number Bj 581, contained weapons and other accoutrement of someone of her rank and she was also buried with gaming pieces, the type she would have used in life to keep her mind sharp and battle ready. See also, Oliver Elton (trans.), *The First Nine Books of the Danish History of Saxo Grammaticus* (London, David Nutt, 1894), p. 83, Saxo also mentions the young Hother who was just as skilled with the lute or harp as he was in archery and swimming, and Janet Shirley (trans.), *The Song of the Cathar Wars – A History of the Albigensian Crusade* (Farnham, Ashgate Publishing Limited, 1996), p. 163, fn. 4. At later tournaments, such as the one that was held each year on

15 August at Le Puy-en-Velay, cerebral contests such as literary competitions could be found.
7. Caroline Arcini, *The Viking Age: A Time With Many Faces* (Oxford, Oxbow Books, 2018), p. 61, See also, Simpson, *Everyday Life in the Viking Age*, pp. 160 and 161 and Elton (trans.), *The First Nine Books of the Danish History of Saxo Grammaticus*, Introduction, pp. lv and lvi.
8. Rory McTurk (trans.), 'Kormak's Saga', *Sagas of Warrior Poets* (London, Penguin Classics, Penguin Group, 2002), p. 31. See also, Paul Belloni Du Chaillu, *The Viking Age: The Early History Manners & Customs of the Ancestors of the English-Speaking Nations (In Two Volumes)* (London, John Murray, 1889), Vol. II, p. 377, for more on games and injuries.
9. Hermann Pálsson and Paul Edwards (trans), *Seven Viking Romances* (London, Penguin Classics, Penguin Group, 1985), p. 201.
10. McTurk, (trans.), 'Kormak's Saga', p. 33. The two men involved were called Steinar and Bersi.
11. Ibid., pp. 34–6, It was Bersi who received the serious injury.
12. R.W. Eyton, *Court, Household and Itinerary of King Henry II* (London, Taylor and Co., 1878), pp. 91 and 217. See also, Thomas Wright (trans.), *The Historical Works of Giraldus Cambrensis* (London, Warton Club, 1905), p. 237, 'Before he left Ireland, the king appointed these following to be constables or governors of cities and strongholds ... in Waterford, Humphrey de Bohun, Robert Fitz-Bernard and Hugh de Gundeville, with forty men-at-arms ...'.
13. Edmond Albe, *Les miracles de Notre-Dame de Roc-Amadour au XIIe siècle* (Paris, Honoré Champion, 1907), p. 148, '... du climat, le changement de nourriture, l'eau mauvaise les rendirent malades et Dieu permit qu'ils perdissent l'usage de la parole'. '... a change in climate, food and bad water made them sick and God allowed them to lose the use of speech'.
14. Auguste Bouillet and Louis Servières, *Sainte Foy, vierge & martyre* (Rodez, Imprimerie E. Carrère, 1900), p. 534, for Bernard, 'Un brillant chevalier, nommé Bernard, originaire de Granson, en Auvergne, fut atteint d'une grave maladie, à son retour du pèlerinage de Rome.' 'He was a brilliant knight named Bernard, originally from Granson, Auvergne, who suffered from a grave sickness upon his return from a pilgrimage to Rome.'
15. Nancy Siraisi, *Medieval & Early Renaissance Medicine, An Introduction to Knowledge and Practice* (University of Chicago Press, 1990), pp. 181 and 182.
16. W.C. Pandya, 'Icon of this issue: Sir Archibald McIndoe', *Indian Journal of Plastic Surgery*, official publication of the Association of Plastic Surgeons of India, 48[3] (2015), pp. 234 and 235.
17. Eldridge Campbell and James Colton (trans), *The Surgery of Theodoric, ca. 1267 – Volumes I and II* (New York, Appleton-Century Crofts, Inc., 1955), Vol. I, Introduction, p. xix.
18. Revd Oswald Cockayne, *Leechdoms, Wortcunning and Starcraft of Early England, Volumes I–III* (Longman, Green, Longman, Roberts and Green, 1864–6), Vol. II, p. 91.
19. Annette Frölich and Anne Mette Kristiansen, 'Er det vikinge-lægens instrument?' ('Is this the instrument of a Viking doctor?'), *Vikingetid i Danmark (Viking Age in Denmark)*, Forhistorisk arkæologi, SAXO-instituttet på Københavns Universitet (2013), p. 103.
20. Ibid., p. 102.

21. Thomas A. DuBois, *Nordic Religions in the Viking Age* (Philadelphia, University of Pennsylvania Press, 1999), p. 98, DuBois notes the certainty of captured British healers acting as both teachers and practitioners.
22. Marjory Scott Wardrop (trans.), *The Man in the Panther's Skin* (London, Royal Asiatic Society, 1912), p. 92.
23. Revd Joseph Stevenson, *The Church Historians of England – Volumes I through V* (London, Seeleys, 1853–8), Vol. III, Part II, p. 457, Simeon of Durham's *History of the Kings*.
24. Ibid., p. 458.
25. William M. Hennessy, *Annals of Ulster – A Chronicle of Irish Affairs From A.D. 431–A.D. 1540, Vol. 1* (Dublin, Alexander Thom and Co., 1887), pp. 383 and 385.
26. Nirmal Dass (trans.), *Viking Attacks on Paris: The Bella parisiacae urbis of Abbo of Saint-Germain-des-Prés* (Leuven, Peeters, 2007), pp. 29 and 109, n. 22, exaggeration was common among chroniclers. Abbo of Saint-German-des-Prés, who chronicled the ninth-century Viking attacks on Paris, is another example claiming that more than 700 of their ships arrived in 885. See also, Conell Mageoghagan, *The Annals of Clonmacnoise Being Annals of Ireland from the Earliest Period to A.D. 1408 – Translated into English A.D. 1627*, ed. Revd Denis Murphy (Dublin, University Press, 1896), p. 156 Other accounts like *Annals of Clonmacnoise* include large numbers of people, '… about 3,000 captives …' taken by the Danes of Dublin in raids all across Ireland, and Paul Lunde and Caroline Stone (trans), *Ibn Fadlān and the Land of Darkness – Arab Travellers in the Far North* (London, Penguin Classics, Penguin Group, 2012), p. 106, Rūs Vikings were said to have captured 10,000 slaves, men, women and children during an attack on the city of Bardha'a in the year 943.
27. Jesch, p. 117, Judith Jesch makes the valid point that in the Vikings and Arabs, 'two such expansionist peoples' were bound to cross paths. See also, Oliver, *Vikings*, pp. 178–83, for information on the Vikings, especially Swedish or Rūs Vikings and Byzantium, and Lunde and Stone (trans), *Ibn Fadlān and the Land of Darkness*, pp. 105–9, for attacks on Spain in 844.
28. Jacqueline Simpson, *Everyday Life in the Viking Age* (London, B.T. Batsford Ltd, 1967), pp. 102–4, also referred to as Abraham ben Jacob. Simpson is of the belief that he must have travelled to Hedeby for the slave trade.
29. George Webbe Dasent (trans.), *Icelandic Sagas, Volume IV, The Saga of Hacon* (London, Her Majesty's Stationery Office, 1894), p. 301, 'Then a leech came to him who had come from abroad out of Spain with Sira Ferant, and gave advice as to the cause of his sickness.' While perhaps not a slave it helps to make the point around the sharing of ideas of medicine from far afield.
30. M.L. Cameron, *Anglo-Saxon Medicine* (Cambridge University Press, 1993), p. 30, held in the British Library, Royal 12. D. XVII is the official designation of the manuscript containing these books.
31. Cockayne, *Leechdoms, Wortcunning and Starcraft of Early England*, Vol. II, p. 121, for Oxa and p. 293, for Dun. See also, Preface, p. xxiii, 'I assume that Oxa and Dun were natives, either of this country (England) or some land inhabited by a kindred people.'
32. Cameron, *Anglo-Saxon Medicine*, pp. 42–5, for more on the Greek and Latin texts within *Bald's*.
33. Cockayne, *Leechdoms, Wortcunning and Starcraft of Early England*, Vol. II, Preface, p. xxv, for Scandinavian influence see p. 145, 'If a man be too salacious …, and Irish, p. 113, 'For flying venom and every venomous swelling …'.

34. Ibid., p. 35. See also, Freya Harrison et al., 'A 1,000-Year-Old Antimicrobial Remedy with Antistaphylococcal Activity', *mBio*, Vol. 6, 4 e01129, 11 August 2015, p. 4.
35. Harrison et al., 'A 1,000-Year-Old Antimicrobial Remedy with Antistaphylococcal Activity', p. 4, MRSA (Methicillin-resistant Staphylococcus aureus).
36. Cameron, *Anglo-Saxon Medicine*, p. 35. See also, Cockayne, *Leechdoms, Wortcunning and Starcraft of Early England*, Vol. II, p. 343, for an example of Scandinavian influence within *Leechbook III*, 'Against temptation of the fiend ...'.
37. Cockayne, *Leechdoms, Wortcunning and Starcraft of Early England*, Vol. II, p. 341.
38. Ibid., p. 345.
39. Dr Leonard D. Rosenman (trans.), *The Surgery of Lanfranchi of Milan* (Xlibris Corporation, 2003), p. 32.
40. Cockayne, *Leechdoms, Wortcunning and Starcraft of Early England*, Vol. II, p. 83, see also, p. 223 '... first clear the wamb with them, and then work light emetic drinks of radish, as leeches ken how to do it.'; *ken* = know.
41. Frances Watkins, Barbara Pendry, Alberto Sanchez-Medina and Olivia Corcoran, 'Antimicrobial assays of three native British plants used in Anglo-Saxon medicine for wound healing formulations in 10th century England', Medicines Research Group, School of Health, Sport and Bioscience, University of East London, 2012, p. 17. See also, Harrison et al., 'A 1,000-Year-Old Antimicrobial Remedy with Antistaphylococcal Activity', p. 5, for similar.
42. Cockayne, *Leechdoms, Wortcunning and Starcraft of Early England*, Vol. II, p. 213, italics are my own to highlight the point. See also, Vol. II, p. 203, 'Form also into a potion an adder, wrought so as leeches ken how to work it ...', and p. 91, 'Again, if thou find a fish within another fish, take and roast it thoroughly, and break it to bits into a draught give it to the sick man to drink in such a manner that he know it not.' Here the knowledge of the leech is again being presumed, something that was seemingly unknown to the common person.
43. John J. Contreni, 'Masters and Medicine in Northern France During the Reign of Charles the Bald', *Charles the Bald: Court and Kingdom*, ed. Margaret Gibson and Janet Nelson (2nd rev. edn, Aldershot, Variorum, 1990), pp. 267–82.
44. John C. Hemmeter and Fielding H. Garrison (trans), 'Salerno – A Mediaeval Health Resort and Medical School on the Tyrrhenian Sea', *Essays in the History of Medicine by Karl Sudhoff* (Hemmeter, Medical Life Press, 1926), p. 246.
45. Siraisi, *Medieval and Early Renaissance Medicine*, pp. 13–16.
46. Dr Pietro Capparoni, *Magistri Salneritani Nondum Cogniti – A Contribution of the History of the Medical School of Salerno – Wellcome Historical Medical Museum* (London, John Bale, Sons & Danielsson Ltd, 1923), p. 12. See also, Matthew Moran, 'San Vincenzo in the Making: The Discovery of an Early Medieval Production Site on the East Bank of the Volturno', *Markets in Early Medieval Europe – Trading and 'Productive' Sites, 650—850* (Macclesfield, WINDgather Press, 2003), p. 262, Salerno benefitted from having one of the largest markets in central and southern Italy since at least the ninth century and by the eleventh century its port was made much larger enabling it to handle more trade and support an even larger marketplace.
47. Siraisi, *Medieval and Early Renaissance Medicine*, p. 13, See also, Monica H. Green, *The Trotula* (Philadelphia, University of Pennsylvania, 2001), pp. 13 and 14.
48. Green, *The Trotula*, p. 10, Dr Green notes that he may have been a drug merchant.
49. Ibid., pp. 10 and 11.

50. Thomas Forester (trans.), *The Ecclesiastical History of England and Normandy by Orderic Vitalis, Volumes I–IV* (London, Henry G. Bohn, 1853–6), Vol. II, p. 366. See also, Ralph Bailey Yewdale, 'Bohemond I, Prince of Antioch – A Dissertation Presented to the Faculty of Princeton University' (accepted by the Faculty of Princeton June 1917), p. 23, different sources indicate that it was illness rather than injury that sent Bohemond to Salerno after a plague broke out among the Norman army.
51. Capparoni, *Magistri Salneritani Nondum Cogniti*, pp. 9 and 12. See also, Hemmeter and Garrison (trans), 'Salerno – A Mediaeval Health Resort and Medical School on the Tyrrhenian Sea', p. 245, '… many a returning warrior found a convenient haven of rest, for healing of wounds or illness, in this well known and highly esteemed medical center, on his way home'.
52. Stevenson, *Church Historians of England*, Vol. IV, Part I, p. 273, the chronicle of Jordan Fantosme, *Chronicle of the war between the English and the Scots, AD 1173, 1174*, written to record the war between Henry II of England and William Scotland in the years 1173 and 1174, includes a reference to Salerno in speaking about the men of Roger d'Estutevile. See also, William Wistar Comfort (trans.), *Erec and Enide*, Everyman's Library (London, J.M. Dent & Sons Ltd, 1913), p. 166, Chrétien de Troyes' twelfth-century *Cligés* includes physicians from Salerno, although they turn out to be terribly evil in this tale, see also, p. 372, for note on Salerno and Montpellier.
53. Siraisi, *Medieval and Early Renaissance Medicine*, pp. 59 and 60, for more on the influences of places such as Montpellier.
54. Lynn Thorndike, *University Records and Life in the Middle Ages* (New York, Columbia University Press, 1944), p. 10, words that apparently apply to Adelbert II of Saarbrücken, bishop of Mainz in Germany who died in 1141 and who had studied at Montpellier. See also, Comfort (trans.), *Erec and Enide*, p. 314, from Lancelot, "… he was more skilled in the cure of wounds than all the doctors of Montpellier'.
55. Dr Leonard D. Rosenman (trans.), *The Surgery of William of Saliceto* (Xlibris Corporation, 1998), pp. 13 and 14. See also, Dr Leonard D. Rosenman (trans.), *The Chirurgia of Roger Frugard* (Xlibris Corporation, 2002), p. 16 for the 1170 to 1180 date range for Roger's work.
56. Rosenman (trans.), *Chirurgia of Roger Frugard*, p. 14, fn. 1, Rosenman acknowledges the competing views on Roger's identity, origin and education. For the purposes of this text Roger Frugard or occasionally just Roger will be used. See also, Siraisi, *Medieval and Early Renaissance Medicine*, p. 59, for more on Roger at Parma.
57. Rosenman (trans.), *Chirurgia of Roger Frugard*, pp. 14 and 15.
58. Ibid., p. 16, the author of the *Bamberg Surgery* that came before Roger is unknown. It is named after the Bamberg Royal Library where two copies of the manuscript were uncovered. See also, George W. Corner, 'On Early Salernitan Surgery and Especially the "Bamberg Surgery" – With an Account of a Previously Undescribed Manuscript of the Bamberg Surgery in the Possession of Dr. Harvey Cushing', *Bulletin of the Institute of the History of Medicine*, Johns Hopkins University, Vol. V, No. 1, January 1937, p. 14, it is clear that parts of the *Bamberg Surgery* were made up of some translations of Constantine the African, including pieces from the *Pantegni*.
59. Rosenman (trans.), *Chirurgia of Roger Frugard*, p. 46.
60. Ibid., p. 44.
61. Ibid., p. 16.
62. Tony Hunt, *The Medieval Surgery* (Woodbridge, Boydell Press, first published 1992), xiii, Books 1–3 of Roger's surgery were converted into Occitan verse.

63. Irina Metzler, *Disability in Medieval Europe – Thinking about physical impairment during the high Middle Ages, c. 1100–1400* (Abingdon, Routledge, 2006), p. 119. See also, Linda M. Paterson, 'Military Surgery: Knights, Sergeants, and Raimon of Avignon's Version of the Chirurgia of Roger of Salerno (1180–1209)', *The Ideals and Practice of Medieval Knighthood II – Papers from the Third Strawberry Hill Conference, 1986* (Woodbridge, Boydell & Brewer, 1988), p. 144, like Roger Frugard, there is no evidence that Raimon of Avignon practised medicine on the battlefield.
64. Hunt, *The Medieval Surgery*, Introduction, pp. xii and xiii.
65. Horton and Bell (trans), *The Lay of the Nibelungs*, p. 44.
66. Piers D. Mitchell, *Medicine in the Crusades – Warfare, Wounds and the Medieval Surgeon* (Cambridge University Press, 2004), p. 26. See also, Alan O.Whipple, *The Story of Wound Healing and Wound Repair* (Springfield, IL, Charles C. Thomas, 1963), p. 46, 'He (Hugo) had been the surgeon in the Bolognese army during the Crusades where he had seen and treated many of the wounded.'
67. Campbell and Colton, *The Surgery of Theodoric*, Vol. I, pp. 93, 199 and 218, Roger too received similar treatment.
68. Ibid., pp. 119–21 and 149, as examples.
69. Nancy Siraisi, *Taddeo Alderotti and his Pupils – Two Generations of Italian Medical Learning* (Princeton University Press, 1981), p. 15.
70. Nancy Siraisi, 'How to write a Latin book on surgery: organizing principles and authorial devices in Guglielmo de Saliceto and Dino del Garbo', *Practical medicine from Salerno to the Black Death* (Cambridge University Press, 1994), pp. 63 and 64, for more on William of Saliceto (Guglielmo da Saliceto).
71. Mitchell, *Medicine in the Crusades*, p. 43, there is some thought that William may also have participated as a doctor during the Crusades.
72. Paul Pifteau (trans.), *Chirurgie de Guillaume de Sâlicet, Achevée en 1275* (Toulouse, Imprimerie Saint-Cyprien, 1898), p. 261.
73. Ibid.
74. Rosenman (trans.), *Surgery of William of Saliceto*, p. 110.
75. Cockayne, *Leechdoms, Wortcunning and Starcraft of Early England*, Vol. I, it is a translation of a combination of much earlier works, which describe the uses for plants and animals. Vol. I of Cockayne contains the 'Herbarium'.
76. Gösta Frisk (ed.), *A Middle English Translation of Macer Floridus De Viribus Herbarum* (Uppsala, Almqvist & Wiksells Boktryckeri AB, 1949), pp. 187 and 188.
77. Campbell and Colton, *The Surgery of Theodoric*, Vol. I, pp. 116 and 133, as examples of Theodoric's inclusion of Macer in his text.
78. Henning Larsen, *An Old Icelandic Medical Miscellany, MS Royal Irish Academy 23 D43 with supplement from MS Trinity College (Dublin) L-2-27* (Oslo, Jacob Dybwad, 1931), pp. 26 and 27.
79. Rosenman (trans.), *Chirurgia of Roger Frugard*, p. 14.

Chapter 2 – Chronicles, Songs and Saints
1. J.A. Giles (trans.), *Matthew Paris's English History – Volumes I, II and III* (London, Henry G. Bohn, 1852–3), Vol. I, p. 167.
2. Giles, *Matthew Paris's English History*, Vol. I, pp. 422 and 423, for further comments made by Matthew Paris on the bravery of John Mansel.
3. Ibid, Vol. I, pp. 440 and 441.
4. Forester (trans.), *The Ecclesiastical History of England and Normandy by Orderic Vitalis*, Vol. II, pp. 121 and 122, an example of this humour can be found the passage below written by the Anglo-Norman chronicler Orderic Vitalis. He begins by providing a

scathing report of Gilbert Maminot, bishop of Lisieux and physician to William the Conqueror. On one hand he noted his brilliance at medicine, but then explained, 'Ease and leisure were his great objects, and he indulged frequently in dice and other games of hazard. Negligent and slothful in his ecclesiastical duties, he was ready and active enough in hunting and hawking'. Vitalis continued like this before seeming to remember, 'I could write more about him, but I check my pen, because it was by him that I was admitted to the order of subdeacon ...'.

5. Richard Cusimano and John Moorhead (trans), *The Deeds of Louis the Fat* (Washington DC, The Catholic University Press, 1992), p. 157, Suger noted that the king referred to him as 'his intimate friend'.
6. Ibid., p. 145.
7. Ibid., for other wounds like the loss of an eye, see also, p. 141 for torture, p. 136 for maiming and p. 153 for disease.
8. Janet L. Nelson (trans.), *The Annals of St-Bertin, Ninth-Century Histories, Volume 1* (Manchester and New York, Manchester University Press, 1991), p. 57, the winter of 844, for example, was very mild. See also, Bernhard Walter Scholz, *Carolingian Chronicles* (Ann Arbor, The University of Michigan Press, 1972), p. 82, *The Royal Frankish Annals* for the years 801 and 802 concerning an elephant being delivered to Charlemagne, a gift from the Persian king, Nelson (trans.), *The Annals of St-Bertin*, p. 37, for an example of a Viking attack on Frisia (now the Netherlands and North-Western Germany) in the year 837, and Timothy Reuter (trans.), *The Annals of Fulda – Ninth-Century Histories, Volume II* (Manchester University Press, 1992), p. 23, for another attack by the Northmen, this time in 845 along the Seine to Paris and again in Frisia.
9. Reuter, *The Annals of Fulda*, p. 84.
10. Lunde and Stone (trans), *Ibn Fadlān and the Land of Darkness*, pp. 150 and 152.
11. Phillip K. Hitti (trans.), *An Arab-Syrian Gentleman & Warrior in the Period of the Crusades* (New York, Columbia University Press, 1929), pp. 151 and 163.
12. W.A. Sibley and M.D. Sibley (trans), *The History of the Albigensian Crusade – Peter of les Vaux-de-Cernay* (Woodbridge, Boydell & Brewer Ltd, 1998), p. 53.
13. Ibid., pp. 83 and 169, for weapon injuries and torture.
14. Comfort (trans.), *Erec and Enide*, p. 265, from Chrétien de Troyes' *The Knight with the Lion, Yvain*.
15. Dass (trans.), *Viking Attacks on Paris*, pp. 71 and 101, see also, p. 63 for prosthesis. More is discussed in Chapter 6 here, section on Prostheses and Devices.
16. N. Kershaw (trans.), *Anglo-Saxon and Norse Poems* (Cambridge University Press, 1922), p. 91.
17. Michael Alexander (trans.), *Beowulf* (London, Penguin Classics, Penguin Group, 1973), p. 145.
18. George Webbe Dasent (trans.), *The Story of Burnt Njal or Njal's Saga – In Two Volumes* (Edinburgh, Edmonston and Douglas, 1861), Vol. II, p. 337.
19. Ibid., Vol. I, p. 185.
20. Ibid., Vol. II, p. 387.
21. Gwyn Jones (trans.), *Eirik the Red and Other Icelandic Sagas* (World's Classics, 1980, repr. of Oxford University Press edn, 1961), p. 66.
22. Ibid., p. 67.
23. Ibid., pp. 74 and 75.
24. Ibid., p. 75.
25. McTurk (trans.), 'Kormak's Saga', pp. 57 and 58, see also, p. 273, n. 48, which explains the nature of this reference to a sacrifice to the elves.

26. Keneva Kunz (trans.), 'Eirik the Red's Saga', *The Sagas of the Icelanders* (London, Penguin Books, Penguin Group, 2001), p. 658 and Pálsson and Edwards (trans), *Seven Viking Romances*, p. 250.
27. National Museum of Denmark website, 'A seeress from Fyrkat?', https://en.natmus.dk/historical-knowledge/denmark/prehistoric-period-until-1050-ad/the-viking-age/religion-magic-death-and-rituals/a-seeress-from-fyrkat/.
28. DuBois, *Nordic Religions in the Viking Age*, p. 116, for more on magic, witchcraft and healing.
29. Cockayne, *Leechdoms, Wortcunning and Starcraft of Early England*, Vol. I, p. 95 and Vol. II, pp. 43 and 69.
30. Ainslie Hight (trans.), *The Saga of Grettir the Strong* (London, J.M. Dent & Sons Ltd, 1913), Introduction, p. x, 'The important thing to remember is that they are at least in the first instance, apart from accretions, truthful accounts of the events narrated, so far as they were known to the narrator.'
31. Keneva Kunz (trans.), 'The Saga of the Greenlanders', *The Sagas of the Icelanders* (London, Penguin Books, Penguin Group, 2001), p. 630, preface to the saga outlines some the details of the Viking base found at L'Anse aux Meadows in Newfoundland, Canada.
32. Glyn S. Burgess and Keith Busby (trans), *The Lais of Marie de France* (London, Penguin Books, 1986), p. 83.
33. Ibid., p. 48, see also, p. 78, for the author's recognition of issues around mental health, in the *lai* called *Lanval*.
34. William W. Kibler (trans.), 'The Knight of the Cart (Lancelot)', 'The Knight with the Lion (Yvain)' and 'The Story of the Grail (Perceval)', *Chrétien de Troyes – Arthurian Romances* (London, Penguin Books, Penguin Group, 1991), p. 249.
35. Ibid., p. 513, n. 15 for more on the popularity of this ointment. The three Marys are usually considered to be Mary Magdalene, Mary the mother of James and Mary Salome. See also, Holy Bible, New Testament, p. 73, the Gospel of Mark 16:1, the women intended to anoint the body of Christ after his death.
36. Urban Holmes, *A History of Old French Literature; from the origins to 1300* (New York, Russell and Russell, 1962), p. 81. See also, Comfort (trans.), *Erec and Enide*, p. 372. *Mort Aimeri de Narbonne* is apparently another source where this particular ointment is mentioned.
37. Holy Bible, New Testament, p. 145, Gospel of John, 19:39, is the only Gospel of the four to name the elements that were to be used, aloes and myrrh, although here it is Joseph and Nicodemus doing the anointing.
38. Campbell and Colton, *The Surgery of Theodoric*, Vol. II, p. 16, '... mix in powder of myrrh and aloes, and apply ...', see also, Vol. II, p. 108. See also, Frisk (ed.), *A Middle English Translation of Macer Floridus De Viribus Herbarum*, p. 187, see also, pp. 188 and 189 for the other uses of aloes. See also, Rosenman (trans.), *Surgery of William of Saliceto*, p. 220 #19 (aloes) and p. 243 #299 (myrrh).
39. Shirley (trans.), *The Song of the Cathar Wars*, p. 4, for discussion on the use of eyewitnesses by the chronicler. See also, pp. 1 and 2 of the same volume for more on William of Tudela.
40. Sibley and Sibley (trans), *The History of the Albigensian Crusade*, Introduction, p. xxii, the second writer is identified as possibly hailing from Toulouse.
41. Meyer, *La chanson de la croisade contre les Albigeois*, p. 331.
42. Flores (ed.), *An Anthology of Medieval Lyrics*, trans. James J. Wilhelm, p. 56, 'Helmets, swords, shields and mail, And bodies, spear-split from belt to brain, And stallions running unmounted, unreined, And many a lance through thigh and chest.'

43. Ibid., trans. William M. Davis, p. 58.
44. Jessie L. Weston (trans.), *Parzival – A Knightly Epic by Wolfram von Eschenbach, Volumes I and II* (London, David Nutt, 1894), Vol. I, p. 276, this method of retracting the weapon falls in line with surgeons such as Theodoric. See also, Campbell and Colton, *The Surgery of Theodoric*, Vol. I, pp. 147 and 148, weapons lodged in the body were always to be drawn out by the same path that had seen them enter, and Alison Adams (trans.), *The Romance of Yder* (Cambridge, D.S. Brewer, 1983), pp. 115 and 117, this is contradicted by the method outlined in the Arthurian epic *The Romance of Yder*, in which the title character has a broken lance lodged in his chest. It is pushed out through his back, creating a second wound and considerable blood loss.
45. Ross G. Arthur and Noel L. Corbett (trans), *The Knight of the Two Swords, A Thirteenth-Century Arthurian Romance* (Gainesville, University Press of Florida, 1996), pp. 31 and 32, strung between two poles and mounted through loops hanging from either side of a pair of horses, one in front of the other, these could be simple cots or much more elaborate couches draped and covered in fine cloth. Removed from the horses, they could then be carried quite easily to the place of treatment.
46. Clair Hayden Bell (trans.), *Peasant Life in Old German Epics* (New York, Columbia University Press, 1931), pp. 97 and 98.
47. Ibid., pp. 125 and 126.
48. Albe, *Les miracles de Notre-Dame de Roc-Amadour au XIIe siècle*, p. 224, 'Ne trouvant aucun médecin capable de le guérir, il résolut de venir à Notre-Dame de Rocamadour.' 'When he was unable to find a doctor who could cure him, he resolved to come to Notre-Dame de Rocamadour.'
49. Marcus Graham Bull, *The Miracles of Our Lady of Rocamadour: Analysis and Translation* (Woodbridge, Boydell & Brewer Ltd, 1999), pp. 11 and 12.
50. S.B. Edgington, *The Life and Miracles of St. Ivo* (Edgington, Norris Library and Museum, 1985), pp. 55–8, for Pagan Peverel, see also, p. 90, note for Chapter 8, regarding further research on this knight, and p. 62, for a list of knight's armour and equipment.
51. Bull, *The Miracles of Our Lady of Rocamadour*, pp. 192 and 193, see also, p. 181, fnn. 1 and 2.
52. Albe, *Les miracles de Notre-Dame de Roc-Amadour au XIIe siècle*, p. 298.
53. Edgington, *The Life and Miracles of St. Ivo*, pp. 91 and 92. See also, Metzler, *Disability in Medieval Europe*, p. 185 for further discussion and explanation around medieval miracle healings.
54. Pamela Sheingorn (trans.), *The Book of Sainte Foy* (Philadelphia, University of Pennsylvania Press, 1995), p. 148, for Hugh, the son of Siger, freed from torture and captivity, see also, pp. 88–90, for a lost falcon that was recovered.
55. Edgington, *The Life and Miracles of St. Ivo*, pp. 39 and 40, Miracle of St Ivo for a leprous woman whose cure was not instant.
56. Bull, *The Miracles of Our Lady of Rocamadour*, pp. 36 and 37.
57. Sheingorn (trans.), *The Book of Sainte Foy*, p. 24.
58. Irina Metzler, *A Social History of Disability in the Middle Ages – Cultural Considerations of Physical Impairment* (New York, Routledge, 2013), p. 199. See also, Edwin A. Abbott, *St. Thomas of Canterbury – His Death and Miracles, Volumes I and II* (London, Adam and Charles Black, 1898), Vol. II, p. 52, after being cured of leprosy, John of Salisbury was called to testify in front of a panel to prove he was now clean from the disease, 'The Bishop had begged him to come to the council in order to manifest the glory of the Martyr.'

59. D.H. Farmer, (trans.), 'The Canonization of St. Hugh of Lincoln', *Lincolnshire Architectural and Archaeology Society Reports and Papers*, Vol. 6, Part 2 (1956), p. 88.
60. Sheingorn (trans.), *The Book of Sainte Foy*, p. 130.
61. Bouillet and Servières, *Sainte Foy, vierge & martyre*, p. 515.
62. Sheingorn (trans.), *The Book of Sainte Foy*, pp. 130 and 131.
63. Bouillet and Servières, *Sainte Foy, vierge & martyre*, p. 517, '… un mince filet rouge marquant la trace du glaive'. On Raymond's first journey to St Foy he did not know enough to tell anyone about the miraculous healing. It was only after Peter had related the story to the monks at St Foy that Raymond made another trip to verify the details.
64. Ibid., the entry notes that Raymond, though asleep, could see the saint repairing the damage to his mouth and face. The portion of the miracle, where the saint was said to have touched his face and mouth, does have a dreamy, drug-induced quality about it.
65. Harvard Program in Placebo Studies – Beth Israel Deaconess Medical Center/ Harvard Medical School.
66. William Hunt, *Two Chartularies of the Priory of St. Peter at Bath* (London, Harrison and Sons, 1893), Introduction, p. xxii, the Second Lateran Council of 1139 would try to forbid those involved with the church from practising medicine, but in the end it did little to change things.
67. Forester (trans.), *The Ecclesiastical History of England and Normandy by Orderic Vitalis*, Vol. IV, p. xxvii.
68. Hunt, *Two Chartularies of the Priory of St. Peter at Bath*, Introduction, p. xlii.
69. C.H. Talbot and E.A. Hammond, *The Medical Practitioners in Medieval England, A Biographical Register* (London, Wellcome Historical Medical Library, 1965), pp. 252 and 253.
70. Abbott, *St. Thomas of Canterbury*, Vol. I, p. 262. See also, Brian Kemp (trans.), 'The Miracles of the Hand of St. James', *Berkshire Archaeological Journal*, Vol. 65, 1970, p. 17, Miracle xxiv and Miracle xxiva, this may have been true for some twelfth-century pilgrims, among them two named knights, who attended at Reading Abbey where the miracle-inducing hand of St James was said to be kept. The first, called Robert of Stanford, had struggled for a long time with a severe fever. Once at the abbey he was given a drink that also made him ill, but it soon caused the fever to dissipate. The second knight from this record, called Ralph Gibuin, was suffering from the same thing. The entry notes that Gibuin was cured in the same manner as were many men and women. Apparently, the number of people made well was so large that the scribe could not list them all. These entries give the sense that this crowd of people had contracted a contagious illness for which the monks had a remedy. If they were secretly helping the sick by lacing a drink with a cure it would certainly have seemed like a miracle to those pilgrims who were made well when nothing they had tried had worked for them.
71. Francis J. Tschan, *History of the Archbishops of Hamburg-Bremen – Adam of Bremen* (New York, Columbia University Press, 2002), p. 213, see also, pp. 97 and 128 for more on the miracles.
72. Hamre S. Suppersberger, G.A. Ersland, V. Daux, W. Parson and C. Wilkinson, 'Three individuals, three stories, three burials from medieval Trondheim, Norway', *PLOS ONE*, 3 July 2017, p. 2, see notes on the possible sites of this burial.
73. Ibid., p. 17.
74. Ibid., p. 19.

75. Ibid., p. 21. See also, Nelson (trans.), *The Annals of St-Bertin*, p. 120, for an example from the Frankish *Annals of St. Bertin* for the year 864. King Louis of Germany fell from his horse while hunting near Frankfurt, causing damage to his ribs. The injury was severe enough that he was taken to a neighbouring monastery where he was bedridden for a time, before making a full recovery thanks to the monks who treated him.
76. Edgington, *The Life and Miracles of St. Ivo*, p. 46, Edgington provides some commonsense elucidation around miracle cures. Recoveries were often nothing more than a 'happy coincidence' and they could easily be short-lived or take time to heal the pilgrim. See also, Francis Rice, *The Hermit of Finchale – The Life of Saint Godric* (Durham, UK, The Pentland Press Limited, 1994), pp. 320 and 321, for a knight who travelled more than 400km from the north of England to Canterbury only to find no healing for the painful swelling on his leg at the tomb of St Thomas.
77. Joseph McAlhany and Jay Rubenstein (trans), *Guibert of Nogent – Monodies and On the Relics of Saints – The Autobiography and a Manifesto of a French Monk from the Time of the Crusades* (London, Penguin Books, 2011), p. 205.
78. Ibid., p. 206, Guibert did not stop there, mentioning another absurdity that again he had observed. After the cathedral of Laon, France was destroyed by fire during a riot at Easter in 1112 the church organized tours of its holy relics to raise money for the rebuilding. Guibert pointed out one swindler who was apparently acting on the church's behalf and claiming to have around his neck, in a small reliquary box called a philacterium, a miraculous piece of bread that had been chewed by Jesus himself. Guibert went on to call this sort of thing 'dirty profit', something certainly not uncommon in his time. See also, p. 324, n. 32 for more on Laon.
79. Bull, *The Miracles of Our Lady of Rocamadour*, pp. 36 and 37, for more on wax and silver offerings.
80. Sheingorn (trans.), *The Book of Sainte Foy*, p. 290, n. 26.
81. Ralph Jackson, *Doctors and Diseases in the Roman Empire* (London, British Museum Press, 1988), pp. 157–61.
82. Richard Strange, *The Life and Gests of St. Thomas of Hereford – From the Original 1674 Printing* (repr. London, Burns and Oates, 1879), pp. 171 and 172.
83. Ibid., p. 172, it is a remarkable list of items recorded at the shrine of St Thomas. There were 170 little silver ships and 41 of the wax variety, presumably for a safe journey. They found 3 little wooden, votive carts and 1 made of wax, like the type used by those who were unable to walk. There were 108 full-sized crutches discovered. Heartbreakingly, there were 95 children's coats, some made of silk and others of linen. Unusual and valuable items such as silk cloth and cloth of gold, 38 in total, were also included in this diverse lot of offerings.
84. Brian Spencer, *Pilgrim Souvenirs and Secular Badges* (London, Museum of London, The Stationery Office, 1998), p. 235, the visit of the English king, Henry II in 1170 did help to raise the profile of Rocamadour in the late twelfth century. See also, Bull, *The Miracles of Our Lady of Rocamadour*, p. 89, for more on Henry II's visits to Rocamadour in 1159 and 1170.
85. Spencer, *Pilgrim Souvenirs and Secular Badges*, p.235, the widespread dispersal of pilgrim souvenirs and other documentary evidence are proof of the success of Rocamadour.
86. Albe, *Les miracles de Notre-Dame de Roc-Amadour au XIIe siècle*, pp. 288 and 289.
87. Bull, *The Miracles of Our Lady of Rocamadour*, p. 188.
88. Ibid., pp. 189 and 190.

89. Bull, *The Miracles of Our Lady of Rocamadour*, p. 97, the prologue in the original manuscript notes specifically the many who were made well after being injured by swords and arrows or run through with lances. See also, Albe, *Les miracles de Notre-Dame de Roc-Amadour au XIIe siècle*, p. 148, 'Sur les conseils pressants de ceux de leurs amis qui avaient entendu les merveilles de la Vierge de Rocamadour, ou qui en avaient ressenti eux mêmes les bienfaits …'. Hugh de Gundeville, discussed in the previous chapter, was an Anglo-Norman knight who became unwell while in Ireland. Friends and colleagues who knew about the miracles at Rocamadour or who had personally experienced them apparently told Hugh that he might receive healing through the saint. This supports the idea that it was a place known far and wide and quite popular with soldiers and knights.
90. Albe, *Les miracles de Notre-Dame de Roc-Amadour au XIIe siècle*, p. 252, at Rocamadour, from one of the many miracles involving soldiers, 'Bientôt complètement guérile chevalier fit faire une image d'argent portant fixee sur elle la flèche même dont it avait été blessé, et vint l'offrir à sa Liberatrice …'. 'Soon he was completely healed, so the knight had a silver image made that included the very arrow from which he had been wounded and came to offer it to his Liberator …'.
91. Ibid., p. 224, those who made their way to these places such as Rocamadour were usually accompanied by others who assisted them in making their journeys. This was true of a young knight from the Gascony region of France who suffered from paralysis and epilepsy. It took a small retinue to get him to the Abbey at Rocamadour, which was certainly not uncommon for those among the knightly classes. 'Assisté de quelques compagnons de route, il arrive a l'église dans les meilleurs sentiments de supplication et de piété.' 'He was assisted by a few travelling companions who helped him arrive at the church full of piety and supplication'. See also, Benedicta Ward, *Miracles and the Medieval Mind – Theory, Record and Event – 1000–1215* (Aldershot, Wildwood House Limited, 1987), p. 147 for further discussion on the different groups that arrived with each pilgrim, such as knights arriving with their escorts and retainers.

Chapter 3 – Soldiers, Smiths and Safety

1. Horton and Bell (trans), *The Lay of the Nibelungs*, p. 43.
2. British Medical Association, *Hen feddegyaeth kymrie: (ancient Cymric medicine) and lecture memoranda, British Medical Association meeting, Swansea, 1903* (London, Burroughs Wellcome and Company, 1903), p. 21.
3. Talbot and Hammond, *The Medical Practitioners in Medieval England*, p. 19.
4. Ibid., pp. 231 and 232.
5. *Calendar of Documents Relating to Scotland, Preserved in the Public Record Office and the British Library – Volume V (Supplementary) – 1108–1516* (issued under the direction of the Keeper of the Records of Scotland, Scottish Record Office, 1881), p. 170.
6. Du Chaillu, *The Viking Age*, Vol. II, p. 202, from Chapter 45 of the *Jomsviking Saga*.
7. Cusimano and Moorhead (trans), *The Deeds of Louis the Fat*, p. 129, fn. 'e', see also, p. 203, n. 6, for the way in which figures tended to be inflated by those who chronicled the Middle Ages.
8. G.N. Garmonsway (trans.), *The Anglo-Saxon Chronicle* (London, J.M. Dent & Sons Ltd, 1953), p. 96, *Anglo-Saxon Chronicle* entry for 911, '… slaying many thousands …', p. 204, entry for 1069, '… slaying many hundreds of Frenchmen …'. See also, Lunde and Stone (trans), *Ibn Fadlān and the Land of Darkness*, p. 150, during battle between Rūs and Muslim forces 700 Rūs were killed. See also, Kathleen Tyson (trans.), *Carmen de Triumpho Normannico – The Song of the Norman Conquest*

(CreateSpace Independent Publishing Platform, 2013), p. 67, from *Carmen Wido*, a reference to 10,000 dead.
9. Meyer, *La chanson de la croisade contre les Albigeois*, pp. 98 and 99.
10. Shirley (trans.), *The Song of the Cathar Wars*, pp. 94, 99 and 175 are among the many scenes that recall the brutal details of blood, brains and body parts that littered the ground after the many battles and sieges of this campaign.
11. Ibid., pp. 104 and 134.
12. Paterson, 'Military Surgery', p. 119, see also, p. 145, Guillaume de Congenis included very military specific procedures in his teachings, including how to correct a dislocated shoulder with the use of a knight's saddle and shield.
13. Metzler, *Disability in Medieval Europe*, pp. 119 and 120, Dr Metzler points out that not all armies brought surgeons along with them, so knights and soldiers would have trained themselves to be able to perform simple surgical and first-aid procedures.
14. Canadian Army, *Notes for Instructors in Battle First Aid – June, 1943* (Ottawa, Edmond Cloutier, 1943), p. 2, Sessions 15 and 16 were devoted to self treatment of injuries, including bullet and shell fragment wounds, see also, pp. 32 and 33.
15. Colonel Charles G. Batty, 'Changes in the Care of the Battle Casualty: Lessons Learned from the Falklands Campaign', *Military Medicine*, Vol. 164, May 1999, p. 336.
16. Leo Sherley-Price, *Bede – A History of the English Church and People*, revised by R.E. Latham (London, Penguin, 1986), p. 243. See also, J.A. Giles (trans.), *Roger of Wendover – Flowers of History, In Two Volumes* (London, Henry G. Bohn, 1849), Vol. I, p. 111.
17. Samuel Laing, *The Heimskringla, A History of Norse Kings – Volumes I–III* (London, The Norroena Society, 1907), Vol. II, p. 678, Sturluson goes on to say, '… they all became afterwards the best of doctors. There were two Iceland men among them; the one was Thorkil, a son of Geire, from Lyngar; the other was Atle, father of Bard Svarte of Selardal, from whom many good doctors are descended.' See also, Bernard Scudder (trans.), 'Egil's Saga', *The Sagas of the Icelanders* (London, Penguin Books, Penguin Group, 2001), p. 36, for similar.
18. Elton (trans.), *The First Nine Books of the Danish History of Saxo Grammaticus*, p. 264.
19. Philip E. Bennett (trans.), *La Chanson de Guillaume* (London, Grant & Cutler Ltd, 2000), p. 59, see also, pp. 201 and 202, there are two missing lines in the existing manuscript. Bennett is of the opinion that they could refer to the bandaging of more significant injuries such as head and stomach wounds.
20. Ibid., pp. 59 and 60.
21. Robert Steele, *Huon of Bordeaux: Done into English by Sir John Bourchier, Lord Berners* (London, George Allen Ruskin House, 1895), p. 26.
22. Kibler (trans.), 'The Story of the Grail (Perceval)', *Chrétien de Troyes – Arthurian Romances*, p. 465, according to de Troyes, Gawain knew more about medicine than anyone else.
23. Ibid., p. 461.
24. Ibid., pp. 464 and 465.
25. Ibid., p. 466, the book referenced in this passage is not mentioned, however, the herbal of *Macer Floridus* must be a candidate worthy of consideration. Also written in France, it was certainly a popular and influential herbal throughout the Middle Ages, one that would have been known to many (Frisk (ed.), *A Middle English Translation of Macer Floridus De Viribus Herbarum*, p. 15). Chrétien de Troyes' apparent knowledge of medicine makes it likely that he was at least aware of this text.

26. Kibler (trans.), 'The Story of the Grail (Percival)', *Chrétien de Troyes – Arthurian Romances*, p. 466.
27. Edouard Nicaise, *La grande chirurgie de Guy de Chauliac* (Paris, Ancienne Librairie Germer Ballière, 1890), pp. 15 and 16. See also, Siraisi, *Medieval and Early Renaissance Medicine*, p. 35.
28. Nicaise, *La grande chirurgie de Guy de Chauliac*, p. 16. See Siraisi, *Medieval and Early Renaissance Medicine* for more on Guy de Chauliac's sects.
29. Weston (trans.), *Parzival*, Vol. II, p. 5. See also, Rosenman (trans.), *Chirurgia of Roger Frugard*, p. 117, Roger Frugard's method of drainage was quite different. It involved tying the patient to a plank of wood so that they could be twisted and turned to the best position to allow fluid to flow away from the injury.
30. Weston (trans.), *Parzival*, Vol. II, p. 5.
31. G.O. Sayles (trans.), *Fleta – Volume IV – Book V and Book VI* (London, Selden Society, 1984), p. 129.
32. Siraisi, *Medieval and Early Renaissance Medicine*, p. 176. See also, Campbell and Colton, *The Surgery of Theodoric*, Introduction, Vol. I, p. xxxviii, for reference to Theodoric's insistence regarding the proper preparation of a wound before being sutured.
33. Adams (trans.), *The Romance of Yder*, p. 117.
34. Faye Marie Getz (ed.), *Healing and Society in Medieval England, A Middle English Translation of the Pharmaceutical Writings of Gilbertus Anglicus* (Madison, The University of Wisconsin Press, 1991), Introduction, p. lii, fn. 70. See also, Sharon Turner, *The History of the Anglo-Saxons from the Earliest Period to the Norman Conquest – In Three Volumes* (London, Longman, Brown, Green and Longmans, 1852), pp. 384 and 385, the English historian Sharon Turner also wrote of women and medicine, 'Before men began to take up medicine as a profession, the domestic practice of it would, of course, fall on females, who, in every stage of society, assume the kind of task of nursing sickness …', and Comfort (trans.), *Erec and Enide*, p. 364, note on line 5113, 'Many examples will be met of women skilled in the practice of medicine and surgery.'
35. Monica H. Green, *Making Women's Medicine Masculine – The Rise of Male Authority in Pre-Modern Gynaecology* (Oxford University Press, 2008), p. 120.
36. Edward J. Kealey, 'England's Earliest Women Doctors', *Journal of the History of Medicine and Allied Sciences*, Vol. 40, Issue 4, October 1985, p. 473.
37. Talbot and Hammond, *The Medical Practitioners in Medieval England*, p. 200.
38. Green, *Making Women's Medicine Masculine*, p. 126.
39. Talbot and Hammond, *The Medical Practitioners in Medieval England*, p. 209.
40. Ibid., p. 10, Talbot confirms the unfortunate rarity of those female physicians acknowledged in the records.
41. Michael Alexander (trans.), *The Earliest English Poems* (London, Penguin Classics, Penguin Group, 1991), p. 36.
42. Renée L. Curtis (trans.), *The Romance of Tristan, The Thirteenth-Century Old French 'Prose Tristan'* (Oxford University Press, 1994), p. 42.
43. John Coles (trans.), *The Story of Þórðr Hreða* (Icelandic Saga Database – sagadb.org, translation 1866), Ch. 7.
44. Edmund Head (trans.), *The Saga of Viga-Glum or Viga Glum's Story* (London, Williams and Norgate, 1866), p. 91.
45. Laing, *Heimskringla*, Vol. II, pp. 627–30.
46. Imperial War Museum, 'A Short Guide to Medical Services During the First World War'. Located close to the trenches and battlefields of the First and Second World

Wars, they were part of a system of early intervention in the treatment of wounds. They became extremely important in helping to save the lives of tens of thousands of casualties that passed through them.
47. Laing, *Heimskringla*, Vol. II, p. 630, for further discussion on this scene see the later section on 'Wounds of the Stomach and Intestines' in the chapter that follows.
48. DuBois, *Nordic Religions in the Viking Age*, p. 99, DuBois is of the opinion that Sturluson's references point to women of Anglo-Saxon or Continental origin. See also, Dasent (trans.), *Icelandic Sagas, Volume IV, The Saga of Hacon*, p. 301, for a saga featuring a physician from beyond Scandinavia, 'Then a leech came to him who had come from abroad out of Spain with Sira Ferant, and gave advice as to the cause of his sickness.'
49. Tyson (trans.), *Carmen de Triumpho Normannico*, p. 85, the *Carmen Wido*, written within months of the Battle of Hastings, is clear that King Harold was well and truly killed by soldiers of the Norman army.
50. Walter de Gray Birch, *Vita Haroldi – The Romance of the Life of Harold, King of England* (London, Elliot Stock, 1885), p. 136, from the Harley Manuscript – kept in the British Library – Harley MSS 3776, see also, Birch's introduction, p. v. See also, Edward A. Freeman, *History of the Norman Conquest of England – Its Causes and Its Results – Volumes I to VI* (Oxford, Clarendon Press, 1867–79), Vol. III, p. 515 for more on the same subject.
51. Simon Roffey, Katie Tucker, Kori Filipek-Ogden, Janet Montgomery, Jamie Cameron, Tamsin O'Connell, Jane Evans, Phil Marter, and Michael, G. Taylor, 'Investigation of a Medieval Pilgrim Burial Excavated from the Leprosarium of St Mary Magdalen Winchester, UK', *PLOS Neglected Tropical Diseases*, 26 January 2017, p. 20.
52. Hibbard, *Three Middle English Romances*, p. 138.
53. Comfort (trans.), *Erec and Enide*, pp. 66–8.
54. Adams (trans.), *The Romance of Yder*, p. 115.
55. Thomas Wright (trans.), *The History of Fulk Fitz Warine, an Outlawed Baron in the Reign of King John* (London, George Bell & Sons, 1855), pp. 31 and 32.
56. Louisa May Alcott, *Hospital Sketches* (Boston, James Redpath, 1863), p. 34.
57. Bouillet and Servières, *Sainte Foy, vierge & martyre*, p. 570, '… un fer rouge placé sur la main du blessé ne provoquait aucune sensation'.
58. Faye Getz, *Medicine in the Middle Ages* (Princeton University Press, 1998), p. 7.
59. Lotte Hedeager, *Iron Age Myth and Materiality: An Archaeology of Scandinavia AD 400–1000* (London and New York, Routledge, 2011), p. 139. See also, Elton (trans.), *The First Nine Books of the Danish History of Saxo Grammaticus*, Intro, p. xxviii, 'The smith was the object of a curious prejudice'.
60. *Secrets of the Castle* (BBC and Lion Television, 2014), episode 4, minutes 33 and 34. In an interview with Professor Ronald Hutton he explains the role of the medieval blacksmith as a healer.
61. John Rhys, *Celtic Folklore – Welsh and Manx – Volume 1* (Oxford, Clarendon Press, 1901), p. 295.
62. Sheingorn (trans.), *The Book of Sainte Foy*, pp. 102 and 103, such a mass of iron votive offerings was brought to St Foy that the monks had blacksmiths turn the objects into beautiful doors. These adorned the abbey in large numbers, see also, p. 294, n. 91, for more.
63. *Secrets of the Castle*, episode 4, minutes 33 and 34.
64. Sheingorn (trans.), *The Book of Sainte Foy*, p. 216, although his genitals are at one point described as being diseased, he seems to have been dealing with an inguinal hernia.

65. Bouillet and Servières, *Sainte Foy, vierge & martyre*, pp. 584 and 585.
66. Sheringorn (trans.), *The Book of Sainte Foy*, pp. 216 and 217.
67. Bouillet and Servières, *Sainte Foy, vierge & martyre*, p. 585. In addition, Boulliet mentions in fn. 1 that this may have been Robert, who was the abbot of Issoire, in central France, under the Carolingian king Lothar or Lothair (d. 986), perhaps making this account much earlier than *c.* 1050.
68. Bull, *The Miracles of Our Lady of Rocamadour*, p. 120.
69. Albe, *Les miracles de Notre-Dame de Roc-Amadour au XIIe siècle*, p. 122, 'Aussitôt il fit appeler un simple forgeron qui pouvait l'enlever légèrement et sans douleur.' 'Right away he called a simple blacksmith who could remove it without pain.'
70. Edgar Taylor (trans.), *Master Wace – His Chronicle of the Norman Conquest from the Roman de Rou* (London, William Pickering, 1837) p. 235.
71. Hitti (trans.), *An Arab-Syrian Gentleman & Warrior in the Period of the Crusades*, p. 144.
72. *Calendar of Chancery Warrants Preserved in the Public Record Office – AD 1244–1326* (London, His Majesty's Stationery Office, 1927), p. 64.
73. Ibid.
74. Ibid.
75. Meyer, *La chanson de la croisade contre les Albigeois*, p. 427, 'La lutte et le carnage durèrent jusqu'à la nuit obscure, qui sépara les combattants affaiblis ... Alors vous eussiez entendu gémir les blessés, réclamer les médecins, chercher les onguents, et crier «Dieu aide!» à cause des cuisantes douleurs.' 'The fighting and carnage lasted until the dark night, which then separated the weakened warriors ... Then you would have heard the wounded moan and call for the doctors to bring their ointments, and shout "God help!" Because of the stinging pains.'
76. Ibid., pp. 257 and 258.
77. Taylor (trans.), *Master Wace*, p. 235. See also, Freeman, *History of the Norman Conquest of England*, Vol. III, p. 492, who notes quite a different outcome for some of the English soldiers, 'The slightly wounded could not escape, but were crushed to death by the thick ranks of their comrades.', see also, fn. 1.
78. Taylor (trans.), *Master Wace*, pp. 256 and 257, fn. 8, for William of Jumièges, who noted that William the Conqueror and his men did not return from their harrying of the retreating English until at least midnight, making this sort of escape a possibility. See also, Tyson (trans.), *Carmen de Triumpho Normannico*, p. 89, *Carmen Wido* offers some support of this notion of English soldiers using darkness as cover, along with the densely wooded areas.
79. James Henthorn Todd (trans.), *War of the Gaedhil with the Gaill or The Invasions of Ireland by the Danes and Other Norsemen* (London, Longmans, Green, Reader and Dyer, 1867), pp. 213 and 215, see also, Introduction, p. cxciii, according to Henthorn the wounded were to be placed in a fort at Rath Maisten.
80. Ibid., p. 217.
81. Bennett (trans.), *La Chanson de Guillaume*, p. 59.
82. Cusimano and Moorhead (trans), *The Deeds of Louis the Fat*, p. 130, in the end, this battle, meant to have taken place in 1124 against the ranks of the Holy Roman Emperor Henry V, never happened. See also, p. 136, in another incident that did occur at Clermont, some of the French slept under their shields in order to protect themselves against the constant harassment of arrows.
83. Ibid., pp. 130 and 131.
84. Laing, *Heimskringla*, Vol. II, p. 625, 'The wounded were taken home to the farms, so that every house was full of them; and tents were erected over some.'

85. Goddard Henry Orpen (trans.), *The Song of Dermot and the Earl – An Old French Poem – From the Carew Manuscript No. 596* (Oxford, Clarendon Press, 1892), pp. 61 and 63, lines 802–5 and 814–23. See also, Horton and Bell (trans), *The Lay of the Nibelungs*, p. 43, similarly, in the early thirteenth-century German poem *The Lay of the Nibelungs*, King Gunther welcomed the army of Siegfried, along with those prisoners who had been captured in battle. The warriors and injured alike received the care and hospitality of the townpeople.
86. Metzler, *Disability in Medieval Europe*, pp. 117 and 118.

Chapter 4 – Wounds and Surgery

1. Forester (trans.), *The Ecclesiastical History of England and Normandy by Orderic Vitalis*, Vol. I, p. 483.
2. Sheingorn (trans.), *The Book of Sainte Foy*, p. 230, Unfortunately, the name of the castle that was besieged is not mentioned in the entry.
3. Ibid., p. 231.
4. Bouillet and Servières, *Sainte Foy, vierge & martyre*, p. 598.
5. Ronald C. Finucane, *Miracles and Pilgrims – Popular Beliefs in Medieval England* (New York, St Martin's Press, 1995), pp. 66 and 67, very often in miracle accounts the work of physicians and surgeons is downplayed or condemned outright.
6. Sheingorn (trans.), *The Book of Sainte Foy*, pp. 231 and 232. See 'Family Matters' section of Chapter 8, Tormented Minds, for more on the wife of Mathfred.
7. Ibid., p. 231, there is a perhaps a small clue early on when the scribe claims that Mathfred would not recover until one of the doctors had enough belief in themselves to open the wound up and remove the arrow.
8. Mitchell, *Medicine in the Crusades*, p. 156, see discussion regarding modern research into the relationship between an arrow's velocity and wounds.
9. Wright (trans.), *The Historical Works of Giraldus Cambrensis*, pp. 370 and 371. This was a soldier of William de Braose (d. 1211), the example that follows describes, 'Another soldier had his hip, equally sheathed in armour, penetrated by an arrow quite to the saddle, and on turning his horse round, received a similar wound on the opposite hip, which fixed him on both sides to his seat.'
10. Tyson (trans.), *Carmen de Triumpho Normannico*, Appendix 1, p. 55, the Normans apparently mass-produced four types of '… vicious steel-tipped arrows …' also forging armour piercing crossbow bolts. See also, Shirley (trans.), *The Song of the Cathar Wars*, p. 180, crossbow quarrels were described as 'twice-tempered' to give them a less brittle quality, suitable for piercing armour. See also, Oliver Jessop, 'A New Artefact Typology for the Study of Medieval Arrowheads', *Medieval Archaeology*, Vol. XL (1996) (The Society for Medieval Archaeology, 1996), pp. 194–5 for diagrams of several types of arrowheads, and Campbell and Colton, *The Surgery of Theodoric*, Vol. I, p. 83, Pifteau (trans.), *Chirurgie de Guillaume de Sâlicet*, p. 253, fn. 1 and Joan M. Ferrante (trans.), *Guillaume d'Orange: Four Twelfth-Century Epics* (New York, Columbia University Press, 1991), p. 81, for descriptions of the many shapes and styles of arrowheads.
11. Shirley (trans.), *The Song of the Cathar Wars*, p. 170, see also, fn. 2 on the same page.
12. Pifteau (trans.), *Chirurgie de Guillaume de Sâlicet*, p. 253, fn. 1, 'Quant au fer, il était tantôt inséré et cloué solidement au manche, et tantôt si peu assujetti à dessein, qu'il restait toujours dans la plaie.' 'As for the iron tip, it was sometimes inserted and nailed firmly to the handle, and sometimes by design there was so little used to affix it to the shaft to enable it to remain in the wound.'

13. *Calendar of Documents Relating to Scotland Preserved in Her Majesty's Public Record Office, London – Volume II – 1272–1307* (Edinburgh, Her Majesty's General Register House, 1884), p. 412. See also, Tyson (trans.), *Carmen de Triumpho Normannico*, Appendix 1, p. 111 for more on mass-produced arrows and bolts made by the Norman smiths.
14. Laing, *Heimskringla*, Vol. III, p. 990, from the *Saga of Hakon the Broad-Shouldered* within the *Heimskringla*. 'And no man knows where an arrow may hit, even from the hands of a bad bowman'.
15. Du Chaillu, *The Viking Age*, Vol. II, p. 91.
16. Dass (trans.), *Viking Attacks on Paris*, p. 43, see also, pp. 33 and 41.
17. Freeman, *History of the Norman Conquest of England*, Vol. III, p. 175, for Varaville, and Tyson (trans.), *Carmen de Triumpho Normannico*, p. 59, for Hastings from the *Carmen Widonis*, the earliest account of the Norman Conquest of England, '... bitter plague of death-dealing darts ...'. See also, fn. 54 on the same page for more on the tactics of arrows and javelins at the Battle of Hastings, with the Normans able to easily resupply themselves, while the Anglo-Saxon army was trapped and unable to do so.
18. Comfort (trans.), *Erec and Enide*, p. 111.
19. Elton (trans.), *The First Nine Books of the Danish History of Saxo Grammaticus*, p. 208, see also, pp. 327 and 328, and Laurence Marcellus Larson (trans.), *The King's Mirror – Speculum Regale – Konungs Skuggsja* (Oxford University Press, 1917), p. 215 for a reference to their use onboard ships.
20. Larsen, *Old Icelandic Medical Miscellany*, p. 164, 'If this stone (lodestone) is crushed and applied to wounds it draws out iron if it is therein.', a functional idea for locating arrows and perhaps removing small fragments of iron from the body, provided they were not too deeply embedded. This comes from an earlier Danish source, the author of medicine Henrik Harpestræng (d. 1244), see also, p. 26.
21. Laing, *Heimskringla*, Vol. II, pp. 627 and 630.
22. Ibid., p. 630.
23. Hermann Pálsson and Paul Edwards (trans), *Eyrbyggja Saga* (London, Penguin Classics, Penguin Group, 1989), p. 123.
24. Albe, *Les miracles de Notre-Dame de Roc-Amadour au XIIe siècle*, p. 250, fn. 2, 'Il s'agit de l'ancienne Bourgogne, qui comprenait le Dauphine.' 'This is the old Burgundy that included the Dauphine'. See also, Bull, *The Miracles of Our Lady of Rocamadour*, p. 171, for this entry.
25. Ibid., p. 251, 'Cependant il ne put pas toucher la Dame de miséricorde au point d'obtenir immédiatement la santé.'
26. See Chapter 3, under 'The Blacksmith as a Healer', for other examples of healing involving metalsmiths and their similarities to this case.
27. Albe, *Les miracles de Notre-Dame de Roc-Amadour au XIIe siècle*, p. 251, '... de ses domestiques, homme rustique parfaitement inhabile pour ce qu'il allait lui demander, et lui commanda de faire ce que n'avaient pu faire les médecins, d'extraire de son corps le fer de flèche ...'. '... one of the servants, a rustic man perfectly incompetent for what he was going to ask him to do, which was something the doctors had been unable to do, extract the arrowhead from his body ...'.
28. Ibid., '... car la chair était toute pourrie en dedans ...'. '... the flesh was all rotten inside ...'.
29. Peter of Eboli's *Liber ad Honorem Augusti*, Burgerbibliothek Bern, Cod. 120.II, f. 110r, see copy of the image in the plates.

30. Cockayne, *Leechdoms, Wortcunning and Starcraft of Early England*, Vol. II, p. 95 and p. 327 for *Leechbook III* example.
31. Rosenman (trans.), *Chirurgia of Roger Frugard*, pp. 46 and 47.
32. Mitchell, *Medicine in the Crusades*, p. 155, it was not uncommon to leave a stubborn arrow inside the wound for a few days to allow for the tissues around the site to begin to rot and soften up, making retrieval an easier process. See also, Campbell and Colton, *The Surgery of Theodoric*, Vol. I, p. 85, Theodoric noted something similar regarding arrows that were immediately difficult to remove, '... ought to be let alone for some days until the flesh surrounding it becomes putrid, because from that time on it may be withdrawn with ease'.
33. Rosenman (trans.), *Chirurgia of Roger Frugard*, p. 47.
34. Ibid., pp. 77 and 110, according to his surgery just one piece of bacon was to be placed through the entire path the arrow had taken through the neck, but where a limb was involved a piece was to be pushed into each opening.
35. Ibid., pp. 47 and 48. See also, Rosenman (trans.), *Surgery of William of Saliceto*, p. 99, for the same recommendation.
36. Campbell and Colton, *The Surgery of Theodoric*, Vol. I, p. 84, 'for I have cured some and seen many cured by Master Hugo'.
37. Robert Ignatius Burns, 'The Medieval Crossbow as a Surgical Instrument: An Illustrated Case History', *Bulletin of The New York Academy of Medicine*, Vol. 48, No. 8, September 1972, pp. 986–8, even the crossbow could apparently be used to extract an arrow that was not barbed, using the force of the bow to extract the arrow in the opposite direction. I discovered this useful reference in Mitchell's *Medicine in the Crusades*, p. 156.
38. Campbell and Colton, *The Surgery of Theodoric*, Vol. I, pp. 85 and 87.
39. Ibid., p. 86.
40. Pifteau (trans.), *Chirurgie de Guillaume de Sâlicet*, pp. 298 and 299.
41. Laing, *Heimskringla*, Vol. II, p. 630.
42. Daniel P. Rignault, 'Abdominal trauma in war', *The World Journal of Surgery* (1992), 16, p. 940. By the time of the First World War the mortality rate for abdominal wounds was still as high as 53 per cent, dropping to about half that figure by the Second World War. Certainly, these injuries involved things such as shrapnel and bullets, rather than the stabbing and slicing weapons of the Middle Ages, but they are a useful guide to the dangers of these kinds of injuries.
43. Rosenman (trans.), *Chirurgia of Roger Frugard*, p. 118. See also, Dr Leonard D. Rosenman (trans.), *The Surgery of Roland of Parma* (Xlibris Corporation, 2001), p. 80.
44. The Cambro-Briton, *The Laws of Hywel Dha*, Vol. 2 (1821), p. 396, the other two types were skull fractures and a compound fracture of a limb.
45. Laing, *Heimskringla*, Vol. II, p. 630, triage is the process of separating casualties into three groups: 1. Those requiring only minor attention; 2. Those requiring immediate treatment to save their lives; and 3. Those with little or no chance of survival, even with medical intervention. By its very nature it requires clear and unemotional thinking to be useful.
46. Scudder (trans.), 'Egil's Saga', p. 91, focusing just on warriors who stood a chance of surviving their wounds seems to have been quite normal, as echoed in *Egil's Saga*, 'Afterwards the men who were thought likely to survive had their wounds dressed.' See also, Pálsson and Edwards (trans), *Seven Viking Romances*, p. 226, from *The Saga of Bosi and Herraud* for similar.

47. Stevenson, *Church Historians of England*, Vol. IV, Part I, p. 282. See also, Meyer, *La chanson de la croisade contre les Albigeois*, p. 457, 'Yeux, cervelles, poings, bras, cheveux, mâchoires, membres coupés, foies, entrailles, sang, chair, sont étendus partout.' 'Eyes, brains, fists, arms, hair, jaws, severed limbs, livers, entrails, blood, flesh are to be found everywhere.'
48. Bennett (trans.), *La Chanson de Guillaume*, p. 58.
49. Rice, *The Hermit of Finchale*, p. 315.
50. Ibid., p. 316.
51. Cockayne, *Leechdoms, Wortcunning and Starcraft of Early England*, Vol. II, p. 359.
52. Rosenman (trans.), *Chirurgia of Roger Frugard*, p. 119.
53. Ibid. See also, Corner, 'On Early Salernitan Surgery and Especially the "Bamberg Surgery"', p. 16, the idea of a wooden cannula sewn inside a wounded soldier seems so odd to the modern mind, but it is there in earlier works such as the *Bamberg Surgery*. What is not clear from the Bamberg text is whether the cannula was meant to be a support to keep the shape of the intestine as it was being repaired before being removed as the last stitches were put in or if it was to be left inside as Roger described.
54. Ibid., pp. 119 and 120, see also, n. 66 at the bottom of p. 119.
55. Leonard D. Rosenman (trans.), *The Surgery of Bruno da Longoburgo – An Italian Surgeon of the Thirteenth Century, by Mario Tabanelli* (Pittsburgh, Dorrance Publishing Co., Inc., 2003), p. 11.
56. Campbell and Colton, *The Surgery of Theodoric*, Vol. I, p. 159.
57. Ibid., p. 158.
58. Pifteau (trans.), *Chirurgie de Guillaume de Sâlicet*, p. 303.
59. Rosenman (trans.), *Surgery of Lanfranchi of Milan*, p. 103.
60. Pifteau (trans.), *Chirurgie de Guillaume de Sâlicet*, p. 304, see also, p. 302, '... que ce mode est plus avantageux tant parce qu'à cause de la continuité du fil et des points la suture durera davantage ...'. William preferred this stitch because it would last longer.
61. Rosenman (trans.), *Surgery of William of Saliceto*, p. 128, see also, example on p. 127 where enlarging the opening with a razor was recommended if the original opening was too small to return the intestines to their rightful place.
62. Charles Scott Moncrieff, *The Song of Roland* (London, Chapman & Hall Ltd, 1919), pp. 64 and 65.
63. Du Chaillu, *The Viking Age*, Vol. II, pp. 89 and 79, multiple names for axes and swords can be found on these pages.
64. Alexander (trans.), *The Earliest English Poems*, p. 36, both were healed by Waltharius' wife, Hiltgunt, who looked after their wounds.
65. L.J. Gardiner (trans.), *Cligés – Chrétien de Troyes* (London, Chatto & Windus, 1912), p. 173, Cligés '... raises his [Cligés] sword, and strikes him, so that beneath the knee he has cut off his leg as clean as a stalk of fennel'.
66. Bennett (trans.), *La Chanson de Guillaume*, p. 68.
67. Meyer, *La chanson de la croisade contre les Albigeois*, p. 426. See also, Giles (trans.), *Roger of Wendover*, p. 590, the chronicle of Roger of Wendover explains how quickly something like this could occur. He recalled how in 1234 a knight of gigantic size, who was mistaken for another, had both of his hands cut off with the single stroke of a sword, despite the fact he was wearing armour.
68. Keneva Kunz (trans.), 'The Saga of the People of Laxardal', *The Sagas of the Icelanders* (London, Penguin Books, Penguin Group, 2001), p. 371.

69. Dasent (trans.), *The Story of Burnt Njal or Njal's Saga*, Vol. II, p. 71. See also, John F. Benton (ed.), *Self and Society in Medieval France – The Memoirs of Abbot Guibert of Nogent* (New York, Harper & Row, 1970), p. 185, Guibert of Nogent provides another in his memoirs. Describing Thomas of Marle's treatment of a wounded prisoner who struggled to keep up, in a rage Thomas '… cut off both the man's feet, and of that he died'. While the outcome was perhaps obvious, this incident recalls the sort of injuries that were common in battle.
70. Dr James Greive (trans.), *A. Cornelius Celsus of Medicine. In Eight Books* (London, D. Wilson and T. Durham, 1756), p. 462.
71. Ibid., p. 463.
72. Cameron, *Anglo-Saxon Medicine*, p. 44.
73. Ibid., pp. 43 and 44, *Passionaris Galeni* is one source containing this procedure, see also, pp. 70 and 71 for more on these sources.
74. Cockayne, *Leechdoms, Wortcunning and Starcraft of Early England*, Vol. II, p. 85.
75. Rosenman (trans.), *Surgery of William of Saliceto*, p. 31.
76. Campbell and Colton, *The Surgery of Theodoric*, Vol. II, p. 37. See also, Frisk, *A Middle English Translation of Macer Floridus De Viribus Herbarum*, p. 85. The use of leeks and salt is also recommended in *Macer Floridus*, 'Stampe leek and salt and ley hem to a newe and fressh wounde; this wole close it a-non.'
77. Mitchell, *Medicine in the Crusades*, p. 153.
78. Cameron, *Anglo-Saxon Medicine*, p. 171, Cameron suggests that a cautery may well have been used to control the bleeding during the procedure, see also, p. 173 for more on the lack of sterile conditions, etc.
79. Cockayne, *Leechdoms, Wortcunning and Starcraft of Early England*, Vol. III, p. 23. See also, Cameron, *Anglo-Saxon Medicine*, p. 173.
80. Campbell and Colton, *The Surgery of Theodoric*, Vol. II, pp. 212–13.
81. Cockayne, *Leechdoms, Wortcunning and Starcraft of Early England*, Vol. II, pp. 95 and 97.
82. Ibid., p. 97.
83. Brian Moffat, *SHARP Practice 6, The Sixth Report on Researches into the Medieval Hospital at Soutra Scottish Borders/Lothian, Scotland* (Pathhead, SHARP, 1998), p. 12, page heading – II.e, Black Henbane *plus* Hemlock *plus* Poppy: a final word.
84. Brian Moffat and Other Participants in SHARP, *SHARP Practice 4, Fourth Report on Researches into the Medieval Hospital at Soutra, Lothian/Borders Region Scotland* (Edinburgh, SHARP, 1992), Section 65a.
85. Don Walker, *Disease in London, 1st–19th centuries – An illustrated guide to diagnosis* (London, Museum of London Archaeology, 2012), pp. 154 and 155, the date range of the individual was *c.* 1250–*c.* 1400. See also, *Calendar of the Close Rolls Preserved in the Public Record Office for Edward II – A.D. 1313–1319* (printed for Her Majesty's Stationery Office by Erye and Spottiswoode, 1893), p. 192, for examples of extant documentation such as William son of Thomas le Charetter of Grove and those like him who survived losing their hands. More is discussed in Chapter 6 here regarding disability.
86. Caroline Arcini, *Health and Disease in Early Lund – Osteo-Pathologic Studies of 3,305 Individuals Buried in the Cemetery Area of Lund 990-1536* (Department of Community Health Sciences Medical Faculty Lund University, 1999), pp. 145 and 146.
87. Campbell and Colton, *The Surgery of Theodoric*, Vol. I, p. 93.
88. Terry Jones, *Terry Jones – Medieval Lives*, 2 discs (BBC Video, 2008), Disc 2, *Philosopher*, see interview with Dr Faye Getz in Scene 2 for discussion on the value of food in the medieval healing process.

89. Coles (trans.), *The Story of Thórðr Hreða*, Ch. 7.
90. Comfort (trans.), *Erec and Enide*, p. 67.
91. Campbell and Colton, *The Surgery of Theodoric*, Vol. I, p. 90, for Theodoric and Rosenman (trans.), *Surgery of William of Saliceto*, p. 115.
92. Comfort (trans.), *Erec and Enide*, p. 68. See also, Hibbard, *Three Middle English Romances*, p. 113, 'When he had eaten enough, he stopped his wound with a kerchief ...'.
93. Cockayne, *Leechdoms, Wortcunning and Starcraft of Early England*, Vol. II, p. 359.
94. Rosenman (trans.), *Chirurgia of Roger Frugard*, p. 115.
95. Campbell and Colton, *The Surgery of Theodoric*, Vol. I, p. 25.
96. Ibid., pp. 92 and 93, see also, p. 142, for diet when the jugular vein was injured, as an example.
97. Rosenman (trans.), *Surgery of William of Saliceto*, pp. 80–2, especially D 1 and 2, and pp. 16 and 17, in his English translation Rosenman wisely chose to exclude much of the duplication in William's text, such as those things that helped to remove the bad humours from a wound (diet, evacuation of the bowels, etc.). Pifteau's earlier French version kept them in their entirety, see Pifteau, *Chirurgie de Guillaume de Sâlicet*, pp. 217 and 218, Head Wounds, as an example.
98. Terry Jones, *Medieval Lives* (London, BBC Books, 2004), p. 135. See also, Siraisi, *Medieval and Early Renaissance Medicine*, pp. 104–6, Rosenman (trans.), *Surgery of Lanfranchi of Milan*, pp. 127–9, for Lanfranchi's piece on the four humours and digestion.
99. Rosenman (trans.), *Surgery of Lanfranchi of Milan*, p. 34.
100. Bloodletting: Cockayne, *Leechdoms, Wortcunning and Starcraft of Early England*, Vol. II, pp. 233 and 341, Campbell and Colton, *The Surgery of Theodoric*, Vol. I, p. 70. Cupping: Cockayne, *Leechdoms, Wortcunning and Starcraft of Early England*, Vol. II, p. 207, Campbell and Colton, *The Surgery of Theodoric*, Vol. I, p. 27, Pifteu, p. 221, 'Et remarque que cette phlébotomie ou cette ventousation se fait pour que les humeurs du sang soient détournées, par l'écoulement, de la partie lésée'. 'And notice how this bloodletting or this sucking is done so that the humours of the blood are moved away from the injured part.' Evacuation: Campbell and Colton, *The Surgery of Theodoric*, Vol. I, p. 28, Pifteau, *Chirurgie de Guillaume de Sâlicet*, p. 314, 'Qu'on ne néglige pas non plus l'évacuation naturelle ou artificielle du ventre.' 'Do not neglect the evacuation of the bowels, either by natural or artificial means.'
101. Cockayne, *Leechdoms, Wortcunning and Starcraft of Early England*, Vol. II, pp. 23 and 53. See also, Cameron, *Anglo-Saxon Medicine*, p. 127, Campbell and Colton, *The Surgery of Theodoric*, Vol. I, p. 74, honey used in treating cuts through the muscles, and Rosenman (trans.), *Surgery of William of Saliceto*, p. 237, No. 20.
102. Ben Waggoner (trans.), *Norse Magical and Herbal Healing – A Medical Book from Medieval Iceland* (New Haven, CT, Troth Publications, 2011), Introduction, pp. xxvi and xxvii, for references to henbane being found in excavations across the Viking world, and Rosenman (trans.), *Surgery of William of Saliceto*, p. 116, as an example of a topical pain relief ointment containing henbane (*Surgery* written c. 1275).
103. Pálsson and Edwards (trans), *Seven Viking Romances*, p. 245.
104. Campbell and Colton, *The Surgery of Theodoric*, Vol. II, p. 21. See also, Chapter 6 here, section on 'Burn Injuries'.
105. Rosenman (trans.), *Surgery of Lanfranchi of Milan*, p. 59.
106. Rosenman (trans.), *Surgery of William of Saliceto*, p. 138.

Chapter 5 – Broken Bones and Fractured Skulls

1. A.J. Wyatt, *The Lay of Havelok the Dane* (London, W.B. Clive and Co., 1889), p. 42.
2. Weston (trans.), *Parzival*, Vol. I, p. 168, 'Right arm, and left leg had he broken – so mighty his overthrow.'
3. Mitchell, *Medicine in the Crusades*, p. 117.
4. Meyer, *La chanson de la croisade contre les Albigeois*, p. 440, '… mais ce n'est point merveille s'ils ont eu le dessus, car ils ont reçu et donné de tels coups que les os leur en craquent sous les armures'. 'No wonder they defeated them, because the blows they received and gave were so strong that their bones were cracked and broken inside their armour.' See also, Edith Rickert (trans.), *Early English Romances in Verse: Done into Modern English* (London, Chatto & Windus, 1908), p. 82, from the fourteenth-century *The Earl of Toulouse*, 'Shields and shafts were splintered, and heads were cracked through their helmets, and many a hauberk torn.'
5. Lucy Allen Paton, *Arthurian Romance* (London, J.M. Dent & Sons, 1912), p. 180, from *Layamon's Brut*.
6. Siraisi, *Medieval and Early Renaissance Medicine*, p. 154.
7. Hitti (trans.), *An Arab-Syrian Gentleman & Warrior in the Period of the Crusades*, p. 144.
8. Katherine Park, *Doctors and Medicine in Early Renaissance Florence* (Princeton University Press, 1985), p. 67, see also, pp. 91 and 92. Also cited by Dr Irina Metzler in *Disability in Medieval Europe*, p. 118.
9. Anne Russcher and Rolf H. Bremmer Jr '"For a Broken Limb": Fracture Treatment in Anglo-Saxon England', *Amsterdamer Beiträge zur älteren Germanistik*, 69, 1 January 2012, p. 170. The authors of this paper on the treatment of broken bones in Anglo-Saxon society underline just how little is known about the bonesetters of the time. See also, Siraisi, *Medieval & Early Renaissance Medicine*, p. 20, for more on the hierarchy of medical professionals.
10. Siraisi, *Taddeo Alderotti and his Pupils*, p. 300.
11. Nicaise, *La grande chirurgie de Guy de Chauliac*, Introduction, p. LXXII, 'Les fractures et les luxations étaient abandonnées souvent à des rhabilleurs; dans les siècles suivants, on a vu des chirurgiens refuser de les soigner. Guy s'élève contre cette pratique, dangereuse pour les malades.' 'Fractures and dislocations were often left to dressers; in the following centuries, as surgeons refused to treat them. Guy protested this practice because it was dangerous for the injured.'
12. Giles, *Matthew Paris's English History*, Vol. II, p. 513.
13. Arcini, *Health and Disease in Early Lund*, p. 140, see also, p. 135 for details of the survey. The breakdown of bodies examined is as follows, dating from 990–1100, 1,104 skeletons, 1100–1300, 407 bodies, 1300–1536, 755 burials.
14. Ibid., pp. 149 and 150.
15. Ibid., p. 149. See also, Mitchell, *Medicine in the Crusades*, p. 117.
16. Arcini, *The Viking Age*, p. 63.
17. Du Chaillu, *The Viking Age*, Vol. II, p. 376, 'At night three men had their arms broken, and many were bruised or maimed …'.
18. Walker, *Disease in London*, pp. 125 and 126, for St Mary Spital, and Jean D. Dawes and J.R. Magilton, *The Cemetery of St Helen-on-the-Walls, Aldwark* (York, Council for British Archaeology, 1980), p. 56, for St Helen-on-the-Walls.
19. Thomas Fuller, *The History of the University of Cambridge and of Waltham Abbey with the Appeal of Injured Innocence* (James Nichols, 1840), p. 20.
20. Arthur and Corbett (trans), *The Knight of the Two Swords*, p. 112, '… he pushed him right out of the saddle, knocking him to the ground; and in falling the man broke his arm …', see also, p. 61.

21. Mitchell, *Medicine in the Crusades*, p. 117. See also, Shirley (trans.), *The Song of the Cathar Wars*, p. 186, '... sergeants entered the battle to kill the fallen'.
22. Dasent (trans.), *The Story of Burnt Njal or Njal's Saga*, Vol. I, p. 176, see also, p. 57, 'Then Hrut made a blow with the sword in his right hand at Thiostolfs leg, just above the knee ...'. See also, Vol. II, p. 276, for a spear aimed at the calves of another.
23. Arcini, *The Viking Age*, p. 64.
24. Shirley (trans.), *The Song of the Cathar Wars*, p. 170.
25. *Medieval Dead*, Season 1, Episode 2, *Last Stand at Visby* (Like a Shot Entertainment, 2013), see minutes 29–43 for discussion between osteoarchaeologists Malin Holst (University of York) and Petter Akeson (National Historical Museum, Sweden) on damage to the leg bones discovered in this mass grave. It goes into some detail about the tactics of aiming for a soldier's legs in battle. See also, Metzler, *A Social History of Disability in the Middle Ages*, p. 38, for more facts and figures on the bodies uncovered at Visby in the 1930s. More than 50 per cent of the skeletons had damage to the tibia bone.
26. Cockayne, *Leechdoms, Wortcunning and Starcraft of Early England*, Vol. II, p. 67, see also, another therapy, specific to the repair of a fractured lower leg, offered just prior to this one. It follows the same pattern of limited information, offering only the use of a splint and a salve made from crushed bonewort (daisy?) mixed with egg white.
27. Ibid., p. 69, this type of fracture can cause a shortening of the leg because the strong muscles of the thigh can pull either end of the bone at the fracture site, causing them to overlap, thus reducing the length of the limb. The remedy was to use a trough filled with hot water and curative herbs to make the limb more pliable to allow for it to be straightened and realigned.
28. Arcini, *The Viking Age*, p. 64.
29. Corner, 'On Early Salernitan Surgery and Especially the "Bamberg Surgery"', p. 10.
30. Roseman (trans.), *Chirurgia of Roger Frugard*, p. 140, the healing of the upper arm and forearm are noted as the reference for healing lower leg fractures.
31. Ibid., p. 114. See also, Pifteau, *Chirurgie de Guillaume de Sâlicet*, p. 391, William of Saliceto suggested three assistants when repairing a broken leg, '... tu auras trois servants capables ...', '... you will require three capable assistants ...'.
32. Roseman (trans.), *Chirurgia of Roger Frugard*, p. 114.
33. Campbell and Colton, *The Surgery of Theodoric*, Vol. I, pp. 168 and 180.
34. Larsen, *Old Icelandic Medical Miscellany*, p. 27, the remedy involving a stuffed rooster is from a group of Scandinavian manuscripts *c*. 1300 that are referred to as the *S* group, broken down into sections, *S* 9, *S* 10, etc.
35. Ibid., p. 212, part of *S* 25 that provides cures for sleeplessness and excessive thirst, among other things.
36. Cambro-Briton, *The Laws of Hywel Dha*, p. 396, the other two types of injuries that fell under this category were head wounds where the brain was exposed and, as we have seen already, stomach injuries in which the bowels could be seen.
37. J.A. Riley (trans.), *Annals of Roger de Hoveden, Comprising the History of England and of Other Countries of Europe From A.D. 732 TO A.D. 1201, Volumes I and II* (London, Henry G. Bohn, 1853), Vol. II, pp. 346 and 347. See also, Giles (trans.), *Roger of Wendover*, Vol. II, p. 140 and Stevenson, *Church Historians of England*, Vol. IV, Part II, p. 631, *The History of William of Newburgh*, for similar.
38. Rosenman (trans.), *Chirurgia of Roger Frugard*, p. 115.
39. Campbell and Colton, *The Surgery of Theodoric*, Vol. I, pp. 171–6, infection in the bone itself is also a very real concern and can be life-threatening.
40. Pifteau, *Chirurgie de Guillaume de Sâlicet*, p. 371.

41. D.-A. Hallbäck, 'A medieval(?) bone with a copper plate support, indicating an open surgical treatment', *Ossa*, 3⁴ (1976–7), p. 80, the twelfth century is the earliest possible date for this fix, however, it could very well be from a later medieval date.
42. Christopher J. Knüsel, Richard L. Kemp and Paul Budd, 'Evidence for Remedial Medical Treatment of a Severe Knee Injury from the Fishergate Gilbertine Monastery in the City of York', *Journal of Archaeological Science* (1995), 22, p. 381.
43. Campbell and Colton, *The Surgery of Theodoric*, Vol. I, p. 189, Theodoric noted that the ancient physicians considered the clavicle a difficult bone to fix.
44. Pálsson and Edwards (trans), *Seven Viking Romances*, p. 150.
45. Dasent (trans.), *The Story of Burnt Njal or Njal's Saga*, Vol. II, p. 290, see also, Vol. II, p. 272 and Vol. I, p. 56, '... hewed asunder the shoulderbone and collarbone'.
46. Arcini, *The Viking Age*, p. 63.
47. Ibid., p. 61. See also, Arcini, *Health and Disease in Early Lund*, p. 145, Arcini's large study of medieval bones from Lund, Sweden also included the clavicle in a limited number of cases.
48. Michael A. Newth (trans.), *The Song of Girart of Vienne by Bertrand de Bar-sur-Aube* (Tempe, Arizona Centre for Medieval & Renaissance Studies, 1999), p. 116, '... a blow upon his neck it breaks the collar-bone ...'. See also, Arthur and Corbett (trans), *The Knight of the Two Swords*, pp. 61, 111 and 112.
49. Comfort (trans.), *Erec and Enide*, p. 39.
50. Kibler (trans.), 'The Knight With the Lion (Yvain)', *Chrétien de Troyes – Arthurian Romances*, p. 434.
51. Campbell and Colton, *The Surgery of Theodoric*, Vol. I, p. 187, assistants are not normally named, however, see Pifteau, *Chirurgie de Guillaume de Sâlicet*, p. 426, for a rare inclusion in the surgery of William of Saliceto who named two physicians that assisted him in repairing a dislocated hip, master Gérard Ricius and master Albert Deretilionus, about whom little is known.
52. Campbell and Colton, *The Surgery of Theodoric*, Vol. I, pp. 188 and 189.
53. Pálsson and Edwards (trans), *Seven Viking Romances*, p. 201. See also, Arcini, *The Viking Age*, pp. 61 and 63, for examples of unhealed shoulder separations in two females.
54. Kunz (trans.), 'Eirik the Red's Saga', p. 662.
55. Cockayne, *Leechdoms, Wortcunning and Starcraft of Early England*, Vol. II, p. 327.
56. Bull, *The Miracles of Our Lady of Rocamadour*, p. 112, see n. 19, this was likely Robert III.
57. Shoulder separations are notorious for their recurrence. It is an injury that is common among modern ice-hockey players. Falls and collisions at speed with other players or against the wooden boards that surround the ice surface create impacts with significant force not unlike a fall from a horse. Ice-hockey players often have the same difficulty with repeat separations. Sincere thanks to former under 23 and university ice-hockey player Tyler Mort for his insight into this type of injury. He suffered with recurring shoulder separations, eventually requiring surgery to properly repair the damage.
58. Bull, *The Miracles of Our Lady of Rocamadour*, pp. 112 and 113.
59. Ibid., p. 113. See also, Edgington, *The Life and Miracles of St. Ivo*, pp. 44 and 45 for the eleventh-century account of a monk called Patrick from Coventry who fell from his horse, seemingly breaking his shoulder bones. He was said to have recovered very quickly, which as Edgington notes was more likely a case of a dislocated shoulder than a fracture. This was likely true in other more miraculous sounding cases, as well.

60. Walker, *Disease in London*, p. 120. See also, Dawes and Magilton, *The Cemetery of St Helen-on-the-Walls*, p. 56, for another with chronic dislocation of the shoulder, leaving the individual with a partial disability, and Rosenman (trans.), *Surgery of William of Saliceto*, p. 170, William noted that when it came to recurring separations resulting from damaged ligaments there was nothing that could be done to assist the patient.
61. Francis William Bourdillon (trans.), *Aucassin and Nicolette – Translated from the Old French* (London, Kegan Paul, Trench, Trübner & Co. Ltd, 1903), p. 56.
62. Ibid., p. 58.
63. Paterson, 'Military Surgery', p. 140.
64. Rosenman (trans.), *Surgery of Bruno da Longoburgo*, p. 44.
65. Rosenman (trans.), *Chirurgia of Roger Frugard*, p. 112, for Roger's instruction on the treatment of a dislocated shoulder. See also, Corner, 'On Early Salernitan Surgery and Especially the "Bamberg Surgery"', p. 20 for earlier *Bamberg Surgery* version of the same.
66. Rosenman (trans.), *Surgery of Roland of Parma*, pp. 75 and 76.
67. Michael A.H. Newth (trans.), *Heroes of the French Epic: A Selection of Chansons de Geste* (Woodbridge, Boydell Press, 2005), p. 593, from *The Knights of Narbonne*.
68. John O'Donovan, *Annals of Ireland – Three Fragments, Copied from Ancient Sources – From a Manuscript Preserved in the Burgundian Library at Brussels* (Dublin University Press, 1860), p. 147.
69. Alexander (trans.), *The Earliest English Poems*, pp. 35 and 36.
70. Laing, *Heimskringla*, Vol. III, p. 988.
71. Dasent (trans.), *The Story of Burnt Njal or Njal's Saga*, Vol. II, p. 54.
72. Pálsson and Edwards (trans), *Seven Viking Romances*, p. 268. See also, Du Chaillu, *The Viking Age*, Vol. II, p. 201, from the *Jomsvikings Saga*, 'Bui's teeth flew off at the blow', and Arcini, *The Viking Age*, p. 63, for archaeological evidence of the same, and Rasmus B. Anderson (trans.), *Viking Tales of the North – The Sagas of Thorstein, Viking's Son and Fridthjof the Bold* (Chicago, Scott, Foresman and Company, 1901), p. 8, in an odd reversal of roles Bjorn Blue-Tooth in *The Saga of Thorstein, Viking's Son* used his tooth in battle to kill and injure his enemies.
73. C.I. Matthews, 'The Anglo-Saxon cemetery at Marina Drive', Dunstable, *Bedfordshire Archaeological Journal*, 1 (1962), pp. 30 and 47. See also, T. Anderson, 'Dental treatment in Anglo-Saxon England', *British Dental Journal*, Volume 197, No. 5, 11 September 2004, p. 274 and Sam Lucy, *The Anglo-Saxon Way of Death – Burial Rites in Early England* (Stroud, Sutton Publishing, 2000), p. 94 for other examples, as well.
74. Cockayne, *Leechdoms, Wortcunning and Starcraft of Early England*, Vol. II, p. 53, see also, for more treatments.
75. Ibid., p. 311, see also, Vol. I, p. 95, from the *Old English Herbarium*.
76. Frisk, *A Middle English Translation of Macer Floridus De Viribus Herbarum*, p. 173.
77. Winston Black (trans.), *Henry Huntingdon – Anglicanus ortus – A Verse Herbal of the Twelfth Century* (Oxford, The Bodleian Library, 2012), p. 91.
78. Comfort (trans.), *Erec and Enide*, pp. 77 and 78. See also, Arthur and Corbett (trans), *The Knight of the Two Swords*, p. 116, the title character fights Brien de la Gastine in single combat. Knocking Brien to the ground, the Knight unlaced his helmet, pulled it off of his head, 'Then he fractured and crushed his face with the handle of his sword ...'.
79. Kibler (trans.), 'The Knight of the Cart (Lancelot)', *Chrétien de Troyes – Arthurian Romances*, p. 294. See also, Kibler (trans.), 'The Knight with the Lion (Yvain)',

Chrétien de Troyes – Arthurian Romances, pp. 371, de Troyes described the two knights, Yvain and Gawain, viciously beating each other about the face after their helmets had been knocked off (and p. 372).

80. Edward J. Kealey, *Medieval Medicus – A Social History of Anglo-Norman Medicine* (Baltimore, Johns Hopkins University Press, 1981), pp. 35 and 134.
81. Bull, *The Miracles of Our Lady of Rocamadour*, p. 113.
82. Metzler, *A Social History of Disability in the Middle Ages*, pp. 97 and 98. In twelfth- and thirteenth-century Europe it was not unusual for a knight to be expected to fight well into his 60s, with the age of 70 being the cut-off point in some places.
83. Bull, *The Miracles of Our Lady of Rocamadour*, p. 113. See also, Marlo Willows, 'Health Status in Lowland Medieval Scotland: A Regional Analysis of Four Skeletal Populations – Volume 1 and 2' (University of Edinburgh, Thesis, 2016), p. 250, a recent review of medieval burials from Scotland provides evidence that the concerns of this knight with the missing teeth may well have been justified. The 2016 work, completed by Marlo Willows, looked at four separate populations living in medieval Scotland between 500 and 1500. It was found that 42 per cent of the 385 skeletons examined had some form of dental disease, including tooth loss of some type. Now, this is a single study, but it provides an understanding of why the knight was as concerned as he was.
84. Bull, *The Miracles of Our Lady of Rocamadour*, p. 113, see also, Albe, *Les miracles de Notre-Dame de Roc-Amadour au XIIe siècle*, p. 105, 'Bientôt, ses dents perdues furent remises en place, différentes des autres par leur couleur qui était la blancheur de l'ivoire.' 'Soon the teeth he had lost were put back in place, different from the others by their colour, which was as white as ivory.'
85. Nicaise, *La grande chirurgie de Guy de Chauliac*, p. 510, see also, Introduction, p. LIV, Guy de Chauliac believed that teeth should also be left to the surgeons, rather than tooth pullers and the like, and Simona Minozzi et al., 'A Dental Prosthesis from the Early Modern Age in Tuscany (Italy)', *Clinical Implant Dentistry and Related Research*, 19 (2017), pp. 365–71, one of the oldest sets of dentures made from human teeth was discovered at the S. Francesco monastery in Lucca, Italy. It consists of ten teeth linked together by a band of gold. Its date has been difficult to pin down exactly, between the fourteenth and seventeenth centuries seems the most likely. If it is from the earlier date, it would go a long way to confirm Chauliac's assertion.
86. Walker, *Disease in London*, p. 257, ivory dental prostheses had a tendency to rot in the mouth over time, leading to all sorts of infections and ulcers. By the end of the eighteenth century fewer and fewer of these were being made using ivory.
87. Albe, *Les miracles de Notre-Dame de Roc-Amadour au XIIe siècle*, p. 105, '... il apportait quatre dents d'argent selon le nombre de celles qu'il avait perdues'. '... he brought with him four teeth made of silver, the same number that he had lost'. See also, Strange, *The Life and Gests of St. Thomas of Hereford*, pp. 171 and 172, a request for new teeth or thanksgiving for them seems to have been common at pilgrimage sites.
88. Gardiner (trans.), *Cligés*, p. 23, 'Nature bestowed special pains, so that whoever should see them [teeth] when the mouth opens would never dream that they were not of ivory or silver.' See also, Arthur and Corbett (trans), *The Knight of the Two Swords*, p. 64, teeth are here again compared to polished ivory.
89. Rosenman (trans.), *Chirurgia of Roger Frugard*, p. 66.
90. Campbell and Colton, *The Surgery of Theodoric*, Vol. I, p. 183. See also, Rosenman (trans.), *Surgery of William of Saliceto*, p. 148, for similar.
91. Pifteau, *Chirurgie de Guillaume de Sâlicet*, p. 71. See also, Siraisi, *Taddeo Alderotti*, p. 281, in the late thirteenth century, the doctor and professor of medicine at

Bologna, Taddeo Alderotti, was also treating dental problems, among a multitude of other medical issues, which at times could include things as diverse as hair loss and halitosis.
92. Comfort (trans.), *Erec and Enide*, p. 13.
93. Campbell and Colton, *The Surgery of Theodoric*, Vol. I, p. 124.
94. York Archaeological Trust, *Plague, Poverty, Prayer* (York, York Archaeological Trust, 2009), p. 19.
95. Hight (trans.), *The Saga of Grettir the Strong*, p. 35, Newth (trans.), *The Song of Girart of Vienne by Bertrand de Bar-sur-Aube*, p. 63, 'He splits his head and down spurt all his brains;', Flores (ed.), *An Anthology of Medieval Lyrics*, trans. Paul Blackburn, p. 52, from Bertran de Born's *Un sirventes cui motz no falh*, 'brains mixed with armour, a red mud smearing their heads', and Tyson (trans.), *Carmen de Triumpho Normannico*, p. 75, from *Carmen Widonis*.
96. Rosenman (trans.), *Surgery of Bruno da Longoburgo*, p. 51, fn. 19.
97. Terence Wise, *Men-at-Arms, Saxon, Viking and Norman* (Oxford, Osprey Publishing Ltd, 1979), p. 15. See also, Simpson, *Everyday Life in the Viking Age*, pp. 121–3, Logan Thompson, *Ancient Weapons in Britain* (Barnsley, Pen & Sword Military, 2004), p. 138, Ian Mortimer, *The Time Traveller's Guide to Medieval England – A Handbook for Visitors of the Fourteenth Century* (London, The Bodley Head, 2008), p. 120, among some of the many discussions on helmets or the lack of them in medieval warfare, and Bernard S. Bachrach and David S. Bachrach (trans), *Widukind of Corvey – Deeds of the Saxons* (Washington DC, The Catholic University of America Press, 2014), p. 128, Widukind of Corvey noted how dangerous it could be for those without a helmet in medieval battle. Duke Conrad the Red was killed in 955 after he was struck by an arrow in the neck, '… when he loosened the clasps of his helmet and sucked in air, he was struck by arrows …'.
98. Taylor (trans.), *Master Wace*, p. 209.
99. *Medieval Dead*, Season 1, Episode 2, *Last Stand at Visby*, see minutes 28–30. Most of the soldiers who died defending the island of Gotland in Sweden, at the Battle of Visby in 1361, were buried with the armour still on their bodies, all except their helmets. No helmet has ever been recovered from the more than 1,000 skeletons excavated at the battle site. These were no doubt taken by the conquering army, as both helmets and weapons were easily portable and reusable or could be recycled into something else.
100. Newth (trans.), *The Song of Girart of Vienne by Bertrand de Bar-sur-Aube*, p. 96. See also, Newth (trans.), *Heroes of the French Epic*, p. 667, from the *The Knights of Narbonne*, 'The coif was strong and saved the skull beneath'.
101. Nelson (trans.), *The Annals of St-Bertin*, Preface, p. xiii, Genealogy III, at the time of the death of Charles the Child, Charles the Bald was King of Francia.
102. Ibid., p. 112.
103. Ibid., p. 134.
104. Dasent (trans.), *The Story of Burnt Njal or Njal's Saga*, Vol. II, p. 207, saga after saga contain such references, see also, Anderson (trans.), *Viking Tales of the North*, p. 56, from *The Saga of Thorstein Viking's Son*, 'The sword hit the helmet, split the whole body and the byrnie-clad man from head to foot …', and Alexander (trans.), *Beowulf*, p. 145, the Swedish king Ongentheow struck a return blow at the head of Wulf the son of Wonred, managing to '… cut through the casque [helmet] on his head …'.
105. Elton (trans.), *The First Nine Books of the Danish History of Saxo Grammaticus*, pp. 68 and 69, see also, pp. 137, 317 and 326 for more of the same.

106. Knut Wester, 'The mystery of the missing Viking helmets', *Neurosurgery*, Vol. 47, Issue 5 (November 2000), pp. 1216–29, a compelling article on the subject of Viking helmets or the lack of them. In Norway alone, 10,000-plus weapons have been recovered from Viking graves, but in all of Scandinavia just one complete Viking helmet has ever been found.
107. Chris Caple, 'The Yarm Helmet', *Medieval Archaeology*, Vol. 64 (2020), Issue 1, pp. 31–64.
108. Arcini, *Health and Disease in Early Lund*, pp. 147–50, see also, p. 135 for more on the survey. See also, Arcini, *The Viking Age*, p. 61 for more on this study, as well.
109. Arcini, *Health and Disease in Early Lund*, p. 146, within the date range of 990–1100 there were 1,104 skeletons and only 407 between 1100–1300.
110. Ibid., p. 149. See also, Arcini, *The Viking Age*, p. 67. Burials between 500 and 900 tended to have been cremations, leaving little in the way of buried clues.
111. Arcini, *The Viking Age*, p. 63.
112. Ibid., Arcini offers a number of plausible suggestions around this unusual fact.
113. Cockayne, *Leechdoms, Wortcunning and Starcraft of Early England*, Vol. II, p. 23.
114. Ibid., p. 93.
115. Ibid., p. 343.
116. Cameron, *Anglo-Saxon Medicine*, p. 39.
117. Sheingorn (trans.), *The Book of Sainte Foy*, p. 301, n. 47, for more on the castle and its exact location.
118. Ibid., p. 201.
119. Bouillet and Servières, *Sainte Foy, vierge & martyre*, p. 573.
120. Sheingorn (trans.), *The Book of Sainte Foy*, p. 301, n. 48, this was quite likely water which had been used to wash the reliquary statue of St Foy and would have been seen to have taken on the healing powers of the saint.
121. Ibid., p. 202.
122. Meyer, *La chanson de la croisade contre les Albigeois*, p. 419, Simon de Montfort was killed by a large stone hurled from a mangonel, his helmet being of no use to him, 'Et la pierre vint tout droit là où il fallait, et frappa si juste le comte sur le heaume d'acier qu'elle lui mit en morceaux les yeux, la cervelle, les dents, le front, la mâchoire …'. 'And the rock came right to where it needed to be, and directly hit the count right on his steel helmet, smashing his eyes, his brain, his teeth, forehead, jaw …'.
123. Wright (trans.), *The Historical Works of Giraldus Cambrensis*, pp. 191 and 192.
124. Ibid., p. 192.
125. Arthur and Corbett (trans), *The Knight of the Two Swords*, pp. 30–5.
126. Rosenman (trans.), *Chirurgia of Roger Frugard*, p. 42, fn. 11.
127. Ibid., pp. 40 and 41.
128. Ibid., p. 37.
129. Ibid., pp. 39, 44, 48 and 49, as examples of trepanation within Roger's surgery. See also, Paterson, 'Military Surgery', p. 125, an interesting side note from Raimon of Avignon, in his thirteenth-century version of Roger Frugard's surgery. He claimed that sergeants were in fact the soldiers most susceptible to head injuries during battle, especially if they were '… without an iron hat …', a fact seemingly confirmed in the story of Fulk Fitz Warine, Wright (trans.), *The History of Fulk Fitz Warine*, p. 76, 'Then a sergeant sprang forward, and struck John a great blow with a sword. John struck him again on the head, that he fell to the ground insensible.'
130. Walker, *Disease in London*, p. 151.
131. Ibid., pp. 91 and 92.

132. Campbell and Colton, *The Surgery of Theodoric*, Vol. I, pp. 110 and 111.
133. Rosenman (trans.), *William of Saliceto*, p. 106. See also, Pifteau, *Chirurgie de Guillaume de Sâlicet*, p. 251, '… et l'enlèvement de quelques parties de l'os coupé, séparées de l'os sain et non lésé, étant faite par moi avec mes instruments, lorsque j'ai vu clairement et ouvertement toute la plaie …'. '… and the removal of some of the slivers of bone, separated from the healthy part of the skull, which had not been damaged, as done by me with my instruments, when I saw the whole wound clearly and openly …'.
134. Pifteau, *Chirurgie de Guillaume de Sâlicet*, pp. 251 and 252.
135. Rosenman (trans.), *Surgery of William of Saliceto*, p. 107, Saliceto is careful to note that it was the help of God and Nature that resulted in Lazarino's return to good health.

Chapter 6 – Disfigured and Disabled
1. Ferrante (trans.), *Guillaume d'Orange*, p. 94.
2. Michael C.C. Adams, *Living Hell – The Dark Side of the Civil War* (Baltimore, Johns Hopkins University Press, 2014), p. 146.
3. Julie Anderson, '"Jumpy Stump": amputation and trauma in the first world War', *First World War Studies*, 6 (2015), p. 9.
4. Mortimer, *The Time Traveller's Guide to Medieval England*, p. 36, see his discussion on the number of disfigured and disabled who would have existed within the population from injuries received during war. While Mortimer is discussing the fourteenth century, the same holds true for these five centuries, particularly after extended periods of war. See also, Metzler, *A Social History of Disability in the Middle Ages*, pp. 19 and 218, n. 62 for similar, and Helen J. Nicholson (trans.), *The Chronicle of the Third Crusade* (Farnham, Ashgate Publishing Limited, 2001), p. 193, from the Third Crusade (1187–92) the captured were mutilated by having one eye put out or their nose cut off or a hand or foot maimed.
5. Tschan, *History of the Archbishops of Hamburg-Bremen*, p. 76. See also, Garmonsway (trans.), *The Anglo-Saxon Chronicle*, p. 145 for similar.
6. Wright (trans.), *The History of Fulk Fitz Warine*, p. 70.
7. Meyer, *La chanson de la croisade contre les Albigeois*, p. 363, as the men of Toulouse attacked the Crusaders '… et la chair, le carnage, les membres, les os, les bras, les jambes, les cheveux et les mentons …'. '… and the flesh and carnage, limbs, bones, arms, legs, hair and chins'.
8. Du Chaillu, *The Viking Age*, Vol. II, p. 438, Ari the One-Eyed and Haki the Cheek-Cut One and Dasent (trans.), *The Story of Burnt Njal or Njal's Saga*, Vol. II, p. 115, for Kettle Flatnose.
9. Irina Metzler, 'Medieval Bynames and Nicknames that Relate to "Disability"', *The Treatment of Disabled Persons in Medieval Europe* (Lewiston, NY, The Edwin Mellen Press, 2010), p. 378, see Appendix, pp. 353–85 for a large list of similar names compiled by Dr Metzler.
10. Ibid., p. 373. See also, Irina Metzler, 'What's in a name? Considering the Onomastics of Disability in the Middle Ages', *The Treatment of Disabled Persons in Medieval Europe* (Lewiston, NY, The Edwin Mellen Press, 2010), p. 33, for Hamal.
11. Elton (trans.), *The First Nine Books of the Danish History of Saxo Grammaticus*, p. 245. see also, p. 144, '… for his unscarred face and his brow, ploughed by no marks of battle, showed that his knowledge of such matters was but slender'.
12. Bouillet and Servières, *Sainte Foy, vierge & martyre*, p. 598, see also, p. 597, the scribe recalled heroes of the ancient world and their scars of battle being something desirable.

13. Hitti, *An Arab-Syrian Gentleman & Warrior in the Period of the Crusades*, p. 79.
14. Ibid., pp. 80 and 81.
15. Benton (ed.), *Self and Society in Medieval France*, p. 181, see fn. 9, Benton notes the frequency of a secret mark used to identify a corpse in medieval literature, although this does not always represent the types of scars noted here. See also, Freeman, *History of the Norman Conquest of England*, p. 514.
16. Elton (trans.), *The First Nine Books of the Danish History of Saxo Grammaticus*, p. 218.
17. Kibler (trans.), 'The Knight with the Lion (Yvain)', *Chrétien de Troyes – Arthurian Romances*, p. 331, one of the women who found the knight was alerted to the fact that it was Yvain by seeing the scar, when frankly nothing else could identify him.
18. Ferrante (trans.), *Guillaume d'Orange*, p. 92.
19. Ibid., p. 96.
20. Ibid., p. 236, see also, p. 281.
21. Bull, *The Miracles of Our Lady of Rocamadour*, pp. 35 and 36. See Chapter 2 here for more on the process for establishing a miracle.
22. Albe, *Les miracles de Notre-Dame de Roc-Amadour au XIIe siècle*, p. 160, 'En effet il est guéri: il se rend au sanctuaire de la Vierge, il montre ses cicatrices ...'. 'He was healed and so he returned to the sanctuary of the Virgin, where he showed his scars ...'.
23. Bouillet and Servières, *Sainte Foy, vierge & martyre*, p. 530, 'En peu de temps le jeune homme se trouva si bien guéri qu'il ne conserva de sa plaie qu'une légère cicatrice visible à tous les regards ...'.
24. Rice, *The Hermit of Finchale*, p. 317.
25. John Jay Parry (trans.), *The Art of Courtly Love by Andreas Capellanus* (New York, Columbia University Press, 1941), p. 174.
26. Ibid.
27. Cockayne, *Leechdoms, Wortcunning and Starcraft of Early England*, Vol. II, p. 57. See also, Cameron, *Anglo-Saxon Medicine*, p. 169 for more. See also, Kenneth Young (trans.), *Handbook to the Cultural History of the Middle Ages – Supplementary to displays in Bryggens Museum* (Bergen, Bryggens Museum, 1978), p. 63, around 1248, a German barber-surgeon called Vilhjalmr apparently performed an operation to fix a cleft lip in Norway in the presence of King Hakon Hakonsson.
28. Giles, *Matthew Paris's English History*, Vol. I, p. 39.
29. Campbell and Colton, *The Surgery of Theodoric*, Vol. I, p. 135. See also, Rosenman (trans.), *Surgery of Lanfranchi of Milan*, p. 90. Other surgeons were also cognizant of leaving unsightly scars. Lanfranchi noted more than once that doctors should be especially careful around the face to avoid leaving disfiguring scars when repairing damage.
30. Campbell and Colton, *The Surgery of Theodoric*, Vol. I, p. 135.
31. Larson (trans.), *The King's Mirror*, p. 226.
32. Sibley and Sibley (trans), *The History of the Albigensian Crusade*, p. 164.
33. Larson (trans.), *The King's Mirror*, p. 224, this thirteenth-century Norwegian text notes, 'Boiling water, molten glass, and molten lead are also useful in defending walls.'
34. Dass (trans.), *Viking Attacks on Paris*, p. 33.
35. Dasent (trans.), *The Story of Burnt Njal or Njal's Saga*, Vol. II, p. 179. See also, Martin S. Regal (trans.), 'Gisli Sursson's Saga', *The Sagas of the Icelanders* (London, Penguin Books, Penguin Group, 2001), p. 503, *Gisli Sursson's Saga* is another story in which twelve were burned to death in an attack while ten others managed to escape the smoke and flames, and Jones (trans.), *Eirik the Red and Other Icelandic Sagas*, p. 232, for a similar tale from *King Hrolf and his Champions*.

36. Hight (trans.), *The Saga of Grettir the Strong*, pp. 18 and 242, n. 18, the character of Svidukari 'Scorched Kari' (Kari Solmund) appears in this saga.
37. Dasent (trans.), *The Story of Burnt Njal or Njal's Saga*, Vol. II, p. 207, from a song sung by Kari, 'Listen men unto my moaning, Mark the telling of my grief.' See also here, section on 'Nightmares' in Chapter 8 for more on psychological damage done to Kari.
38. Larson (trans.), *The King's Mirror*, p. 225, see also, p. 215 for another reference to coal and sulphur. See also, Meyer, *La chanson de la croisade contre les Albigeois*, p. 240, 'Et lorsque le soufre fut enflammé et liquéfié, l'odeur et la flamme ont tellement suffoqué les mineurs, qu'aucun d'eux ne put y rester et n'y resta.' 'And when the sulphur was set alight, the smell and flames choked the miners so much that none of them could remain there.'
39. Meyer, *La chanson de la croisade contre les Albigeois*, p. 257, '... l'eau et la chaux bouillante qu'on jette du mur dans le fossé, ...'. '... water and boiling lime thrown from the wall into the ditch ...'.
40. Giles (trans.), *Roger of Wendover*, Vol. II, pp. 399 and 400.
41. Mitchell, *Medicine in the Crusades*, p. 174.
42. Ferrante (trans.), *Guillaume d'Orange*, p. 173.
43. Nicholson (trans.), *The Chronicle of the Third Crusade*, p. 88.
44. Ibid., p. 109.
45. Giles, *Matthew Paris's English History*, Vol. III, p. 415.
46. Giles (trans.), *Roger of Wendover*, Vol. II, p. 409.
47. Samuel Hazzard Cross and Olgerd P. Sherbowitz-Wetzor (trans), *The Russian Primary Chronicle – Laurentian Text* (Cambridge, MA, The Mediaeval Academy of America, 1953), p. 72. See also, Giles (trans.), *Roger of Wendover*, Vol. I, p. 409 for similar description of Greek fire as 'lightning'.
48. Cross and Sherbowitz-Wetzor (trans), *The Russian Primary Chronicle*, p. 72.
49. Giles (trans.), *Roger of Wendover*, Vol. I, pp. 92, 104 and 407. See also, Forester (trans.), *The Ecclesiastical History of England and Normandy by Orderic Vitalis*, Vol. III, p. 156 and Giles, *Matthew Paris's English History*, Vol. II, pp. 374, 385, just a few of the many references to Greek fire that can be found within the contemporary chronicles.
50. Larson (trans.), *The King's Mirror*, p. 226, even as far north as Norway this text references a siege weapon described as '... a stooping shield-giant which breathes forth flame and fire'. In his note on the same page Larson suggests that it may be a reference to Greek fire seen by Norwegians during the Crusades.
51. Riley (trans.), *Annals of Roger de Hoveden*, Vol. II, p. 372, Dieppe in Normandy was a part of English territory at this time.
52. Samuel Bentley (ed.), *Excerpta Historica or Illustrations of English History* (London, Samuel Bentley, 1860), p. 428, the entry comes from Pipe Roll 6 of Richard I (London and Middlesex). 'Pro carriandis targiis et quarellis et pilettis et *igne greco* a Lond. usque Notingeham.'
53. *Calendar of Documents Relating to Scotland, Preserved in the Public Record Office and the British Library – Volume V (Supplementary)*, p. 183.
54. Revd Joseph Stevenson, *Documents Illustrative of the History of Scotland from the Death of King Alexander the Third to the Assession of Robert Bruce, Volumes I and II* (Edinburgh, HM General Register House, 1870), Vol. II, pp. 479 and 480.
55. Nicholson (trans.), *The Chronicle of the Third Crusade*, p. 88.
56. Wright (trans.), *The Historical Works of Giraldus Cambrensis*, p. 289. See also, Forester (trans.), *The Ecclesiastical History of England and Normandy by Orderic Vitalis*, Vol. II,

pp. 517 and 519, Orderic Vitalis relates a burn scar on the face of a priest called Walkelin, Stevenson, *Church Historians of England*, Part I, Vol. V, p. 300, Gervase of Canterbury, a monk of the late twelfth and early thirteenth centuries wrote, 'Odo sent soldiers, who violently dragged from the king's court the woman of fornication, and having seared her face with a hot iron, he banished her.'
57. Cockayne, *Leechdoms, Wortcunning and Starcraft of Early England*, Vol. II, p. 131. See also, Cameron, *Anglo-Saxon Medicine*, p. 128 for more specifics on burn remedies in *Leechbook III*.
58. Larsen, *Old Icelandic Medical Miscellany*, p. 159.
59. Priscilla Throop (trans.), *Hildegard von Bingen's Physica – The Complete English Translation of her Classic Work on Health and Healing* (Rochester, VT, Healing Arts Press, 1998), p. 68.
60. Rosenman (trans.), *Chirurgia of Roger Frugard*, p. 143.
61. Rosenman (trans.), *Surgery of Roland of Parma*, p. 100.
62. Rosenman, *Chirurgia of Roger Frugard*, p. 143.
63. Campbell and Colton, *The Surgery of Theodoric*, Vol. II, p. 135.
64. Ibid.
65. Rosenman (trans.), *Surgery of William of Saliceto*, p. 77.
66. Giles (trans.), *Roger of Wendover*, Vol. II, p. 352.
67. Ibid. See also, Mitchell, *Medicine in the Crusades*, pp. 124 and 125 for more on torture methods like these.
68. Forester (trans.), *The Ecclesiastical History of England and Normandy by Orderic Vitalis*, Vol. III, p. 30, '... his great delight was, like Phalaris the Sicilian, to invent new and unheard of modes of torturing his wretched victims'.
69. Hennessy, *Annals of Ulster*, p. 207. See also, John O'Donovan, *Annals of the Kingdom of Ireland – By the Four Masters – From the Earliest Period to the Year 1616 – Volumes I and II* (Dublin, Hodges, Smith and Co., 1856), p. 343, this chronicle indicates that some of these six were crucified.
70. Mageoghagan, *Annals of Clonmacnoise*, p. 133, the chronicle does not name any specific means of torture, simply '... all manner of crueltyes ...'.
71. Ibid., p. 160, 'Moylekyeran o'Mayney was cruelly tortured and martyred to death by the Danes of Dublin.'
72. Laing, *Heimskringla*, Vol. I, p. 45. See also, Joseph Anderson (ed.), *Orkneyinga Saga* (Edinburgh, Edmondston and Douglas, 1873), Introduction, p. xxiv, including n. 2, for more on the Blood-Eagle. See also, George Stephens (trans.), 'Tegner's Fridthjof's Saga', *Viking Tales of the North – The Sagas of Thorstein, Viking's Son and Fridthjof the Bold* (Chicago, Scott, Foresman and Company, 1901), p. 299 from *Fridthjof's Saga*, 'Fall'st thou, war-brother, I'll 'venge thee well; Blood-eagle lines on thy foe shall be flowing.'
73. Tschan, *History of the Archbishops of Hamburg-Bremen*, p. 208, 'Even dogs and horses hang there with men', fn. 'b' has more.
74. Lunde and Stone (trans), *Ibn Fadlān and the Land of Darkness*, p. 53, see also, p. 127 for Ibn Rusta's account of a woman who is buried alive, 'When a leading man dies ...', being placed inside his tomb.
75. Sheingorn (trans.), *The Book of Sainte Foy*, pp. 190 and 191.
76. Bouillet and Servières, *Sainte Foy, vierge & martyre*, p. 563.
77. A. Jessopp and M.R. James (trans), *The Life and Miracles of St. William of Norwich by Thomas of Monmouth* (Cambridge University Press, 1896), p. 198. See also, McAlhany and Rubenstein (trans), *Guibert of Nogent*, p. 275, in his early twelfth-

century work *On the Inner World* the monk, Guibert of Nogent, recalled other tortures including those who were hung up by the genitals, some who had their teeth pulled out with iron tools and an odd one that had been developed centuries earlier in the Roman world. It involved continuously coating a prisoner's heels in salt and allowing a goat to lick away the salt and flesh from the feet of the unfortunate captive, see also, pp. 338 and 339, n. 16 for more on this torture method. See also, Benton (ed.), *Self and Society in Medieval France*, p. 185, Nogent speaks again about those who were hung by the testicles or penis. Nogent explains Thomas of Marle's mistreatment of prisoners, '... he hung them up by their testicles, and as these often tore off from the weight of the body, the vitals soon burst out'. In some cases, a stone was placed on the shoulders of the prisoner to create more tearing force. See also, Sibley and Sibley (trans), *The History of the Albigensian Crusade*, p. 169 for similar. Captive crusaders were subjected to torture by the Cathars who '... tied cords to their genitals and pulled them violently'.
78. Sibley and Sibley (trans), *The History of the Albigensian Crusade*, p. 127, n. 49 regarding Walter Langton.
79. Ibid.
80. Rosenman (trans.), *Surgery of William of Saliceto*, p. 140.
81. Ibid., p. 142.
82. Ibid., p. 140, fn. 132, Rosenman notes that some types of damage would have been beyond the medicine of the time. No doubt true, there are any number of injuries associated with this sort of abuse that would have been outside the capability of the doctors of the time, for example, dental, damage to internal organs, etc.
83. Ibid., pp. 140 and 141.
84. Ibid., p. 142.
85. Ibid., p. 140, fn. 131.
86. Dr Leonard D. Rosenman (trans.), *The Surgery of Henri De Mondeville – Volume II* (Xlibris Corporation, 2003), pp. 742 and 743.
87. Ibid., p. 741.
88. Ibid., pp. 741 and 742.
89. Ibid., p. 742.
90. Ibid.
91. Ibid., p. 539, Henri de Mondeville died before his treatise on bones could be written.
92. Bessel van der Kolk, *The Body Keeps Score – Mind, Brain and Body in the Transformation of Trauma* (London, Penguin Books, 2014), pp. 79, 80 and 190.
93. Rosenman (trans.), *Surgery of William of Saliceto*, p. 141.
94. Rosenman (trans.), *Surgery of Henri De Mondeville*, p. 742.
95. Hight (trans.), *The Saga of Grettir the Strong*, p. 3.
96. Rosenman (trans.), *Surgery of Lanfranchi of Milan*, p. 89.
97. Patricia Skinner, *Living with Disfigurement in Early Medieval Europe* (New York, Palgrave MacMillan, 2017), pp. 75 and 76, see also, p. 112, one source claims it was both his nose and ears that were removed and later replaced with ones made of gold.
98. Guibert of Nogent, *The Deeds of God through the Franks* (Teddington, Echo Library, 2008), p. 72.
99. G. Sperati, 'Amputation of the nose throughout history or L'amputazione del naso nella storia', *Acta Otorhinolaryngol Ital* (2009), 29, p. 48, see sixteenth-century example made from papier mâché. While well out of the date range and available material here, it does represent the sort of homemade prosthesis that could have been constructed from a piece of shaped and hardened leather or carved wood.

100. David M. Lubin, 'Masks, Mutilation, and Modernity: Anna Coleman Ladd and the First World War', *Archives of American Art Journal*, Vol. 47, No. 3/4 (2008), pp. 4–6. See also, Julie Anderson, 'Mutilation and Disfiguration', 3 August 2017, *International Encyclopedia of the First World War*, https://encyclopedia.1914-1918-online.net/article/mutilation_and_disfiguration. She notes that many disfigured French soldiers did not wear a mask after the war, but instead chose to tie a cloth around the mutilated portion of their faces.
101. Pálsson and Edwards (trans), *Seven Viking Romances*, p. 230.
102. Ileana Micarelli, Robert Paine, Caterina Giostra, Mary Anne Tafuri, Antonio Profico, Marco Boggioni, Fabio Di Vincenzo, Danilo Massani, Andrea Papini and Giorgio Manzi, 'Survival to amputation in pre-antibiotic era: a case study from a Longobard necropolis (6th–8th centuries AD)', *Journal of Anthropological Sciences*, Vol. 96 (2018), p. 193, see also, pp. 194 and 195 for further evidence of the same.
103. Ibid., p. 192.
104. Ibid., p. 196.
105. Dass (trans.), *Viking Attacks on Paris*, p. 63, Oddo was perhaps the Lord of Dunois and Chartrain, see also, p. 114, n. 100, for more on his possible identity.
106. Forester (trans.), *The Ecclesiastical History of England and Normandy by Orderic Vitalis*, Vol. III, p. 15, fn. 1. 'There seems no reason to doubt the truth of these accounts', and Kealey, *Medieval Medicus*, p. 189, there are those who do doubt the veracity of this story, but it must be said that some of the other artificial limbs and appendages already seen seem only to strengthen Forester's view.
107. M. Binder, J. Eitler, J. Deutschmann, S. Ladstätter, F. Glaser and D. Fiedler, 'Prosthetics in antiquity – An early medieval wearer of a foot prosthesis (6th century AD) from Hemmaberg/Austria', *International Journal of Paleopathology*, Vol. 12, March 2016, p. 31, see also, p. 33, another skeleton, an adult male dating to the sixth century, was found at Hemmaberg in Southern Austria missing his lower left leg and foot. The remnants of a prosthesis of some sort were found constructed using an iron ring, which was attached to the stump and secured a replacement leg perhaps made of wood.
108. Ibid.
109. Hight (trans.), *The Saga of Grettir the Strong*, p. 3, Onund Treefoot, and Pálsson and Edwards (trans), *Eyrbyggja Saga*, p. 52, for Thorir Wood-Leg.
110. Pálsson and Edwards (trans), *Eyrbyggja Saga*, p. 52.
111. Ibid., p. 54.
112. Bennett (trans.), *La Chanson de Guillaume*, p. 137.
113. Kibler (trans.), 'The Story of the Grail (Percival)', *Chrétien de Troyes – Arthurian Romances*, pp. 474 and 475.
114. Jessopp and James (trans), *The Life and Miracles of St. William of Norwich by Thomas of Monmouth*, p. 275, see also, p. 205, for another pilgrim, a poor woman who used this trestle method to transport herself around.
115. Ibid.
116. Ibid., p. 245 for handbarrow, and p. 242 for horse.
117. Stevenson, *Church Historians of England*, Vol. III, Part II, p. 562, Simeon of Durham.
118. Ivo Štefan, Petra Stránská and Hana Vondrová, 'The archaeology of early medieval violence: the mass grave at Budeč', *Czech Republic. Antiquity*, 90 (2016), pp. 766, 771 and 772.
119. Carole Rawcliffe, *Medicine & Society in Later Medieval England* (Stroud, Sutton Publishing Ltd, 1995), p. 3.

120. BBC, *History Cold Case*, Series Two, Episode Three, *The York 113* (Shine TV Limited and Red Planet Pictures, 2011), see especially minutes 37–9 for discussion on the role of the disabled in early armies.
121. Metzler, *A Social History of Disability in the Middle Ages*, p. 40.
122. Rawcliffe, *Medicine & Society in Later Medieval England*, pp. 3 and 4.
123. Tyson (trans.), *Carmen de Triumpho Normannico*, pp. 107 and 109, see fn. 98. See also, Thierry, Vol. I, p. 185, who names him as Ansgar, '... an old soldier, named Ansgar, whose legs were paralyzed with fatigue and wounds, and who was carried on a litter wherever his duty called him'. William the Conqueror may have consulted with him secretly to try and secure a peaceful surrender of the city to the Normans. Once again see Tyson (trans.), *Carmen de Triumpho Normannico*, p. 110, fn. 'a' regarding the possible confusion in Thierry around the name and individual called Ansgar.
124. Giles, *William of Malmesbury*, p. 437.
125. Forester (trans.), *The Ecclesiastical History of England and Normandy by Orderic Vitalis*, Vol. III, p. 450, fn. 2, Forester notes that Baldwin died on 17 June 1119.
126. Rosenman (trans.), *Surgery of William of Saliceto*, p. 35, William explained to his readers and students that it was important to collect a proper fee from a patient, because he believed that it strengthened a patient's respect for the surgeon, which helped him to heal better. See also, p. 111 for a fee taken. See also, p. 36, William seems to have had a slightly misguided sense of charity. He spoke of the importance of treating paupers, but only because it improved the surgeon's image, which would bring with it more patients and higher fees. See also, Roseman (trans.), *Surgery of Lanfranchi of Milan*, p. 32, William's student Lanfranchi was more generous in his approach suggesting that the fees of the rich should be such that they cover the cost of treating the poor.
127. Ibid., p. 107.
128. Metzler, *A Social History of Disability in the Middle Ages*, p. 40.
129. Forester (trans.), *The Ecclesiastical History of England and Normandy by Orderic Vitalis*, Vol. II, pp. 79 and 80. They do not appear to have been able to fight any further, because within a few sentences Vitalis noted that the largest part of William's forces was fighting overseas and the inference may be that these men were not included among them.
130. Ibid., p. 80, Vitalis wrote about William's inhuman treatment of his own soldiers, 'Many of those who shed their blood in his service have been treated with ingratitude, and on slight pretexts have been sentenced to death, as if they were his enemies.' See also, p. 79, it is important to note that Vitalis, who had been born in England, had a great dislike for William's conquest, which is certainly clear from his writing.
131. Skinner, *Living with Disfigurement in Early Medieval Europe*, p. 120. See also, Metzler, *Disability in Medieval Europe*, p. 119, regarding Harvey de Cornubia, a valet of Edward I. He was wounded fighting the Scots at Galway and was provided with expenses for his return home and to cover medical costs.
132. *Calendar of Documents Relating to Scotland Preserved in Her Majesty's Public Record Office, London – Volume II*, p. 369, taken from the Exchequer Q. R. Miscellanea (Wardrobe) Nos 28 and 24.
133. *Calendar of Documents Relating to Scotland, Preserved in the Public Record Office and the British Library – Volume V (Supplementary)*, p. 230, Documents Illustrative of English History in the Thirteenth and Fourteenth Centuries, from the Records of the Queen's Remembrancer in the Exchequer, ed. H. Cole (Rec. Comm., 1844) [fo. 4 v.]

134. *Calendar of the Close Rolls Preserved in the Public Record Office for Edward II – A.D. 1313–1319*, p. 192. See also, Moffat et al., *SHARP Practice 4*, pp. 65a, the suggestion is made that he was a carter, as his name indicates, almost certainly a part of the English war effort.
135. *Calendar of the Close Rolls Preserved in the Public Record Office for Edward II – A.D. 1313–1319*, p. 192.
136. Ibid., p. 193.
137. Skinner, *Living with Disfigurement in Early Medieval Europe*, p. 120, for a similar point on the rarity of payments such as these. See also, Moffat et al., *SHARP Practice 4*, pp. 65b for more about the last three on the list who lost their hands, and Metzler, *Disability in Medieval Europe*, p. 119, also discusses the rarity of such cases of soldiers being compensated for their injuries.
138. BBC, *History Cold Case*, Series One, Episode One, *Ipswich Man* (Shine TV Limited and Red Planet Pictures, 2011), see especially minutes 27–32 for more on the monastery itself, and 42–6 for more on the types of individuals that ended up in this medieval hospital because of serious disease or injury. Interestingly, the episode focuses on the skeleton of an African man living in England during the thirteenth century. It seems quite likely that he returned to England with Tiptoth after the Ninth Crusade. Like the others found in this grave site, he was seriously disabled, meaning that he was likely cared for by the Grey Friars before his death and burial at this monastery.
139. Kealey, *Medieval Medicus*, p. 155, no. 39.
140. Rotha Mary Clay, *The Mediaeval Hospitals of England* (London, Methuen & Co., 1909), p. 8.
141. Metzler, 'What's in a name? Considering the Onomastics of Disability in the Middle Ages', p. 45.
142. Norman Moore, *The History of the Study of Medicine in the British Isles* (Oxford, Clarendon Press, 1908), pp. 21 and 22.
143. Wilfred Owen, *Poems* (London, Penguin Classics, 2017), p. 35, Wilfred Owen, *Disabled*.
144. Ibid., pp. 36 and 37.

Chapter 7 – Illness and Infection

1. Giles (trans.), *Roger of Wendover*, Vol. II, pp. 15 and 16, from addition inserted into Roger's chronicle by Matthew Paris.
2. John Schofield and Alan Vince, *Medieval Towns – The Archaeology of British Towns in Their European Setting* (New York, Continuum, 1994), p. 240. See also, Mindy Weisberger, 'Medieval Germans Riddles with Tapeworms', Live Science, 5 October, 2018, livescience.com.
3. Hennessy, *Annals of Ulster*, p. 303.
4. I.S. Robinson (trans.), *Eleventh-Century Germany – The Swabian Chronicles* (Manchester University Press, 2008), pp. 78, 103 and 104 as examples.
5. Forester (trans.), *The Ecclesiastical History of England and Normandy by Orderic Vitalis*, Vol. III, p. 369.
6. Lunde and Stone (trans), *Ibn Fadlān and the Land of Darkness*, pp. 48 and 49.
7. Tschan, *History of the Archbishops of Hamburg-Bremen*, pp. 207 and 208.
8. Siraisi, *Medieval and Early Renaissance Medicine*, p. 8, for brief discussion on the subject.
9. Reginald of Durham, *Reginaldi Monachi Dunelmensis Libellus de Admirandis* (London, J.B. Nichols and Son, 1835), p. 295.

10. Flavius Vegetius Renatus, *De Re Militari – Concerning Military Affairs* (Leonaur, 2012), p. 68.
11. Ibid., p. 7.
12. Nelson (trans.), *The Annals of St-Bertin*, p. 129.
13. Robinson (trans.), *Eleventh-Century Germany*, p. 63.
14. Ibid., p. 71.
15. Adams, *Living Hell*, p. 24, until disease and germs began to be understood by medical science these things would remain far more lethal than the weapons of their time. Adams notes that during the Crimean War of the 1850s four out of every five deaths of British soldiers were the result of disease and infection.
16. Meyer, *La chanson de la croisade contre les Albigeois*, p. 69, 'Si Dieu ne leur envoie quelque plaie, comme il fit après leur donnant la dyssenterie, ils ne pourraient être pris.'
17. Dr H. Winter Griffith, *Complete Guide to Symptoms, Illness & Surgery* (New York, The Body Press, 1985), p. 256, there are two major forms of dysentery, bacillary and amebic.
18. Adams, *Living Hell*, p. 25.
19. A.W. Wheen (trans.), *All Quiet on the Western Front*, by Erich Maria Remarque (New York, Ballentine Books edn, 1982), p. 280.
20. Scholz, *Carolingian Chronicles*, p. 107.
21. Lunde and Stone (trans), *Ibn Fadlān and the Land of Darkness*, p. 147.
22. Ibid., p. 150.
23. Ibid., p. 151.
24. Stevenson, *Church Historians of England*, Vol. III, Part II, p. 517, from Simeon of Durham's *History of the Kings of England*.
25. Ibid., Vol. II, Part I, p. 260, *The Chronicle of Florence of Worcester*. See also, Forester (trans.), *The Ecclesiastical History of England and Normandy by Orderic Vitalis*, Vol. I, p. 488, regarding some of William the Conqueror's men not long after the Battle of Hastings, 'A great number of soldiers, who devoured flesh-meat half raw and drank too much water, died of dysentery, and many more felt the effects to the end of their days. The duke, leaving a garrison in the castle, with those who were suffering from dysentery.'
26. Cusimano and Moorhead (trans), *The Deeds of Louis the Fat*, pp. 153–5, Louis VI of France died of dysentery on 1 August 1137. See also, Giles (trans.), *Roger of Wendover*, Vol. II, p. 378, King John died on 19 October 1216.
27. Getz (ed.), *Healing and Society in Medieval England*, Introduction, p. xix.
28. Albert Way, 'Bill of Medicines Furnished for the Use of Edward I, 1306–1307', *Archaeological Journal* 14 (1857), pp. 267–9.
29. Cockayne, *Leechdoms, Wortcunning and Starcraft of Early England*, Vol. II, pp. 291 and 293. See also, Cameron, *Anglo-Saxon Medicine*, pp. 38 and 39, Cameron has suggested that in some cases the recitation of the paternoster was used, in the absence of clocks, as a timekeeping method for these recipes, which certainly makes sense. Reviewing this particular remedy, the use of Psalm 51 and the paternoster do not appear integral to the timing of the brewing process, as the mark of the liquid being ready was the milk turning a red colour. The nine wood chips held in the left hand while reciting the psalm and paternoster may form a link between Christian and pagan. The number nine appears very frequently in Norse and Germanic mythologies. See also, Andy Orchard (ed.), *The Elder Edda: A Book of Viking Lore* (London, Penguin Classics, Penguin Group, 2011), p. 35, Odin hung from the tree for nine nights before receiving wisdom, Du Chaillu, *The Viking Age*, Vol. I, p. 2,

the nine worlds of Norse mythology, Jesse Byock (trans.), *Snorri Sturluson – The Prose Edda* (London, Penguin Classics, Penguin Group, 2005), p. 73, at Ragnarok, after Thor killed the Midgard Serpent he walked back 9ft, Du Chaillu, *The Viking Age*, Vol. I, p. 35, 'Heimdall ... nine maidens bore him as son, and they were all sisters', along with numerous other examples of the use of the number nine. See also, Cockayne, *Leechdoms, Wortcunning and Starcraft of Early England*, Vol. II, p. 323, the same number appears over and over in other Anglo-Saxon concoctions such as in *Leechbook III*, 'For joint pain; sing nine times this incantation thereon, and spit thy spittle on the joint: "Malignus' obligavit; angelus curavit; dominus salvavit." It will soon be well with him.', see also, pp. 315, 347 and 349.

30. Cockayne, *Leechdoms, Wortcunning and Starcraft of Early England*, Vol. II, p. 279, for *Bald's*, see also, Frisk, *A Middle English Translation of Macer Floridus De Viribus Herbarum*, p. 91, for *Macer Floridus*, remedies using rose water are still prescribed in modern homeopathic therapies for similar issues.
31. Getz (ed.), *Healing and Society in Medieval England*, p. 193.
32. Stevenson, *Church Historians of England*, Vol. IV, Part II, p. 686, from the Norman chronicler Robert de Monte, for the year 1109, made reference to St Anthony's fire.
33. George Barger, *Ergot and Ergotism – A Monograph – Based on the Dohme Lectures Delivered in Johns Hopkins University, Baltimore* (London, Gurney and Jackson, 1931), p. 43, see also, M.R. Lee, 'The history of ergot of rye (Claviceps purpurea) I: From antiquity to 1900', *R Coll Physicians Edinb* (2009), 39, p. 182, and Torbjørn Alm and Brita Elvevag, 'Ergotism in Norway. Part 1: Symptoms and their interpretation from the late Iron Age to the seventeenth century', *History of Psychiatry*, 24 ^{1} (2012), p. 21, the word *ergot* itself comes from an older French word *argot* meaning a rooster's spur, referring to the shape of the hook at the end of the infected grains. This form was reflected in some translations of the Old Norse poem *Hávamál* or *The lay of the High One (Odin)*. They included 'spurred rye' as a remedy for a hernia, and Du Chaillu, *The Viking Age*, Vol. II, p. 411, 'And fire against constipation. The (corn) ear against spells, The spurred rye against hernia'.
34. Alm and Elvevag, 'Ergotism in Norway. Part 1', pp. 15–17. See also, Merriam-Webster, *Merriam-Webster's Medical Dictionary* (Springfield, MA, Merriam-Webster Inc., 2006), p. 232.
35. Shirley (trans.), *The Song of the Cathar Wars*, p. 103. See also, fn. 1, Meyer, *La chanson de la croisade contre les Albigeois*, p. 253, 'Et pour peu que cet infernal péril dure nous aurons plus souffert qu'un ardent de saint Martial'. 'And if this blasted danger continues it will be worse than St. Martial's Fire.', also fn. 2.
36. Nelson (trans.), *The Annals of St-Bertin*, p. 81.
37. Barger, *Ergot and Ergotism*, p. 43.
38. Nelson (trans.), *The Annals of St-Bertin*, pp. 82–7, for attacks between 856 and 858. See also, Barger, *Ergot and Ergotism*, p. 43, for the sack of Xanten.
39. Neil Oliver, *Vikings – A History* (London, Orion Publishing Group, 2013), p. 197.
40. Barger, *Ergot and Ergotism*, p. 44.
41. Alm and Elvevag, 'Ergotism in Norway. Part 1', p. 22.
42. Barger, *Ergot and Ergotism*, p. 45, contains a useful map that shows the major outbreaks throughout the centuries.
43. Ward, *Miracles and the Medieval Mind*, p. 142, see also, p. 145 for record of disfiguring damage to the face, and Barger, *Ergot and Ergotism*, p. 54, who mentions it as well, with breasts and faces both being harmed.
44. Barger, *Ergot and Ergotism*, p. 48, there are many examples like the one found in this section, 'Many were tortured and twisted by a contraction of the nerves; others died

miserably, their limbs eaten up by the holy fire and blackened like charcoal.' From the Lorraine area in France 1085.
45. Sheingorn (trans.), *The Book of Sainte Foy*, p. 28.
46. Bouillet and Servières, *Sainte Foy, vierge & martyre*, p. 617, 'Dans ces conjonctures, notre jeune soldat, après un long jeûne, n'eut pour sa part qu'un pain de seigle; il s'en nourrit avidement ... Pour apaiser sa faim, il en vint jusqu'à dévorer des aliments malsains qui, en trompant la nature, causaient les maux les plus funestes ...'. 'In these circumstances, our young soldier, after a long fast, only had rye bread; he fed on it greedily ... To appease his hunger, he had gone so far as to devour unhealthy foods which, by deceiving nature, caused the most fatal ailments ...'.
47. Ibid., '... les autres membres éprouvent une contraction extraordinaire'. '... his limbs experienced extraordinary contractions'.
48. Ibid., p. 618. See also, Sheingorn (trans.), *The Book of Sainte Foy*, pp. 254–6, according to the balance of the story he remained paralysed for four years before receiving healing at St Foy.
49. Bull, *The Miracles of Our Lady of Rocamadour*, p. 117, see also, p. 46, for further discussion of ergotism during this period.
50. Ibid., p. 118.
51. Barger, *Ergot and Ergotism*, p. 44, for similar details about the loss of limbs.
52. Lee, 'The history of ergot of rye (Claviceps purpurea) I', p. 182.
53. Capparoni, *Magistri Salneritani Nondum Cogniti*, p. 11.
54. Metzler, *A Social History of Disability in the Middle Ages*, p. 46, see also, p. 174, Dr Metzler explores the other side of this argument, in the thirteenth century, at hospitals in Angers and Troyes, those suffering from symptoms of ergotism were not welcome.
55. Frisk, *A Middle English Translation of Macer Floridus De Viribus Herbarum*, p. 123.
56. Ibid., p. 133, for other examples see pp. 70, 74, 125 and 146.
57. Pifteau (trans.), *Chirurgie de Guillaume de Sâlicet*, p. 145, '... lorsque quelque indice de corruption future commence à se montrer après le coït avec une femme infectée ...'.
58. Kevin Brown, *The Pox – The Life and Near Death of a Very Social Disease* (Stroud, Sutton Publishing, 2006), p. 123.
59. Ibid., pp. 184 and 185.
60. Adams, *Living Hell*, p. 24.
61. Ibid., p. 16.
62. Brown, *The Pox*, p. 63.
63. Francis Beaumont and John Fletcher, *The Knight of the Burning Pestle* (London, J.M. Dent and Co., 1898), p. 88, Act III, Sc. iv.
64. N. Bailey (trans.), *The Colloquies of Desiderius Erasmus – Concerning Men Manners and Things, Volume I* (London, Gibbings and Company, Limited, 1900), p. 284.
65. Brown, *The Pox*, pp. 8 and 9, Brown discusses some of the medieval references to gonorrhoea, including Richard II of England's surgeon, John of Arderne, who suggested using a syringe to send a lead solution down the urethra.
66. Ibid., pp. 1 and 2, see also, pp. 8 and 9, and J.D. Rolleston, 'Venereal Disease in Literature', *British Journal of Venereal Diseases*, 1 July 1934, pp. 151 and 152. Dr Rolleston and many others concur with Brown that any accounts of syphilis in Europe before the end of the fifteenth century are apocryphal and likely recorded in error or just simply unreliable. He also raises the valid point that were it a prevalent disease during the Middle Ages, writers such as Chaucer, Gower, Langland and many others would have almost certainly included a character like Sassoon's Bert who had 'gone syphilitic'.

67. Brown, *The Pox*, p. 24.
68. Nicholson, (trans.), *The Chronicle of the Third Crusade*, pp. 126 and 299, during the Third Crusade Christian soldiers were accused of spending far too much of their time in taverns and brothels, chasing pursuits of the flesh.
69. Giles, *William of Malmesbury – Chronicle of the Kings of England*, p. 469, see footnote regarding the large number of crusaders who came back from the Holy Land having given up their faith.
70. Ibid., he built the brothel near a castle called Niort.
71. Jacques Rossiaud, *Medieval Prostitution or La Prostituzione Nel Medioevo* (New York, Barnes and Noble, 1996), p. 4.
72. William Becket, *A Collection of Chirurgical Tracts* (London, E. Curll, 1740), p. 77, Appendix One, credited to Richard Rawlinson. See also, Arthur Burrell (trans.), *Piers Plowman, The Vision of a People's Christ by William Langland* (London and Toronto, Everyman's Library, 1912), p. 107, the character of Janet of the Stews, in William Langland's famous fourteenth-century tale *Piers Plowman*, would have been identifiable as a prostitute to later medieval readers by the second part of her name.
73. Becket, *A Collection of Chirurgical Tracts*, pp. 77 and 78.
74. Ibid., p. 78.
75. Joseph and Frances Gies, *Life in a Medieval City* (New York, Harper & Row Publishers, 1981), p. 86.
76. Stevenson, *Church Historians of England*, Vol. V, Part I, p. 281, Richard of Devizes.
77. Fuller, *The History of the University of Cambridge*, p. 20.
78. Ibid., p. 21.
79. Gies and Gies, *Life in a Medieval Castle*, pp. 178–82. See also, Giles, *Matthew Paris's English History*, Vol. III, p. 17, for a tournament in France in 1253 for specific examples.
80. Cockayne, *Leechdoms, Wortcunning and Starcraft of Early England*, Vol. II, p. 71, see also, Vol. III, p. 384, the index lists these cures under diseased genitals.
81. Franjo Gruber, Jasna Lipozenčić and Tatjana Kehler, 'History of Venereal Diseases from Antiquity to the Renaissance', *Acta Dermatovenerol Croat* (2015); 23^1, p. 7.
82. Green, *The Trotula*, p. 95.
83. Campbell and Colton, *The Surgery of Theodoric*, Vol. 2, p. 109, see also, p. 71, for a chapter on abscesses of the penis.
84. Rosenman (trans.), *Surgery of William of Saliceto*, p. 68, Chapter 48, 'Infections of the Penis'.
85. Jospeh Bédier, *The Romance of Tristan and Iseult* (New York, Random House Inc. Vintage Edition, 1965), p. 64, from the twelfth-century romance *Tristan and Iseult*, an example of the atrocious damage to the human form that this disease could cause, leaving so many with hideous disfigurements and impairments.
86. Forester (trans.), *The Ecclesiastical History of England and Normandy by Orderic Vitalis*, Vol. I, p. 394, in his capacity as a monk Vitalis must have seen many examples of leprosy, in both France and England.
87. Cameron, *Anglo-Saxon Medicine*, pp. 96 and 97. It certainly speaks to the incredible fear that leprosy brought with it that so many skin diseases were lumped into that same category, see also, Finucane, *Miracles and Pilgrim*, p. 105, Kealey, *Medieval Medicus*, p. 4 and Rosenman (trans.), *Chirurgia of Roger Frugard*, p. 144, fn. 82, who notes this 'waste-basket diagnosis' that was used for leprosy to account for just about any disease of the skin.

88. M.G. Belcastro, V. Mariotti, F. Facchini and O. Dutour, 'Leprosy in Skeleton from the 7th Century Necropolis of Vienne-Campochin (Molise, Italy)', *International Journal of Osteoarchaeology*, 15 (2005), pp. 433 and 434.
89. Ibid., p. 443. See also, Giles (trans.), *Roger of Wendover*, Vol. II, p. 44, 'That leprous persons, who are excluded from society shall have an oratory and priest of their own.'
90. Stevenson, *Church Historians of England*, Vol. II, Part II, p. 462, Asser's *Annals of King Alfred*.
91. Ibid., p. 463.
92. Arcini, *The Viking Age*, p. 67.
93. Ibid., pp. 68 and 69.
94. Hennessy, *Annals of Ulster*, p. 469, 'A great leprosy upon the Foreigners of Ath-cliath [Vikings of Dublin] ...'.
95. Peter Richards, *The Medieval Leper and His Northern Heirs* (Cambridge, D.S. Brewer, 1977), p. 5.
96. Anderson (trans.), *Viking Tales of the North*, pp. 11 and 12.
97. Ibid., p. 14. See also, Ármann Jakobsson and David Clark (trans), *The Saga of Bishop Thorlak* (Exeter, Short Run Press Limited, 2013), p. 24, another that mentions a man called Tjorvi the Leprous who had hands that were especially damaged by the disease.
98. Forester (trans.), *The Ecclesiastical History of England and Normandy by Orderic Vitalis*, Vol. I, pp. 423 and 424.
99. Ibid., p. 424.
100. John B. Cullen, 'The Ancient Churches of the Town of Wexford', *The Journal of the Royal Society of Antiquaries of Ireland Vol. V – Fifth Series* (Dublin, University Press, 1895), p. 375.
101. Wright (trans.), *The Historical Works of Giraldus Cambrensis*, pp. 207 and 208, 'His body was weak, but his spirit resolute; for being diseased with leprosy, which threatened his life, he sought to anticipate the effects of a disease by a premature, though glorious, death.'
102. Abbott, *St. Thomas of Canterbury*, Vol. II, pp. 51 and 52, see also, Finucane, *Miracles and Pilgrims*, pp. 149 and 150 for same and Abbott, Vol. I, p. 323, another miracle from the shrine St Thomas of Canterbury shows just how pitiful leper victims could be. It involved a man called Richard Sunieve, who was the herdsman of a knight of Edgeworth in Gloucestershire. When Richard began to find spots and swelling on his face he was still permitted to stay on the knight's estate, but the sores and ulcers became so pronounced that he was forced to leave not only the knight's house, but also the village. Pitifully his mother continued to feed him either by leaving food for him where he could find it or feeding him with the use of a long stick.
103. Abbott, *St. Thomas of Canterbury*, p. 52.
104. Bell (trans.), *Peasant Life in Old German Epics*, p. 96.
105. Ibid., p. 126. See also, Edward E. Foster, *Amis and Amiloun, Robert of Cisyle, and Sir Amadace* (Kalamazoo, Medieval Institute Publications, 2nd edn, 2007), pp. 2–6, another story called *Amis and Amiloun* is a tangled tale in which the character Amiloun becomes stricken with leprosy. The cure is made possible by the death of Amis' two children and Amiloun being anointed with their blood. These pages provide a good understanding of the plot in Modern English.
106. David Marcombe, *Leper Knights – The Order of St. Lazarus of Jerusalem in England, c. 1150–1544* (Woodbridge, Boydell & Brewer Ltd, 2003), p. 11.
107. Mitchell, *Medicine in the Crusades*, p. 106.

108. Giles, *Matthew Paris's English History*, Vol. II, p. 409.
109. Marcombe, *Leper Knights*, p. 14.
110. Roffey et al., 'Investigation of a Medieval Pilgrim Burial Excavated from the Leprosarium of St Mary Magdalen Winchester', p. 20.
111. Kealey, *Medieval Medicus*, pp. 108 and 109.
112. Cockayne, *Leechdoms, Wortcunning and Starcraft of Early England*, Vol. II, p. 79, for *Bald's*, and Larson (trans.), *The King's Mirror*, p. 124, for *The King's Mirror*, or *Konungs skuggsjá*, a rorqual whale is any one of the large baleen types.
113. Albe, *Les miracles de Notre-Dame de Roc-Amadour au XIIe siècle*, p. 100, '... et la gangrène se mit aux intestins'.
114. Adams, *Living Hell*, p. 74, at the time of the American Civil War, 1861–5, '... many patients regressed despite successful surgery, succumbing to secondary complications'. It was not until the latter part of the nineteenth century that such wound-contaminating bacteria were even understood in any meaningful way. See also, Harry Schütze, 'Iodine and Sodium Hypochlorite as Wound Disinfectants', *British Medical Journal*, Vol. 2, No. 2869 (25 December 1915), p. 922, the First World War would see more useful antiseptic solutions like Dakin's (also Carrell-Dakin's) begin to have some success, but more effective options like antibiotics and sulfa drugs would not arrive until even later in the twentieth century.
115. Laing, *Heimskringla*, Vol. I, p. 37. See also, McTurk (trans.), 'Kormak's Saga', pp. 27 and 28, *Kormak's Saga* contains a duel between the title character and a man called Bersi. The two warriors met with their bands of supporters and fought with swords in single combat. During the fighting Kormak cut his hand at the joint of his thumb. Being a fairly minor injury, he refused any immediate treatment, but instead decided to travel to his mother for help. By the time he reached her his hand was badly infected. His mother was able to resolve the contamination, but because he had left it so long he ended up with permanent damage to the appendage.
116. Holmes, *A History of Old French Literature*, p. 248. See also, William D. Paden and Frances Freeman (trans), *Troubadour Poems From the South of France* (Cambridge, D.S. Brewer, 2007), p. 28, the crusader and troubadour William IX, Duke of Aquitaine spoke about the value of finding a good physician who could heal, because the result of finding the opposite only meant being made worse. See also, Giles, *Matthew Paris's English History*, Vol. I, p. 77, Matthew of Paris was another who made similar comments when he said, '... it is no light matter for a physician to be ignorant of the business of healing', and Vol. III, p. 276, '... we should not attend to the orders of a quack ...'.
117. Bouillet and Servières, *Sainte Foy, vierge & martyre*, p. 576, 'Les médecins inexpérimentés ...'. 'The inexperienced doctors ...'.
118. Siraisi, *Medieval and Early Renaissance Medicine*, p. 176. The cause of the infection here is similar to that recorded by the student of Guillaume de Congenis in Chapter 3 here where soldiers mistreated the wounds of a fellow knight, causing his death.
119. Sheingorn (trans.), *The Book of Sainte Foy*, p. 206, while miracle accounts do repeatedly downplay the work of physicians and surgeons, there is enough information in this entry to believe that these were doctors who did get it wrong, causing such a terrible infection.
120. Bouillet and Servières, *Sainte Foy, vierge & martyre*, p. 577.
121. Sheingorn (trans.), *The Book of Sainte Foy*, p. 207. See also, Bull, *The Miracles of Our Lady of Rocamadour*, p. 112, for what is possibly another of these injuries involving the malpractice of doctors. The knight was called William from Redon in Brittany.

122. Forester (trans.), *The Ecclesiastical History of England and Normandy by Orderic Vitalis*, Vol. IV, p. 93, 'Soon afterwards he was compelled to retire to his bed; for what is called the "sacred fire" mingled with the inflammation of the wound, and his whole arm up to the shoulder turned as black as coal. He lay sick for five days, and being penitent for his sins, called for a monk's dress, and, fortified by receiving the Lord's body and by confession, then expired.'
123. Stevenson, *The Church Historians of England*, Vol. IV, Part II, p. 700, Robert de Monte, '… a trifling wound on the hand, which occasioned his death'.
124. Ward, *Miracles and the Medieval Mind*, p. 142.
125. Cockayne, *Leechdoms, Wortcunning and Starcraft of Early England*, Vol. II, pp. 99 and 101.
126. Hitti, *An Arab-Syrian Gentleman & Warrior in the Period of the Crusades*, pp. 162 and 163.
127. Bull, *The Miracles of Our Lady of Rocamadour*, p. 133, fn. 83, the author notes that the name Siger suggests the Low Countries, Rhineland or Lorraine.
128. Ibid., the entry notes that Siger lingered for nearly a year with this infection, perhaps either the length of time may have been embellished somewhat or the wound and resulting contamination were not as severe as first described.
129. Rosenman (trans.), *Chirurgia of Roger Frugard*, pp. 46 and 117, reviewing the texts of surgeons like Roger and Roland, their notes for wound therapy regularly suggested drains be used to wick away the pus that would be formed.
130. Campbell and Colton, *The Surgery of Theodoric*, Vol. I, p. 138, it is important to note that Roger Frugard was likely dead before Theodoric was even born. However, I have included his name because of his influence on Roland's text and the fact that Theodoric called Roger out on his theory. Roland was a contemporary of Theodoric, but the former was extremely disliked by the latter, see also, p. 149, for more on Theodoric's mistrust of Roland.
131. Siraisi, *Medieval and Early Renaissance Medicine*, pp. 169 and 170. See also, Rosenman (trans.), *Chirurgia of Roger Frugard*, p. 109, including fn. 58 regarding white and black pus.
132. Campbell and Colton, *The Surgery of Theodoric*, Vol. I, Foreword, p. xxxix, Campbell relates how far ahead of his time Theodoric was in his thinking. See also, Siraisi, *Taddeo Alderotti and his Pupils*, pp. 256, including fn. 43, and p. 297, for more on dry vs moist healing.
133. Siraisi, *Medieval and Early Renaissance Medicine*, p. 182, see also, p. 170, for more on Henri de Mondeville's endorsement of this practice and the resistance he experienced.
134. Dass (trans.), *Viking Attacks on Paris*, pp. 45 and 112, n. 59. In addition to being made with little to adhere the tip of the arrow to the wooden shaft these weapons could be dipped into poison, excrement or something equally foul, causing infection much more easily. Abbo describes Viking arrows being dipped in hemlock or wolfsbane before they were fired.
135. Rosenman (trans.), *Surgery of William of Saliceto*, p. 107.

Chapter 8 – Tormented Minds

1. Kershaw (trans.), *Anglo-Saxon and Norse Poems*, p. 11.
2. Laura Crawley, 'Archaeology, PTSD, and Happiness: How the Dead are Helping the Living', *TROWEL*, Vol. XVIII, October 2017, pp. 2 and 3, for examples of mental health issues relating to war and violence in the ancient world. See also, George Wither, *Campo-Musae or the Field-Musings of Major George Wither Touching*

his *Military Ingagement for the King and Parliament* (London, R.A., 1661), p. 18, physically Major Wither was left unharmed, but wrote of the terrible torment that conflict had caused to his psyche, being especially haunted by nightmares.
3. Bouillet and Servières, *Sainte Foy, vierge & martyre*, p. 571, 'Deux seigneurs de l'Albigeois se faisaient une guerre acharnée ...'. 'Two lords of the Albigensians waged a bitter war ...'.
4. Sheingorn (trans.), *The Book of Sainte Foy*, pp. 197 and 198.
5. Wheen (trans.), *All Quiet on the Western Front*, p. 185.
6. Peter Bernstein, *Trauma: Healing the Hidden Epidemic* (Petaluma, The Bernstein Institute for Integrative Psychotherapy & Trauma Treatment, 2013), p. 67.
7. Ibid., pp. 21–9, Dr Bernstein provides a very useful explanation of the damage that trauma can cause to the human mind, see also, pp. 7 and 8, for a comprehensive list of the symptoms that can be caused by trauma, including: depression, sexual dysfunction, nightmares, sleep disturbance, chronic pain, low self-esteem, etc. See also, van der Kolk, *The Body Keeps Score*, pp. 1–3, and Dr Edith Eva Eger, *The Choice – Embrace the Possible* (New York, Scribner, 2017), pp. 8 and 9, the eminent psychologist, Dr Eva Eger, who as a teenager experienced the terror and degradation of Auschwitz, is clear that there is no one trauma worse than another. In her practice patients have often feared bringing their issues to someone who experienced so much brutality and pain during the Holocaust. However, as she explains to her patients there is no scale of suffering, no chart that indicates that one individual's suffering is any worse than another's. Each of us deals with trauma differently and is impacted in a manner that is unlike the next person.
8. Anderson, '"Jumpy Stump"', pp. 15 and 16, Anderson's paper stresses the connection between war injury and a wounded psyche.
9. Harold Wiltshire, 'A Contribution to the Etiology of Shell Shock', *The Lancet*, 17 June 1916, pp. 1207, 1208 and 1212, Dr Harold Wiltshire, MA, MD CANTAB, FRCP Lond. See also, Owen, *Poems*, p. 35, this idea of horrible sights causing damage to the mind is explored by Wilfred Owen in his poem *Mental Cases*. He recounts the 'Multitudinous murders ...' and '... sloughs of flesh ...' that these poor men had seen and the terrible toll it took on their minds.
10. Marc-Antoine Crocq and Louis Crocq, 'From shell shock and war neurosis to posttraumatic stress disorder: a history of psychotraumatology', *Dialogues in Clinical Neuroscience*, Vol. 2, No. 1 (2000), p. 49, also noted is the French psychiatrist Emmauel Régis, who was of the same opinion, as well. See also, Adams, *Living Hell*, pp. 92–4, he lists the many generals, on both sides of the American Civil War, whose minds were tormented by things they had seen.
11. Elton (trans.), *The First Nine Books of the Danish History of Saxo Grammaticus*, p. 274, from the seventh book of Saxo Grammaticus' *Gesta Danorum*.
12. Nelson (trans.), *The Annals of St-Bertin*, p. 129.
13. Jon Geir Høyersten, 'Madness in the Old Norse Society. Narratives and ideas', *Nord J Psychiatr* (2007), 61, pp. 330 and 331, Dr Høyersten has written extensively on the numerous mental health issues found throughout the sagas. See also, Jon Geir Høyersten, 'Manifestations of psychiatric illness in texts from the medieval and Viking ear', *Archives of Psychiatry and Psychotherapy*, 17, 57–60, 10.12740/APP/44385 (2015).
14. Anderson (trans.), *Viking Tales of the North*, p. 150, 200 years ago the Swedish professor Esaias Tegnér (1782–1846) also recognized this pervasiveness of melancholy in Scandinavian songs and sagas that had existed for centuries, 'Another peculiarity common to the people of the North is a certain disposition for melancholy and

heaviness of spirit ... its sound pervades all our old national melodies, and generally whatever is expressive in our annals, for it is found in the depths of the nation's heart.'

15. Kershaw (trans.), *Anglo-Saxon and Norse Poems*, p. 127, his sons' deaths were not battle related, one drowned and the other was taken by fever, see also, pp. 130 and 132.
16. Ibid., p. 126, Egil and his brother were fighting on the side of King Aethelstan of England when Thorolf was killed.
17. Ibid., p. 139, verse 22.
18. Du Chaillu, *The Viking Age*, Vol. I, p. 161.
19. Byock, *Snorri Sturluson*, pp. 35 and 36. See also, Orchard (ed.), *The Elder Edda*, p. 170, Verse 6 of *Sigrdrifa's Lay* from *The Elder Edda*. It advised warriors to cut runes into their swords, twice invoking Tyr's name, to be assured of victory in battle.
20. Byock, *Snorri Sturluson*, pp. 39 and 40.
21. Ibid., p. 41.
22. Orchard (ed.), *The Elder Edda*, p. 90, Verse 38 of *Lokasenna*. See also, Byock, *Snorri Sturluson*, p. 36.
23. Hight (trans.), *The Saga of Grettir the Strong*, p. 3. See also, Dasent (trans.), *The Story of Burnt Njal or Njal's Saga*, Vol. I, Introduction, p. xvii, 'He [Northman] might lose a limb. Well! Tyr lost a limb when the Wolf bit off his hand; but it was his duty.'
24. Wiltshire, 'A Contribution to the Etiology of Shell Shock', p. 1208, '... in four [patients] the wounds were completely healed before the onset of symptoms'. Symptoms here being of the damage done to the patient's minds.
25. Hight (trans.), *The Saga of Grettir the Strong*, p. 6.
26. Ibid., p. 15.
27. Van der Kolk, *The Body Keeps Score*, pp. 53–5, 82 and 83, this immobilization or dissociative state caused by trauma is well recognized by psychiatrists. Dr van der Kolk, who has treated large numbers of soldiers (p. 83), 'Once this system takes over, other people, and we ourselves, cease to matter. Awareness is shut down, and we may no longer even register physical pain.' See also, Bernstein, *Trauma: Healing the Hidden Epidemic*, pp. 24 and 25.
28. *Band of Brothers* (HBO Home Video, 1 September 2015).
29. Ibid., Episode 7, *The Breaking Point*, minutes 54–6. The real Lieutenant Dike does not appear to have been at this battle. However, the depiction of this condition is one that rings true. In an earlier episode another soldier called Albert Blithe suffered from severe psychological trauma during battle.
30. H.R. Ellis Davidson, *Gods and Myths of the Viking Age* (New York, Bell Publishing Company, 1981), p. 63.
31. Samuel Laing (trans.), *Heimskringla: The Norse Kings Sagas By Snorre Sturlason, Includes Ynglinga Saga* (London, Everyman's Library, J.M. Dent & Sons Ltd, 1930), p. 11. See also, Pálsson and Edwards (trans), *Seven Viking Romances*, p. 10, the *Ynglinga Saga* is based upon earlier poetry from the ninth century.
32. Du Chaillu, *The Viking Age*, Vol. I, p. 161, 'The third I know, If I am in sore need of Bonds for my foes; I deaden the edges of my foes.'
33. Byock, *Snorri Sturluson*, p. 45.
34. Ibid., p. 44, for the list of each Valkyrie by name, other names include Spear-Waver and Smash. See also, Orchard (ed.), *The Elder Edda*, p. 56, *Grimnismal* within the *Elder Edda* for a similar list of names.
35. J.M. Dent (trans.), *Three Icelandic Outlaw Sagas* (London, Everyman Paperbacks, reissued by Viking Society for Northern Research, 2004), p. 320.

36. Carolyne Larrington (trans.), *The Poetic Edda* (Oxford University Press, 2014), p. 257, this verse from *Groa's Chant*, Verse 10, closely matches Verse 149 of *Hávamál* (*Sayings of the High One*). See, Orchard (ed.), *The Elder Edda*, p. 37, Verse 149.
37. DuBois, *Nordic Religions in the Viking Age*, p. 107.
38. John Jeep, *Medieval Germany: An Encyclopedia* (Routledge, 2001), p. 112.
39. Bernstein, *Trauma: Healing the Hidden Epidemic*, pp. 72 and 73, these form part of the list of symptoms created by those like Dr Bernstein who have treated soldiers suffering from PTSD.
40. Kershaw (trans.), *Anglo-Saxon and Norse Poems*, p. 9, from *The Wanderer*. This manuscript does not actually have a title but has become known by this name over time.
41. Alexander (trans.), *Beowulf*, p. 53, lines 64–7.
42. Ibid., p. 56, lines 170–1.
43. Ibid., p. 57, lines 189–93.
44. Ronald Ganze, 'The Neurological and Physiological Effects of Emotional Duress on Memory in Two Old English Elegies', *Anglo-Saxon Emotions – Reading the Heart in Old English Language, Literature and Culture* (Farnham, Ashgate Publishing, 2015), p. 215, Ganze is of a similar opinion that this former soldier in *The Wanderer* is suffering from PTSD.
45. Kershaw (trans.), *Anglo-Saxon and Norse Poems*, p. 9.
46. Ibid., pp. 9 and 11.
47. Bull, *The Miracles of Our Lady of Rocamadour*, p. 172.
48. Bernstein, *Trauma: Healing the Hidden Epidemic*, p. 72, no. 4 on his list of symptoms of PTSD, 'Distorted speech patterns'. See also, van der Kolk, *The Body Keeps Score*, p. 43, who notes that some victims scream obscenities and as noted we are told that Raymond shouted blasphemies, also Crawley, 'Archaeology, PTSD, and Happiness: How the Dead are Helping the Living', p. 3, Hippocrates example, and Sassoon, *The War Poems*, p. 50, the first couple of lines of Siegfried Sassoon's poem called *Survivors* ring true here:

> No doubt they'll soon get well; the shock and strain
> Have caused their stammering, disconnected talk.

49. J.G. O'Keeffe, *Buile Suibne (The Frenzy of Suibhne) being The Adventures of Suibhne Geilt – A Middle-Irish Romance* (London, Irish Text Society, 1913), Introduction, p. xvi, a later date, after 1200, has also been argued.
50. Ibid., Introduction, p. xxxiv, 'In this connection to Suibhne's madness ... I venture to suggest that the original story attributed the madness to the horrors which he witnessed in the Battle of Magh Rath.' See also, Bernstein, *Trauma: Healing the Hidden Epidemic*, p. 24, who describes this dissociative state as being like '... hitting the brakes and flooring the gas in your car at the same time'. The vehicle remains still, but under the bonnet there is a tornado happening.
51. O'Keeffe, *Buile Suibne*, p. 15.
52. Diane Miller Sommerville, 'Yes, civilians experience PTSD in wartime, as we know from the Civil War', *Washington Post*, 13 January 2020.
53. Giles (trans.), *Roger of Wendover*, Vol. II, p. 391, 'And there everything fell into the hands of these robbers, because the soldiers of the French kingdom being as it were the refuse and scum of that country, left nothing at all untouched.'
54. Farmer (trans.), 'The Canonization of St. Hugh of Lincoln', p. 102.
55. Dasent (trans.), *The Story of Burnt Njal or Njal's Saga*, Vol. II, p. 112.

56. Owen, *Poems*, p. 24, 'In all my dreams before my helpless sight, He plunges at me, guttering, choking, drowning.' See also, www.bl.uk/collection-items/siegfried-sassoon-letters-to-his-uncle, Siegfried Sassoon too, writing to his uncle from hospital on 24 April 1917, explained how the nights were the worst, as he would see the corpses again. Painfully, he wrote how the previous week's nightmares had been worse than anything he had been up against before.
57. Bernstein, *Trauma: Healing the Hidden Epidemic*, p. 7. See also, Owen, *Poems*, p. 31, *Mental Cases*, 'Dawn breaks open like a wound that bleeds afresh.'
58. Van der Kolk, *The Body Keeps Score*, p. 135. See also, Ilana E. Strauss, 'A New Diagnosis for Combat Nightmares', *The Atlantic* magazine, 2 February 2015. It is one of many worthwhile pieces on these awful memories of war that bleed into everyday life, as one soldier put it.
59. Van der Kolk, *The Body Keeps Score*, pp. 187 and 188.
60. Kershaw (trans.), *Anglo-Saxon and Norse Poems*, p. 9.
61. Regal (trans.), 'Gisli Sursson's Saga', pp. 501 and 503 for the fire and some of the violence witnessed by Gisli.
62. Ibid., p. 549.
63. Ibid., pp. 550–2.
64. Crocq and Crocq, 'From shell shock and war neurosis to posttraumatic stress disorder: a history of psychotraumatology', p. 48.
65. Dasent (trans.), *The Story of Burnt Njal or Njal's Saga*, Vol. II, p. 197.
66. Kealey, *Medieval Medicus*, p. 71.
67. Geoffrey Brereton (trans.), *Jean Froissart – Chronicles* (London, Penguin Books, 1978), p. 275.
68. M. Viola-Saltzman and N.F. Watson, 'Traumatic brain injury and sleep disorders', *Neurol Clin.*, (2012), 30 4, pp. 1303 and 1305, Roger's surgery was compiled decades after the life of Henry I (d. 1135) and 200 years before Sir Peter.
69. Rosenman (trans.), *Chirurgia of Roger Frugard*, p. 49.
70. Cockayne, *Leechdoms, Wortcunning and Starcraft of Early England*, Vol. I, p. 71.
71. Ibid.
72. Throop (trans.), *Hildegard von Bingen's Physica*, p. 52.
73. Kibler (trans.), 'The Knight of the Cart (Lancelot)', *Chrétien de Troyes – Arthurian Romances*, p. 259.
74. Elton (trans.), *The First Nine Books of the Danish History of Saxo Grammaticus*, p. 33. See also, Davidson, *Gods and Myths of the Viking Age*, p. 69, for more on tales such as those of Hadding and their legacy.
75. Kibler (trans.), 'The Knight of the Cart (Lancelot)', *Chrétien de Troyes – Arthurian Romances*, pp. 258–60. See also, Wright (trans.), *The History of Fulk Fitz Warine*, pp. 42–7, a young woman called Marion de la Bruere takes her own life during the siege of the castle of Dynan. Deceived by a knight called Sir Arnald de Lys, she unwittingly gave away entry to the castle, which in turn allowed a hundred of his fellow knights and soldiers to besiege the fortress. When she discovered that Sir Arnald had tricked her she killed him before taking her own life.
76. Adams, *Living Hell*, pp. 97 and 98.
77. Sassoon, *The War Poems*, p. 29, 'He put a bullet through his brain. No one spoke of him again.'
78. From an article by Simon Harold Walker, 'The overwhelming number of suicidal military members, and the neglect they face', *Independent*, 8 July 2019.
79. Lunde and Stone (trans), *Ibn Fadlān and the Land of Darkness*, p. 152.

80. Garmonsway (trans.), *The Anglo-Saxon Chronicle*, p. 114, with sincere thanks to the Guides of Wimborne Minster in Dorset, who confirmed that in the 1950s three unmarked graves were discovered in the old Saxon part of the church when flooring was replaced in the Minster. It is thought that one of these may well have been the burial place of King Sigferth, but there is simply no way to be certain.
81. Sheingorn (trans.), *The Book of Sainte Foy*, p. 290, n. 20.
82. Ibid., p. 54, interestingly, *Bald's Leechbook* contains many treatments for wounds and diseases that include fresh goat's milk, see also, Cockayne, *Leechdoms, Wortcunning and Starcraft of Early England*, Vol. II, p. 189, 'For an inward wound of the maw; take goats milk just when it is milked …'.
83. Sheingorn (trans.), *The Book of Sainte Foy*, p. 54, seeming to hallucinate and collapse, he decided he would next take himself to St Foy and so he began to eat again. See also, pp. 51 and 52, the scribe who recorded this case, Bernard of Angers, is vehement that this case is genuine. He added that he managed to obtain so much evidence that it would have been positively boring had he included it all. As it is, this entry is already much lengthier in text than the average record in the books of miracles from St Foy.
84. Forester (trans.), *The Ecclesiastical History of England and Normandy by Orderic Vitalis*, Vol. IV, pp. 75 and 76, in addition to the military action taken against Henry I, Vitalis noted that de la Barre had also 'ridiculed him [Henry I] in his songs'. As Forester notes (fn. 2), it is a shame that these songs have not survived.
85. Pifteau, *Chirurgie de Guillaume de Sâlicet*, p. 260. See also, Rosenman (trans.), *Surgery of William of Saliceto*, p. 111. Pifteau translates the offending weapon as a knife, '… avec un couteau …', while Rosenman calls it a sword. While not specifically noted as a soldier, the assumption here is that this man too was a warrior of some type. The other examples from William's casebook, featured in his chapter on wounds, all involve soldiers or battlefield type wounds.
86. Pifteau, *Chirurgie de Guillaume de Sâlicet*, p. 261.
87. Ibid., p. 303, '… qui se blessa lui-même au ventre avec un couteau …'.
88. Bouillet and Servières, *Sainte Foy, vierge & martyre*, p. 534.
89. Pifteau, *Chirurgie de Guillaume de Sâlicet*, p. 260, '… qui par désespoir …'.
90. Bernstein, *Trauma: Healing the Hidden Epidemic*, pp. 67 and 68, Dr Bernstein is of the opinion that almost every soldier that experiences war harbours at least some trace of psychological trauma, some being able to resolve their issues, while many do not. See also, p. ii, 'As the effects of trauma become more clearly understood, we begin to see its damage on a much larger scale.'
91. Moncrieff, *The Song of Roland*, p. 57.
92. Flores (ed.), *An Anthology of Medieval Lyrics*, trans. J.B. Leishman, pp. 423 and 424.
93. 'The REAL Saving Private Ryan: How bereft sister of four brothers who fought in WWI campaigned to bring one of them home when the others died within six months of one another' by Darren Boyle, *Daily Mail*, 15 September 2017, described how during the First World War the Rea family in England lost three of four brothers before the fourth brother, Harry, was brought home after a request from his sister Beatrice.
94. 'Resolving Repton – A Great Viking winter camp and beyond', *Current Archaeology*, 6 June 2019. The older male was marked G. 511 and the younger G. 295. The two are related in the first degree, meaning that they are either father and son or half-brothers, however, the age difference makes the former much more plausible. See also, C. Jarman, M. Biddle, T. Higham and C. Bronk Ramsey, 'The Viking Great Army in England: New dates from the Repton charnel', *Antiquity*, 92 (361) (2018),

doi:10.15184/aqy.2017.196, pp. 183–6, including Fig. 2 on p. 186, and Garmonsway (trans.), *The Anglo-Saxon Chronicle*, p. 68, for the entry in the *Chronicle* that includes the Great (Heathen) Viking Army that overwintered in England in the 865.
95. Forester (trans.), *The Ecclesiastical History of England and Normandy by Orderic Vitalis*, Vol. III, p. 472, '… soon afterwards died of his wounds and the sufferings to which he had been exposed', see also, fn. 3.
96. Ibid., Vol. III, p. 480, 'Then Enguerrand de Trie, a very brave knight, was wounded in the brow, and some days afterwards, having lost his reason, died miserably.'
97. Shahar Bitton, Rivka Tuval-Mashiach and Sara Freedman, 'Distress Levels among Parents of Active Duty Soldiers during Warfare', *Frontiers in Psychology*, Vol. 8, 26 September 2017, p. 4.
98. Diana Attwood (trans.), 'The Saga of Gunnlaug Serpent-Tongue', *Sagas of Warrior Poets* (London, Penguin Classics, Penguin Group, 2002), pp. 140, 146 and 147.
99. Ibid., pp. 147 and 148, Illugi is said to have maimed Thorgrim after killing another. Also see Diana Whaley, *Sagas of Warrior Poets* (London, Penguin Classics, Penguin Group, 2002), n. 38, p. 282, the act of maiming was apparently very uncommon for sagas set during this time.
100. Dass (trans.), *Viking Attacks on Paris*, p. 49.
101. Charles Dahlberg (trans.), *The Romance of the Rose* (Princeton University Press, 1995), p. 35. See also, Kibler (trans.), 'The Story of the Grail (Percival)', *Chrétien de Troyes – Arthurian Romances*, p. 484, these physical reactions, manifested in the hair loss and self-harm, are detailed by Chrétien de Troyes' in his unfinished work *The Story of the Grail (Perceval)*. Late within the text, as Gawain rode off from the palace to what seemed to be almost certain death, a number of women who had loved and cared for their lord were in great distress and 'tore their hair, and ripped and scratched themselves'.
102. Sheingorn (trans.), *The Book of Sainte Foy*, pp. 257 and 258.
103. Bouillet and Servières, *Sainte Foy, vierge & martyre*, pp. 619 and 620.
104. Sheingorn (trans.), *The Book of Sainte Foy*, p. 259, being a miracle story Bernard was eventually restored to life, but not before a funeral was held for him.
105. Stacy Bannerman, *Homefront 911 – How Families of Wounded Veterans are Wounded by Our Wars* (New York, Arcade Publishing, 2015), p. 50. This book contains many shocking facts and stories regarding the damage that war does to those keeping the home fires burning.
106. Ibid., p. 51.
107. Adams, *Living Hell*, pp. 147 and 148, for examples of the 'Domestic violence and drug abuse …' that damaged families during and after the American Civil War. See also, Canadian Broadcasting Corporation (CBC), 'Domestic violence up in Canadian military families', 31 March 2011, which lays bare the steady increase in domestic violence in homes on military bases, especially those where a soldier had returned from Afghanistan. See also, Renata D'Aliesio, 'Nearly half of soldiers who killed themselves in 2016 were dealing with loved one's suicide', *The Globe and Mail*, 7 December 2017.
108. C.C. Swinton Bland (trans.), *The Miracles of the Blessed Virgin Mary – Johannes Herolt 1435–1440* (New York, Harcourt, Brace and Company, 1928), pp. 27–8, Story Ten, this comes originally from the collection of Caesarius of Heisterbach's *Dialogue of Miracles (Dialogus miraculorum)*. He was a Cisterian Abbot who was born in Cologne *c.* 1170 and died in Lorraine *c.* 1240. His collection of miracles was recorded *c.* 1223. This story appears in Book VII, Chapter III.

109. Bannerman, *Homefront 911*, pp. 98–102, the entirety of this chapter from Bannerman deals with examples that mirror this medieval record, including her own experiences.
110. Sheingorn (trans.), *The Book of Sainte Foy*, pp. 229–32.
111. Ibid., p. 231. See also, Bouillet and Servières, *Sainte Foy, vierge & martyre*, p. 598, '... accablée sous le poids de sa douleur et en proie à une terrible angoisse ...'. '... overwhelmed by the weight of her torment and in the terrible grip of anguish ...'.
112. Sheingorn (trans.), *The Book of Sainte Foy*, pp. 231 and 232, this was the wife of Lord Giselfroy, who led Mathfred and others in the attack on the unnamed castle. See also, pp. 229 and 230.
113. Bull, *The Miracles of Our Lady of Rocamadour*, pp. 106 and 107.
114. Ibid., p. 107.
115. Ibid., p. 63, n. 82, the translator of this miracle collection into English is in some doubt about the validity of this entry because of the lack of detail.
116. Bannerman, *Homefront 911*, pp. 83 and 84, there are numerous examples of these devastating situations involving the families of those in the armed forces who have sadly taken their own lives, as well as those of their children recounted in Chapter 3 of this book. The names of those involved in the instances used in this text have not been included here but are noted in Bannerman's book.
117. Elton (trans.), *The First Nine Books of the Danish History of Saxo Grammaticus*, p. 378.
118. Bannerman, *Homefront 911*, pp. 147 and 148, Bannerman discusses her time looking after chronically homeless veterans. Many of them, because of their mental health issues, no longer had family or friends left to count on, 'After years of burning bridges beyond repair.' See also, Kershaw (trans.), *Anglo-Saxon and Norse Poems*, p. 9, the individual in *The Wanderer* was '... exiled from home and far from my kinsmen'.
119. Nicholson, (trans.), *The Chronicle of the Third Crusade*, p. 379. See also, Adams, *Living Hell*, p. 147, the situation after the American Civil War of the nineteenth century draws another more modern parallel to the plight of so many former soldiers who struggled to re-enter society. They roamed from town to town, pushed on by the police or placed in jail. Described as the 'Tramp System' by the Chief Detective of Massachusetts in 1878, these were ex-soldiers who were unable to return to their pre-war lives. See also, Sassoon, *The War Poems*, p. 77, his poem called *Aftermath* is also of value here. The inability of the soldiers of the First World War to forget their terrible experiences. The narrator continues to ask former soldiers, 'Have you forgotten yet?'
120. Nicholson, (trans.), *The Chronicle of the Third Crusade*, pp. 198, 212 and 215, these are among the many references to warriors who were killed in the most horrific manner.
121. Ibid., p. 379.
122. Article by Vietnam veteran and officer Alan Cutter, 'Learning to come home from war: no one said "thank you" to Vietnam vets', *Guardian*, international edn, 13 April 2013.
123. Nicholson, (trans.), *The Chronicle of the Third Crusade*, p. 9, the suggestion that a crusader was the author of this chronicle is only strengthened by his robust defence of those whose minds had been wounded by their experiences.
124. Ibid., p. 379.
125. Elton (trans.), *The First Nine Books of the Danish History of Saxo Grammaticus*, p. 378, 'Straightway he sought medicine for his grief in loneliness, and patiently confined the grief of his sick soul within the walls of his house.'
126. DuBois, *Nordic Religions in the Viking Age*, p. 97, for more on St John's wort.
127. Moffat, *SHARP Practice 6*, pp. 5, 22 and 23, common valerian has long been used to treat sleep disorders and anxiety.

128. Cockayne, *Leechdoms, Wortcunning and Starcraft of Early England*, Vol. III, p. 51, Number 73.
129. Ibid., Vol. II, p. 335. See also, Cameron, *Anglo-Saxon Medicine*, p. 135, he notes that there must have been a magical element attached to the skin of a porpoise.
130. Adel Omrani, Niki S. Holtzman, Hagop S. Akiskal and Nassir S. Ghaemi, 'Ibn Imran's 10th century Treatise on Melancholy', *Journal of Affective Disorders*, 141 (2012), p. 117.
131. Ibid.
132. Ibid., p. 118.
133. Wardrop (trans.), *The Man in the Panther's Skin*, p. 140.
134. Ibid., p. 140, fn. 1.
135. Charles Burnett, '"Spiritual Medicine": music and healing in Islam and its influence in Western medicine', *Musical Healing in Cultural Contexts* (Farnham, Ashgate Publishing, 2000), p. 87.
136. Wright (trans.), *The Historical Works of Giraldus Cambrensis*, pp. 127–30, see also, van der Kolk, *The Body Keeps Score*, pp. 242 and 243, for more on the arts and their ability to help heal soldiers and the victims of torture, in addition to others struggling with serious psychological injuries.
137. Rosenman (trans.), *Chirurgia of Roger Frugard*, p. 53.
138. Hitti, *An Arab-Syrian Gentleman & Warrior in the Period of the Crusades*, p. 162, here again there is a possibility that we may be up against Usāmah Ibn-Munqidh's propensity for exaggeration in his recollection of this procedure.
139. Robert Steele (ed.), *Medieval Lore: Being Classified Gleanings from the Encyclopedia of Bartholomew Anglicus on the Properties of Things* (London, Elliot Stock, 1893), p. 58.
140. Siraisi, *Taddeo Alderotti and his Pupils*, p. 26, Guglielmo da Brescia died in 1326.
141. Ibid., pp. 232–4.
142. Crawley, 'Archaeology, PTSD, and Happiness: How the Dead are Helping the Living', pp. 3 and 4.
143. Bernstein, *Trauma: Healing the Hidden Epidemic*, pp. 51 and 52.
144. Van der Kolk, *The Body Keeps Score*, p. 188, Dr van der Kolk's 1983 study of Second World War veterans being treated at medical clinics uncovered the fact that a large majority of them were still suffering from what is today known as PTSD. They were only being treated for their physical complaints, while their psychological ailments went undiagnosed for some forty years after their military service experiences.
145. Omrani et al., 'Ibn Imran's 10th century Treatise on Melancholy', p. 117.

Conclusion

1. Forester (trans.), *The Ecclesiastical History of England and Normandy by Orderic Vitalis*, Vol. I, p. 480.
2. Garmonsway (trans.), *The Anglo-Saxon Chronicle*, p. 199.

Bibliography

Studies and Journal Reports

Alm, Torbjørn and Elvevag, Brita, 'Ergotism in Norway. Part 1: Symptoms and their interpretation from the late Iron Age to the seventeenth century', *History of Psychiatry*, 24[1] (2012), pp. 15–33, DOI: 10.1177/0957154X11433960

Anderson, Julie, '"Jumpy Stump": amputation and trauma in the first world War', *First World War Studies*, 6 (2015), pp. 1, 9–19, DOI: 10.1080/19475020.2015.1016581

Anderson, T., 'Dental treatment in Anglo-Saxon England', *British Dental Journal*, Volume 197, No. 5, 11 September 2004, DOI: 10.1038/sj.bdj.4811623

Batty, Colonel Charles G., 'Changes in the Care of the Battle Casualty: Lessons Learned from the Falklands Campaign', *Military Medicine*, Vol. 164, May 1999, pp. 336–40

Belcastro, M.G., Mariotti, V., Facchini, F. and Dutour, O., 'Leprosy in Skeleton from the 7th Century Necropolis of Vienne-Campochin (Molise, Italy)', *International Journal of Osteoarchaeology*, 15 (2005), pp. 431–48, DOI: 10.1002/oa.799

Binder, M., Eitler, J., Deutschmann, J., Ladstätter, S., Glaser, F. and Fiedler, D., 'Prosthetics in antiquity – An early medieval wearer of a foot prosthesis (6th century AD) from Hemmaberg/Austria', *International Journal of Paleopathology*, Vol. 12, March 2016, pp. 29–40, doi.org/10.1016/j.ijpp.2015.11.003

Bitton, Shahar, Tuval-Mashiach, Rivka and Freedman, Sara, 'Distress Levels among Parents of Active Duty Soldiers during Warfare', *Frontiers in Psychology*, Vol. 8, 26 September 2017, doi 10.3389/fpsyg.2017.01679

Burns, Robert Ignatius, 'The Medieval Crossbow as a Surgical Instrument: An Illustrated Case History', *Bulletin of The New York Academy of Medicine*, Vol. 48, No. 8, September 1972, pp. 983–9

Cameron, M.L., 'Bald's "Leechbook": Its Sources and Their Use in Its Compilation', *Anglo-Saxon England*, Vol. 12 (1983), pp. 153–82, JSTOR

Caple, Chris, 'The Yarm Helmet', *Medieval Archaeology*, Vol. 64 (2020), Issue 1, pp. 31–64, doi.org/10.1080/00766097.2020.1755126

Corner, George W., 'On Early Salernitan Surgery and Especially the "Bamberg Surgery" – With an Account of a Previously Undescribed Manuscript of the Bamberg Surgery in the Possession of Dr. Harvey Cushing', *Bulletin of the Institute of the History of Medicine*, Johns Hopkins University, Vol. V, No. 1, January 1937

Crawley, Laura, 'Archaeology, PTSD, and Happiness: How the Dead are Helping the Living', *TROWEL*, Vol. XVIII, October 2017

Crocq, Marc-Antoine and Crocq, Louis, 'From shell shock and war neurosis to posttraumatic stress disorder: a history of psychotraumatology', *Dialogues in Clinical Neuroscience*, Vol. 2, No. 1 (2000)

Cullen, John B., 'The Ancient Churches of the Town of Wexford', *The Journal of the Royal Society of Antiquaries of Ireland Vol. V – Fifth Series*, Dublin, University Press, 1895

Frölich, Annette and Kristiansen, Anne Mette, 'Er det vikinge-lægens instrument?' ('Is this the instrument of a Viking doctor?'), *Vikingetid i Danmark (Viking Age in Denmark)*, Forhistorisk arkæologi, SAXO-instituttet på Københavns Universitet (2013), pp. 101–4

Gruber, Franjo, Lipozenčić, Jasna and Kehler, Tatjana, 'History of Venereal Diseases from Antiquity to the Renaissance', *Acta Dermatovenerol Croat* (2015); 23¹, pp. 1–11

Hallbäck, D.-A., 'A medieval(?) bone with a copper plate support, indicating an open surgical treatment', *Ossa*, 3⁴ (1976–7), pp. 63–82

Harrison, Freya et al., 'A 1,000-Year-Old Antimicrobial Remedy with Antistaphylococcal Activity', *mBio*, Vol. 6, 4 e01129, 11 August 2015, doi:10.1128/mBio.01129-15

Hedenstierna-Jonson, C., Kjellström, A., Zachrisson, T. et al., 'A female Viking warrior confirmed by genomics', *Am J Phys Anthropol* (2017), 164, pp. 853–60, doi.org/10.1002/ajpa.23308

Høyersten, Jon Geir, 'Madness in the Old Norse Society. Narratives and ideas', *Nord J Psychiatr* (2007), 61, pp. 324–31

Høyersten, Jon Geir, 'Manifestations of psychiatric illness in texts from the medieval and Viking ear', *Archives of Psychiatry and Psychotherapy*. 17. 57-60. 10.12740/APP/44385 (2015)

Jarman, C., Biddle, M., Higham, T. and Bronk Ramsey, C., 'The Viking Great Army in England: New dates from the Repton charnel', *Antiquity*, 92 (361) (2018), pp. 183–99, doi:10.15184/aqy.2017.196

Jessop, Oliver, 'A New Artefact Typology for the Study of Medieval Arrowheads', *Medieval Archaeology*, Vol. XL (1996), The Society for Medieval Archaeology, 1996

Kealey, Edward J., 'England's Earliest Women Doctors', *Journal of the History of Medicine and Allied Sciences*, Vol. 40, Issue 4, October 1985, pp. 473–7, https://doi.org/10.1093/jhmas/40.4.473

Knüsel, Christopher J., Kemp, Richard L. and Budd, Paul, 'Evidence for Remedial Medical Treatment of a Severe Knee Injury from the Fishergate Gilbertine Monastery in the City of York', *Journal of Archaeological Science* (1995), 22, pp. 369–84

Lee, M.R., 'The history of ergot of rye (Claviceps purpurea) I: From antiquity to 1900', *R Coll Physicians Edinb* (2009), 39, pp. 179–84

Lubin, David M., 'Masks, Mutilation, and Modernity: Anna Coleman Ladd and the First World War', *Archives of American Art Journal*, Vol. 47, No. 3/4 (2008), pp. 4–15

Matthews, C.I., 'The Anglo-Saxon cemetery at Marina Drive', Dunstable, *Bedfordshire Archaeological Journal*, 1 (1962), pp. 25–47

Micarelli, Ileana, Paine, Robert, Giostra, Caterina, Tafuri, Mary Anne, Profico, Antonio, Boggioni, Marco, Di Vincenzo, Fabio, Massani, Danilo, Papini, Andrea and Manzi, Giorgio, 'Survival to amputation in pre-antibiotic era: a case study from a Longobard necropolis (6th–8th centuries AD)', *Journal of Anthropological Sciences*, Vol. 96 (2018), pp. 1–16

Minozzi, Simona et al. 'A Dental Prosthesis from the Early Modern Age in Tuscany (Italy)', *Clinical Implant Dentistry and Related Research*, 19 (2017), pp. 365–71

Omrani, Adel, Holtzman, Niki S., Akiskal, Hagop S. and Ghaemi, Nassir S., 'Ibn Imran's 10th century Treatise on Melancholy', *Journal of Affective Disorders*, 141 (2012), pp. 116–19, doi:10.1016/j.jad.2012.02.004

Pandya W.C., 'Icon of this issue: Sir Archibald McIndoe', *Indian Journal of Plastic Surgery*, official publication of the Association of Plastic Surgeons of India, 48 (2015), pp. 234–5, https://doi.org/10.4103/0970-0358.173100

Rignault, Daniel P., 'Abdominal trauma in war', *The World Journal of Surgery* (1992), 16, pp. 940–6, doi.org/10.1007/BF02066996

Roffey, Simon, Tucker, Katie, Filipek-Ogden, Kori, Montgomery, Janet, Cameron, Jamie, O'Connell, Tamsin, Evans, Jane, Marter, Phil and Taylor, Michael, G., 'Investigation of a Medieval Pilgrim Burial Excavated from the Leprosarium of St Mary Magdalen

Winchester, UK', *PLOS Neglected Tropical Diseases*, 26 January 2017, DOI: 10.1371/journal.pntd.0005186

Rolleston, J.D., 'Venereal Disease in Literature', *British Journal of Venereal Diseases*, 1 July 1934, pp. 147–74, DOI: 10.1136/sti.10.3.47

Russcher, Anne and Bremmer Jr, Rolf H., '"For a Broken Limb": Fracture Treatment in Anglo-Saxon England', *Amsterdamer Beiträge zur älteren Germanistik*, 69, 1 January 2012, pp. 145–74

Schütze, Harry, 'Iodine and Sodium Hypochlorite as Wound Disinfectants', *British Medical Journal*, Vol. 2, No. 2869, 25 December 1915, pp. 921–2

Sperati, G., 'Amputation of the nose throughout history or L'amputazione del naso nella storia', *Acta Otorhinolaryngol Ital*, 2009, 29, pp. 44–50

Štefan, Ivo, Stránská, Petra and Vondrová, Hana, 'The archaeology of early medieval violence: the mass grave at Budeč', *Czech Republic. Antiquity*, 90 (2016), pp. 759–76, DOI:10.15184/aqy.2016.29

Suppersberger, Hamre S., Ersland, G.A., Daux, V., Parson, W. and Wilkinson, C., 'Three individuals, three stories, three burials from medieval Trondheim, Norway', *PLOS ONE*, 3 July 2017, doi.org/10.1371/journal.pone.0180277

Viola-Saltzman, M. and Watson, N.F., 'Traumatic brain injury and sleep disorders', *Neurol Clin.*, (2012), 30 4, pp. 1299–312, doi:10.1016/j.ncl.2012.08.008

Watkins, Frances, Pendry, Barbara, Sanchez-Medina, Alberto and Corcoran, Olivia, 'Antimicrobial assays of three native British plants used in Anglo-Saxon medicine for wound healing formulations in 10th century England', Medicines Research Group, School of Health, Sport and Bioscience, University of East London, 2012

Way, Albert, 'Bill of Medicines Furnished for the Use of Edward I, 1306–1307', *Archaeological Journal*, 14, pp. 267–71, 1857, archaeologydataservice.ac.uk

Wester, Knut, 'The mystery of the missing Viking helmets', *Neurosurgery*, Vol. 47, Issue 5, November 2000, pp. 1216–29, doi:10.1097/00006123-200011000-00041

Weisberger, Mindy, 'Medieval Germans Riddles with Tapeworms', Live Science, 5 October, 2018, livescience.com

Primary Source Material

Abbott, Edwin A., *St. Thomas of Canterbury – His Death and Miracles, Volumes I and II*, London, Adam and Charles Black, 1898

Adams, Alison (trans.), *The Romance of Yder*, Cambridge, D.S. Brewer, 1983

Albe, Edmond, *Les miracles de Notre-Dame de Roc-Amadour au XIIe siècle*, Paris, Honoré Champion, 1907

Alcott, Louisa May, *Hospital Sketches*, Boston, James Redpath, 1863

Alexander, Michael (trans.), *Beowulf*, London, Penguin Classics, Penguin Group, 1973

Alexander, Michael (trans.), *The Earliest English Poems*, London, Penguin Classics, Penguin Group, 1991

Anderson, Joseph (ed.), *Orkneyinga Saga*, Edinburgh, Edmondston and Douglas, 1873

Anderson, Rasmus B. (trans.), *Viking Tales of the North – The Sagas of Thorstein, Viking's Son and Fridthjof the Bold*, Chicago, Scott, Foresman and Company, 1901

Arthur, Ross G. and Corbett, Noel L. (trans), *The Knight of the Two Swords, A Thirteenth-Century Arthurian Romance*, Gainesville, University Press of Florida, 1996

Attwood, Diana (trans.), 'The Saga of Gunnlaug Serpent-Tongue', *Sagas of Warrior Poets*, London, Penguin Classics, Penguin Group, 2002

Bachrach, Bernard S. and Bachrach, David S. (trans), *Widukind of Corvey – Deeds of the Saxons*, Washington DC, The Catholic University of America Press, 2014

Bailey, N. (trans.), *The Colloquies of Desiderius Erasmus – Concerning Men Manners and Things, Volume I*, London, Gibbings and Company, Limited, 1900

Beaumont, Francis and Fletcher, John, *The Knight of the Burning Pestle*, London, J.M. Dent and Co., 1898

Bédier, Joseph, *The Romance of Tristan and Iseult*, New York, Random House Inc. Vintage Edition, 1965

Bell, Clair Hayden (trans.), *Peasant Life in Old German Epics*, New York, Columbia University Press, 1931

Bennett, Philip E. (trans.), *La Chanson de Guillaume*, London, Grant & Cutler Ltd, 2000

Bentley, Samuel (ed.), *Excerpta Historica or Illustrations of English History*, London, Samuel Bentley, 1860

Benton, John F. (ed.), *Self and Society in Medieval France – The Memoirs of Abbot Guibert of Nogent*, New York, Harper & Row, 1970

Birch, Walter de Gray, *Vita Haroldi – The Romance of the Life of Harold, King of England*, London, Elliot Stock, 1885

Black, Winston (trans.), *Henry Huntingdon – Anglicanus ortus – A Verse Herbal of the Twelfth Century*, Oxford, The Bodleian Library, 2012

Bland, C.C. Swinton (trans.), *The Miracles of the Blessed Virgin Mary – Johannes Herolt 1435–1440*, New York, Harcourt, Brace and Company, 1928

Bouillet, Auguste and Servières, Louis, *Sainte Foy, vierge & martyre*, Rodez, Imprimerie E. Carrère, 1900

Bourdillon, Francis William (trans.), *Aucassin and Nicolette – Translated from the Old French*, London, Kegan Paul, Trench, Trübner & Co. Ltd, 1903

Brereton, Geoffrey (trans.), *Jean Froissart – Chronicles*, London, Penguin Books, 1978

Bull, Marcus Graham, *The Miracles of Our Lady of Rocamadour: Analysis and Translation*, Woodbridge, Boydell & Brewer Ltd, 1999

Burgess, Glyn S. and Busby, Keith (trans), *The Lais of Marie de France*, London, Penguin Books, 1986

Burrell, Arthur (trans.), *Piers Plowman, The Vision of a People's Christ by William Langland*, London and Toronto, Everyman's Library, 1912

Byock, Jesse (trans.), *Snorri Sturluson – The Prose Edda*, London, Penguin Classics, Penguin Group, 2005

Calendar of Chancery Warrants Preserved in the Public Record Office – AD 1244–1326, London, His Majesty's Stationery Office, 1927

Calendar of the Close Rolls Preserved in the Public Record Office for Edward I – A.D. 1272–1279, printed for Her Majesty's Stationery Office by Erye and Spottiswoode, 1900

Calendar of the Close Rolls Preserved in the Public Record Office for Edward I – A.D. 1279–1288, printed for Her Majesty's Stationery Office by Mackie and Co. Ltd, 1902

Calendar of the Close Rolls Preserved in the Public Record Office for Edward II – A.D. 1313–1319, printed for Her Majesty's Stationery Office by Erye and Spottiswoode, 1893

Calendar of Documents Relating to Scotland Preserved in Her Majesty's Public Record Office, London – Volume II – 1272–1307, Edinburgh, Her Majesty's General Register House, 1884

Calendar of Documents Relating to Scotland, Preserved in the Public Record Office and the British Library – Volume V (Supplementary) – 1108–1516, issued under the direction of the Keeper of the Records of Scotland, Scottish Record Office, 1881

Calendar of Inquisitions Miscellaneous (Chancery) – Volume I, published by Authority of His Majesty's Principal Secretary of State for the Home Department, London, 1916

Calendar of the Liberate Rolls Preserved in the Public Record Office – Volumes I–VI, 1226–1272, London, His and Her Majesty's Stationery Office, 1916–64

Cambro-Briton, The, *The Laws of Hywel Dha*, Vol. 2, 1821

Campbell, Eldridge and Colton, James (trans), *The Surgery of Theodoric, ca. 1267– Volumes I and II*, New York, Appleton-Century Crofts, Inc., 1955

Canadian Army, *Notes for Instructors in Battle First Aid – June, 1943*, Ottawa, Edmond Cloutier, 1943

Cockayne, Revd Oswald, *Leechdoms, Wortcunning and Starcraft of Early England, Volumes I–III*, Longman, Green, Longman, Roberts and Green, 1864–6

Coles, John (trans.), *The Story of Þórðr Hreða*, Icelandic Saga Database – sagadb.org, translation 1866

Comfort, William Wistar (trans.), *Erec and Enide*, Everyman's Library, London, J.M. Dent & Sons Ltd, 1913

Cross, Samuel Hazzard and Sherbowitz-Wetzor, Olgerd P. (trans), *The Russian Primary Chronicle – Laurentian Text*, Cambridge, MA, The Mediaeval Academy of America, 1953

Curtis, Renée L. (trans.), *The Romance of Tristan, The Thirteenth-Century Old French 'Prose Tristan'*, Oxford University Press, 1994

Cusimano, Richard and Moorhead, John (trans), *The Deeds of Louis the Fat*, Washington DC, The Catholic University Press, 1992

Dahlberg, Charles (trans.), *The Romance of the Rose*, Princeton University Press, 1995

Dasent, George Webbe (trans.), *Icelandic Sagas, Volume IV, The Saga of Hacon*, London, Her Majesty's Stationery Office, 1894

Dasent, George Webbe (trans.), *The Story of Burnt Njal or Njal's Saga – In Two Volumes*, Edinburgh, Edmonston and Douglas, 1861

Dass, Nirmal (trans.), *Viking Attacks on Paris: The Bella parisiacae urbis of Abbo of Saint-Germain-des-Prés*, Leuven, Peeters, 2007

Dawes, Jean D. and Magilton, J.R., *The Cemetery of St Helen-on-the-Walls, Aldwark*, York, Council for British Archaeology, 1980

Dent, J.M. (trans.), *Three Icelandic Outlaw Sagas*, London, Everyman Paperbacks, reissued by Viking Society for Northern Research, 2004

Elton, Oliver (trans.), *The First Nine Books of the Danish History of Saxo Grammaticus*, London, David Nutt, 1894

Eyton, R.W., *Court, Household and Itinerary of King Henry II*, London, Taylor and Co., 1878

Farmer, D.H. (trans.), 'The Canonization of St. Hugh of Lincoln', *Lincolnshire Architectural and Archaeology Society Reports and Papers*, Vol. 6, Part 2 (1956), pp. 86–117

Ferrante, Joan M. (trans.), *Guillaume d'Orange: Four Twelfth-Century Epics*, New York, Columbia University Press, 1991

Flavius Vegetius Renatus, *De Re Militari – Concerning Military Affairs*, Leonaur, 2012

Flores, Angel (ed.), *An Anthology of Medieval Lyrics*, New York, Modern Library through Random House, 1962

Forester, Thomas (trans.), *The Chronicle of Henry Huntingdon and The Acts of Stephen*, London, Henry G. Bohn, 1853

Forester, Thomas (trans.), *The Ecclesiastical History of England and Normandy by Orderic Vitalis, Volumes I–IV*, London, Henry G. Bohn, 1853–6

Foster, Edward E., *Amis and Amiloun, Robert of Cisyle, and Sir Amadace*, Kalamazoo, Medieval Institute Publications, 2nd edn, 2007

Frisk, Gösta (ed.), *A Middle English Translation of Macer Floridus De Viribus Herbarum*, Uppsala, Almqvist & Wiksells Boktryckeri AB, 1949

Gardiner, L.J. (trans.), *Cligés – Chrétien de Troyes*, London, Chatto & Windus, 1912

Garmonsway, G.N. (trans.), *The Anglo-Saxon Chronicle*, London, J.M. Dent & Sons Ltd, 1953
Getz, Faye Marie (ed.), *Healing and Society in Medieval England, A Middle English Translation of the Pharmaceutical Writings of Gilbertus Anglicus*, Madison, The University of Wisconsin Press, 1991
Giles, J.A. (trans.), *Matthew Paris's English History – Volumes I, II and III*, London, Henry G. Bohn, 1852–3
Giles, J.A. (trans.), *Roger of Wendover – Flowers of History, In Two Volumes*, London, Henry G. Bohn, 1849
Gough, Henry (ed.), *Scotland in 1298 – Documents Relating to the Campaign of King Edward the First in that Year, and Especially to the Battle of Falkirk*, London, Alexander Gardner, Publisher to Her Majesty the Queen, 1888
Green, Monica H., *The Trotula*, Philadelphia, University of Pennsylvania, 2001
Greive, Dr James (trans.), *A. Cornelius Celsus of Medicine. In Eight Books*, London, D. Wilson and T. Durham, 1756
Guibert of Nogent, *The Deeds of God through the Franks*, Teddington, Echo Library, 2008
Head, Edmund (trans.), *The Saga of Viga-Glum or Viga Glum's Story*, London, Williams and Norgate, 1866
Hennessy, William M., *Annals of Ulster – A Chronicle of Irish Affairs From A.D. 431–A.D. 1540, Vol. 1*, Dublin, Alexander Thom and Co., 1887
Hibbard, Laura A., *Three Middle English Romances*, London, David Nutt, 1911
Hight, Ainslie (trans.), *The Saga of Grettir the Strong*, London, J.M., Dent & Sons Ltd, 1913
Hitti, Phillip K. (trans.), *An Arab-Syrian Gentleman & Warrior in the Period of the Crusades*, New York, Columbia University Press, 1929
Holy Bible, Containing the Old and New Testaments, Philadelphia, American Baptist Publication Society, 1913
Horton, Alice and Bell, Edward (trans), *The Lay of the Nibelungs*, London, George Bell & Sons, 1901
Hunt, William, *Two Chartularies of the Priory of St. Peter at Bath*, London, Harrison and Sons, 1893
Jakobsson, Ármann and Clark, David (trans), *The Saga of Bishop Thorlak*, Exeter, Short Run Press Limited, 2013
Jessopp, A. and James, M.R. (trans), *The Life and Miracles of St. William of Norwich by Thomas of Monmouth*, Cambridge University Press, 1896
Jones, Gwyn (trans.), *Eirik the Red and Other Icelandic Sagas*, World's Classics, 1980, repr. of Oxford University Press edn, 1961
Kemp, Brian (trans.), 'The Miracles of the Hand of St. James', *Berkshire Archaeological Journal*, Vol. 65, 1970
Kershaw, N. (trans.), *Anglo-Saxon and Norse Poems*, Cambridge University Press, 1922
Kibler, William W. (trans.), 'The Knight of the Cart (Lancelot)', 'The Knight with the Lion (Yvain)' and 'The Story of the Grail (Perceval)', *Chrétien de Troyes – Arthurian Romances*, London, Penguin Books, Penguin Group, 1991
Kunz, Keneva (trans.), 'Eirik the Red's Saga', *The Sagas of the Icelanders*, London, Penguin Books, Penguin Group, 2001
Kunz, Keneva (trans.), 'The Saga of the Greenlanders', *The Sagas of the Icelanders*, London, Penguin Books, Penguin Group, 2001
Kunz, Keneva (trans.), 'The Saga of the People of Laxardal', *The Sagas of the Icelanders*, London, Penguin Books, Penguin Group, 2001

Laing, Samuel, *The Heimskringla, A History of Norse Kings – Volumes I–III*, London, The Norroena Society, 1907

Laing, Samuel (trans.), *Heimskringla: The Norse Kings Sagas By Snorre Sturlason, Includes Ynglinga Saga*, London, Everyman's Library, J.M. Dent & Sons Ltd, 1930

Larrington, Carolyne (trans.), *The Poetic Edda*, Oxford University Press, 2014

Larsen, Henning, *An Old Icelandic Medical Miscellany, MS Royal Irish Academy 23 D43 with supplement from MS Trinity College (Dublin) L-2-27*, Oslo, Jacob Dybwad, 1931

Larson, Laurence Marcellus (trans.), *The King's Mirror – Speculum Regale – Konungs Skuggsja*, Oxford University Press, 1917

Lunde, Paul and Stone, Caroline (trans), *Ibn Fadlān and the Land of Darkness – Arab Travellers in the Far North*, London, Penguin Classics, Penguin Group, 2012

McAlhany, Joseph and Rubenstein, Jay (trans), *Guibert of Nogent – Monodies and On the Relics of Saints – The Autobiography and a Manifesto of a French Monk from the Time of the Crusades*, London, Penguin Books, 2011

McTurk, Rory (trans.), 'Kormak's Saga', *Sagas of Warrior Poets*, London, Penguin Classics, Penguin Group, 2002

Mageoghagan, Conell, *The Annals of Clonmacnoise Being Annals of Ireland from the Earliest Period to A.D. 1408 – Translated into English A.D. 1627*, ed. Revd Denis Murphy, Dublin, University Press, 1896

Merriam-Webster, *Merriam-Webster's Medical Dictionary*, Springfield, MA, Merriam-Webster Inc., 2006

Meyer, Paul, *La chanson de la croisade contre les Albigeois*, La Société de l'histoire de France, 1879

Moncrieff, Charles Scott, *The Song of Roland*, London, Chapman & Hall Ltd, 1919

Nelson, Janet L. (trans.), *The Annals of St-Bertin, Ninth-Century Histories, Volume 1*, Manchester and New York, Manchester University Press, 1991

Newth, Michael A.H. (trans.), *Heroes of the French Epic: A Selection of Chansons de Geste*, Woodbridge, Boydell Press, 2005

Newth, Michael A. (trans.), *The Song of Girart of Vienne by Bertrand de Bar-sur-Aube*, Tempe, Arizona Centre for Medieval & Renaissance Studies, 1999

Nicaise, Edouard, *La grande chirurgie de Guy de Chauliac*, Paris, Ancienne Librairie Germer Ballière, 1890

Nicholson, Helen J. (trans.), *The Chronicle of the Third Crusade*, Farnham, Ashgate Publishing Limited, 2001

O'Donovan, John, *Annals of the Kingdom of Ireland – By the Four Masters – From the Earliest Period to the Year 1616 – Volumes I and II*, Dublin, Hodges, Smith and Co., 1856

O'Donovan, John, *Annals of Ireland – Three Fragments, Copied from Ancient Sources – From a Manuscript Preserved in the Burgundian Library at Brussels*, Dublin University Press, 1860

O'Keeffe, J.G., *Buile Suibne (The Frenzy of Suibhne) being The Adventures of Suibhne Geilt – A Middle-Irish Romance*, London, Irish Text Society, 1913

Orchard, Andy (ed.), *The Elder Edda: A Book of Viking Lore*, London, Penguin Classics, Penguin Group, 2011

Orpen, Goddard Henry (trans.), *The Song of Dermot and the Earl – An Old French Poem – From the Carew Manuscript No. 596*, Oxford, Clarendon Press, 1892

Owen, Wilfred, *Poems*, London, Penguin Classics, 2017

Paden, William D. and Paden, Frances Freeman (trans), *Troubadour Poems From the South of France*, Cambridge, D.S. Brewer, 2007

Pálsson, Hermann and Edwards, Paul (trans), *Eyrbyggja Saga*, London, Penguin Classics, Penguin Group, 1989

Pálsson, Hermann and Edwards, Paul (trans), *Seven Viking Romances*, London, Penguin Classics, Penguin Group, 1985

Parry, John Jay (trans.), *The Art of Courtly Love by Andreas Capellanus*, New York, Columbia University Press, 1941

Paton, Lucy Allen, *Arthurian Romance*, London, J.M. Dent & Sons, 1912

Pifteau, Paul, (trans.), *Chirurgie de Guillaume de Sâlicet, Achevée en 1275*, Toulouse, Imprimerie Saint-Cyprien, 1898

Regal, Martin S. (trans.), 'Gisli Sursson's Saga', *The Sagas of the Icelanders*, London, Penguin Books, Penguin Group, 2001

Reginald of Durham, *Reginaldi Monachi Dunelmensis Libellus de Admirandis*, London, J.B. Nichols and Son, 1835

Reuter, Timothy (trans.), *The Annals of Fulda – Ninth-Century Histories, Volume II*, Manchester University Press, 1992

Rickert, Edith (trans.), *Early English Romances in Verse: Done into Modern English*, London, Chatto & Windus, 1908

Riley, J.A. (trans.), *Annals of Roger de Hoveden, Comprising the History of England and of Other Countries of Europe From A.D. 732 TO A.D. 1201, Volumes I and II*, London, Henry G. Bohn, 1853

Robinson, I.S. (trans.), *Eleventh-Century Germany – The Swabian Chronicles*, Manchester University Press, 2008

Rosenman, Dr Leonard D. (trans.), *The Chirurgia of Roger Frugard*, Xlibris Corporation, 2002

Rosenman, Dr Leonard D. (trans.), *The Surgery of Bruno da Longoburgo – An Italian Surgeon of the Thirteenth Century, by Mario Tabanelli*, Pittsburgh, Dorrance Publishing Co., Inc., 2003

Rosenman, Dr Leonard D. (trans.), *The Surgery of Henri De Mondeville – Volume II*, Xlibris Corporation, 2003

Rosenman, Dr Leonard D. (trans.), *The Surgery of Lanfranchi of Milan*, Xlibris Corporation, 2003

Rosenman, Dr Leonard D. (trans.), *The Surgery of Roland of Parma*, Xlibris Corporation, 2001

Rosenman, Dr Leonard D. (trans.), *The Surgery of William of Saliceto*, Xlibris Corporation, 1998

Sassoon, Siegfried, *The War Poems of Siegfried Sassoon*, ReadaClassic, 2011

Sayles, G.O. (trans.), *Fleta – Volume IV – Book V and Book VI*, London, Selden Society, 1984

Scholz, Bernhard Walter, *Carolingian Chronicles*, Ann Arbor, The University of Michigan Press, 1972

Scudder, Bernard (trans.), 'Egil's Saga', *The Sagas of the Icelanders*, London, Penguin Books, Penguin Group, 2001

Sheingorn, Pamela (trans.), *The Book of Sainte Foy*, Philadelphia, University of Pennsylvania Press, 1995

Sherley-Price, Leo, *Bede – A History of the English Church and People*, revised by R.E. Latham, London, Penguin, 1986

Shirley, Janet (trans.), *The Song of the Cathar Wars – A History of the Albigensian Crusade*, Farnham, Ashgate Publishing Limited, 1996

Sibley, W.A. and Sibley, M.D. (trans), *The History of the Albigensian Crusade – Peter of les Vaux-de-Cernay*, Woodbridge, Boydell & Brewer Ltd, 1998

Steele, Robert, *Huon of Bordeaux: Done into English by Sir John Bourchier, Lord Berners*, London, George Allen Ruskin House, 1895

Steele, Robert (ed.), *Medieval Lore: Being Classified Gleanings from the Encyclopedia of Bartholomew Anglicus on the Properties of Things*, London, Elliot Stock, 1893

Stephens, George (trans.), 'Tegner's Fridthjof's Saga', *Viking Tales of the North – The Sagas of Thorstein, Viking's Son and Fridthjof the Bold*, Chicago, Scott, Foresman and Company, 1901

Stevenson, Revd Joseph, *The Church Historians of England – Volumes I through V*, London, Seeleys, 1853–8

Stevenson, Revd Joseph, *Documents Illustrative of the History of Scotland from the Death of King Alexander the Third to the Assession of Robert Bruce, Volumes I and II*, Edinburgh, HM General Register House, 1870

Strange, Richard, *The Life and Gests of St. Thomas of Hereford – From the Original 1674 Printing*, repr. London, Burns and Oates, 1879

Taylor, Edgar (trans.), *Master Wace – His Chronicle of the Norman Conquest from the Roman de Rou*, London, William Pickering, 1837

Thorndike, Lynn, *University Records and Life in the Middle Ages*, New York, Columbia University Press, 1944

Throop, Priscilla (trans.), *Hildegard von Bingen's Physica – The Complete English Translation of her Classic Work on Health and Healing*, Rochester, VT, Healing Arts Press, 1998

Todd, James Henthorn (trans.), *War of the Gaedhil with the Gaill or The Invasions of Ireland by the Danes and Other Norsemen*, London, Longmans, Green, Reader and Dyer, 1867

Tschan, Francis J., *History of the Archbishops of Hamburg-Bremen – Adam of Bremen*, New York, Columbia University Press, 2002

Tyson, Kathleen (trans.), *Carmen de Triumpho Normannico – The Song of the Norman Conquest*, CreateSpace Independent Publishing Platform, 2013

Von Fleischhacker, Robert (ed.), *Lanfrank's 'Science of Cirurgie'*, Early English Text Society, Original Series, 102, Berlin, New York and Philadelphia, 1894

Waggoner, Ben (trans.), *Norse Magical and Herbal Healing – A Medical Book from Medieval Iceland*, New Haven, CT, Troth Publications, 2011

Wardrop, Marjory Scott (trans.), *The Man in the Panther's Skin*, London, Royal Asiatic Society, 1912

Weston, Jessie L. (trans.), *Parzival – A Knightly Epic by Wolfram von Eschenbach, Volumes I and II*, London, David Nutt, 1894

Whaley, Diana, *Sagas of Warrior Poets*, London, Penguin Classics, Penguin Group, 2002

Wiltshire, Harold, MA MD, 'A Contribution to the Etiology of Shell Shock', *The Lancet*, 17 June 1916, pp. 1207–12

Wither, George, *Campo-Musae or the Field-Musings of Major George Wither Touching his Military Ingagement for the King and Parliament*, London, R.A., 1661

Wright, Thomas (trans.), *The Historical Works of Giraldus Cambrensis*, London, Warton Club, 1905

Wright, Thomas (trans.), *The History of Fulk Fitz Warine, an Outlawed Baron in the Reign of King John*, London, George Bell & Sons, 1855

Wyatt, A.J., *The Lay of Havelok the Dane*, London, W.B. Clive and Co., 1889

Secondary Source Material

Adams, Michael C.C., *Living Hell – The Dark Side of the Civil War*, Baltimore, Johns Hopkins University Press, 2014

Arcini, Caroline, *Health and Disease in Early Lund – Osteo-Pathologic Studies of 3,305 Individuals Buried in the Cemetery Area of Lund 990-1536*, Department of Community Health Sciences Medical Faculty Lund University, 1999

Arcini, Caroline, *The Viking Age: A Time With Many Faces*, Oxford, Oxbow Books, 2018
Band of Brothers, HBO Home Video, 1 September 2015
Bannerman, Stacy, *Homefront 911 – How Families of Wounded Veterans are Wounded by Our Wars*, New York, Arcade Publishing, 2015
Barger, George, *Ergot and Ergotism – A Monograph – Based on the Dohme Lectures Delivered in Johns Hopkins University, Baltimore*, London, Gurney and Jackson, 1931
BBC, *History Cold Case*, Series One, Episode One, *Ipswich Man*, Shine TV Limited and Red Planet Pictures, 2011
BBC, *History Cold Case*, Series Two, Episode Three, *The York 113*, Shine TV Limited and Red Planet Pictures, 2011
Becket, William, *A Collection of Chirurgical Tracts*, London, E. Curll, 1740
Bernstein, Peter, *Trauma: Healing the Hidden Epidemic*, Petaluma, The Bernstein Institute for Integrative Psychotherapy & Trauma Treatment, 2013
British Medical Association, *Hen feddegyaeth kymrie: (ancient Cymric medicine) and lecture memoranda, British Medical Association meeting, Swansea, 1903*, London, Burroughs Wellcome and Company, 1903
Brown, Kevin, *The Pox – The Life and Near Death of a Very Social Disease*, Stroud, Sutton Publishing, 2006
Burnett, Charles, '"Spiritual Medicine": music and healing in Islam and its influence in Western medicine', *Musical Healing in Cultural Contexts*, Farnham, Ashgate Publishing, 2000
Cameron, M.L., *Anglo-Saxon Medicine*, Cambridge University Press, 1993
Capparoni, Pietro Dr, *Magistri Salneritani Nondum Cogniti – A Contribution of the History of the Medical School of Salerno – Wellcome Historical Medical Museum*, London, John Bale, Sons & Danielsson Ltd, 1923
Clay, Rotha Mary, *The Mediaeval Hospitals of England*, Methuen & Co. London, 1909
Contreni, John J., 'Masters and Medicine in Northern France During the Reign of Charles the Bald', *Charles the Bald: Court and Kingdom*, ed. Margaret Gibson and Janet Nelson, 2nd rev. edn, Aldershot, Variorum, 1990, pp. 267–82
Davidson, H.R. Ellis, *Gods and Myths of the Viking Age*, New York, Bell Publishing Company, 1981
DuBois, Thomas A., *Nordic Religions in the Viking Age*, Philadelphia, University of Pennsylvania Press, 1999
Du Chaillu, Paul Belloni, *The Viking Age: The Early History Manners & Customs of the Ancestors of the English-Speaking Nations (In Two Volumes)*, London, John Murray, 1889
Edgington, S.B., *The Life and Miracles of St. Ivo*, St Ives, Cambridgeshire, Norris Library and Museum, 1985
Eger, Dr Edith Eva, *The Choice – Embrace the Possible*, New York, Scribner, 2017
Finucane, Ronald C., *Miracles and Pilgrims – Popular Beliefs in Medieval England*, New York, St Martin's Press, 1995
Freeman, Edward A., *History of the Norman Conquest of England – Its Causes and Its Results – Volumes I to VI*, Oxford, Clarendon Press, 1867–79
Fuller, Thomas, *The History of the University of Cambridge and of Waltham Abbey with the Appeal of Injured Innocence*, James Nichols, 1840
Ganze, Ronald, 'The Neurological and Physiological Effects of Emotional Duress on Memory in Two Old English Elegies', *Anglo-Saxon Emotions – Reading the Heart in Old English Language, Literature and Culture*, Farnham, Ashgate Publishing, 2015
Getz, Faye, *Medicine in the Middle Ages*, Princeton University Press, 1998
Gies, Joseph and Frances, *Life in a Medieval Castle*, New York, Harper & Row Publishers, 1981

Gies, Joseph and Frances, *Life in a Medieval City*, New York, Harper & Row Publishers, 1981

Green, Monica H., *Making Women's Medicine Masculine – The Rise of Male Authority in Pre-Modern Gynaecology*, Oxford University Press, 2008

Griffith, Dr H. Winter, *Complete Guide to Symptoms, Illness & Surgery*, New York, The Body Press, 1985

Hedeager, Lotte, *Iron Age Myth and Materiality: An Archaeology of Scandinavia AD 400–1000*, London and New York, Routledge, 2011

Hemmeter, John C. and Garrison, Fielding H. (trans), 'Salerno – A Mediaeval Health Resort and Medical School on the Tyrrhenian Sea', *Essays in the History of Medicine by Karl Sudhoff*, New York, Medical Life Press, 1926

Holmes, Urban, *A History of Old French Literature; from the origins to 1300*, New York, Russell and Russell, 1962

Hunt, Tony, *The Medieval Surgery*, Woodbridge, Boydell Press, England, first published 1992

Jackson, Ralph, *Doctors and Diseases in the Roman Empire*, London, British Museum Press, 1988

Jarman, Thomas Leckie, *William Marshal First Earl Of Pembroke And Regent Of England (1216–1219)*, Oxford, Basil Blackwell, 1930

Jeep, John. *Medieval Germany: An Encyclopedia*, Routledge, 2001

Jesch, Judith, *Women in the Viking Age*, Woodbridge, Boydell Press, 2001

Jones, Terry, *Medieval Lives*, London, BBC Books, 2004

Jones, Terry, *Terry Jones – Medieval Lives*, 2 discs, BBC Video, 2008.

Kealey, Edward J., *Medieval Medicus – A Social History of Anglo-Norman Medicine*, Johns Hopkins University Press, 1981

Lucy, Sam, *The Anglo-Saxon Way of Death – Burial Rites in Early England*, Stroud, Sutton Publishing, 2000

Marcombe, David, *Leper Knights – The Order of St. Lazarus of Jerusalem in England, c. 1150–1544*, Woodbridge, Boydell & Brewer Ltd, 2003

Medieval Dead, Season 1, Episode 2, *Last Stand at Visby*, Like a Shot Entertainment, 2013

Metzler, Irina, *Disability in Medieval Europe – Thinking about physical impairment during the high Middle Ages, c. 1100–1400*, Abingdon, Routledge, 2006

Metzler, Irina, 'Medieval Bynames and Nicknames that Relate to "Disability"', *The Treatment of Disabled Persons in Medieval Europe*, Lewiston, NY, The Edwin Mellen Press, 2010, Appendix

Metzler, Irina, *A Social History of Disability in the Middle Ages – Cultural Considerations of Physical Impairment*, New York, Routledge, 2013

Metzler, Irina, 'What's in a name? Considering the Onomastics of Disability in the Middle Ages', *The Treatment of Disabled Persons in Medieval Europe*, The Edwin Mellen Press, 2010

Mitchell, Piers D., 'Anatomy and surgery in Europe and the Middle East during the Middle Ages', *Anatomy and Surgery from Antiquity to the Renaissance*, Amsterdam, Adolf Hakkert, 2016

Mitchell, Piers D., *Medicine in the Crusades – Warfare, Wounds and the Medieval Surgeon*, Cambridge University Press, 2004

Moffat, Brian, *SHARP Practice 6, The Sixth Report on Researches into the Medieval Hospital at Soutra Scottish Borders/Lothian, Scotland*, Pathhead, SHARP, 1998

Moffat, Brian and Other Participants in SHARP, *SHARP Practice 4, Fourth Report on Researches into the Medieval Hospital at Soutra, Lothian/Borders Region Scotland*, Edinburgh, SHARP, 1992

Moore, Norman, *The History of the Study of Medicine in the British Isles*, Oxford, Clarendon Press, 1908

Moran, Matthew, 'San Vincenzo in the Making: The Discovery of an Early Medieval Production Site on the East Bank of the Volturno', *Markets in Early Medieval Europe – Trading and 'Productive' Sites, 650—850*, Macclesfield, WINDgather Press, 2003

Mortimer, Ian, *The Time Traveller's Guide to Medieval England – A Handbook for Visitors of the Fourteenth Century*, London, The Bodley Head, 2008

Murray, Alexander, *Suicide in the Middle Ages – Volume I and II*, Oxford University Press, 1998

Oliver, Neil, *Vikings – A History*, London, Orion Publishing Group, 2013

Park, Katherine, *Doctors and Medicine in Early Renaissance Florence*, Princeton University Press, 1985

Paterson, Linda M., 'Military Surgery: Knights, Sergeants, and Raimon of Avignon's Version of the Chirurgia of Roger of Salerno (1180–1209)', *The Ideals and Practice of Medieval Knighthood II – Papers from the Third Strawberry Hill Conference, 1986*, Woodbridge, Boydell & Brewer, 1988

Rawcliffe, Carole, *Medicine & Society in Later Medieval England*, Stroud, Sutton Publishing Ltd, 1995

Rhys, John, *Celtic Folklore – Welsh and Manx – Volume 1*, Oxford, Clarendon Press, 1901

Rice, Francis, *The Hermit of Finchale – The Life of Saint Godric*, Durham, UK, The Pentland Press Limited, 1994

Richards, Peter, *The Medieval Leper and His Northern Heirs*, Cambridge, D.S. Brewer, 1977

Rossiaud, Jacques, *Medieval Prostitution or La Prostituzione Nel Medioevo*, New York, Barnes and Noble, 1996

Schofield, John and Vince, Alan, *Medieval Towns – The Archaeology of British Towns in Their European Setting*, New York, Continuum, 1994

Secrets of the Castle, BBC and Lion Television, 2014

SHARP, *SHARP Practice 1, The First Report into the Medical Hospital at Soutra, Lothian Region*, Edinburgh, SHARP, 1986

Simpson, Jacqueline, *Everyday Life in the Viking Age*, London, B.T. Batsford Ltd, 1967

Siraisi, Nancy, 'How to write a Latin book on surgery: organizing principles and authorial devices in Guglielmo de Saliceto and Dino del Garbo', *Practical medicine from Salerno to the Black Death*, Cambridge University Press, 1994

Siraisi, Nancy, *Medieval and Early Renaissance Medicine, An Introduction to Knowledge and Practice*, University of Chicago Press, 1990

Siraisi, Nancy, *Taddeo Alderotti and his Pupils – Two Generations of Italian Medical Learning*, Princeton University Press, 1981

Skinner, Patricia, *Living with Disfigurement in Early Medieval Europe*, New York, Palgrave MacMillan, 2017

Spencer, Brian, *Pilgrim Souvenirs and Secular Badges*, London, Museum of London, The Stationery Office, 1998

Stenton, Lady Doris Mary, *English Society in the Early Middle Ages (1066–1307)*, London, Penguin Books Ltd, 1986

Talbot, C.H. and Hammond, E.A., *The Medical Practitioners in Medieval England, A Biographical Register*, London, Wellcome Historical Medical Library, 1965

Thierry, Augustine, *History of the Conquest of England by the Normans, Its Causes and Its Consequences, in England, Scotland, Ireland & on the Continent, Volumes I and II*, London, David Bogue, 1847

Thompson, Logan, *Ancient Weapons in Britain*, Barnsley, Pen & Sword Military, 2004

Turner, Sharon, *The History of the Anglo-Saxons from the Earliest Period to the Norman Conquest – In Three Volumes*, London, Longman, Brown, Green and Longmans, 1852

Turner, Wendy J. and Pearman, Tory Vandeventer, *The Treatment of Disabled Persons in Medieval Europe – Examining Disability in the Historical, Legal, Literary, Medical and Religious Discourses of the Middle Ages*, Lewiston, NY, The Edwin Mellen Press, 2010

Van Der Kolk, Bessel, *The Body Keeps Score – Mind, Brain and Body in the Transformation of Trauma*, London, Penguin Books, 2014

Walker, Don, *Disease in London, 1st–19th centuries – An illustrated guide to diagnosis*, London, Museum of London Archaeology, 2012

Ward, Benedicta, *Miracles and the Medieval Mind – Theory, Record and Event – 1000–1215*, Aldershot, Wildwood House Limited, 1987

Wheen, A.W. (trans.), *All Quiet on the Western Front, by Erich Maria Remarque*, New York, Ballentine Books edn, 1982

Whipple, Alan O., *The Story of Wound Healing and Wound Repair*, Springfield, IL, Charles C. Thomas, 1963

Willows, Marlo A., 'Health Status in Lowland Medieval Scotland: A Regional Analysis of Four Skeletal Populations – Volume 1 and 2', University of Edinburgh, Thesis, 2016

Wise, Terence, *Men-at-Arms, Saxon, Viking and Norman*, Oxford, Osprey Publishing Ltd, 1979

Yewdale, Ralph Bailey, 'Bohemond I, Prince of Antioch – A Dissertation Presented to the Faculty of Princeton University', accepted by the Faculty of Princeton June 1917

York Archaeological Trust, *Plague, Poverty, Prayer*, York, York Archaeological Trust, 2009

Young, Kenneth (trans.), *Handbook to the Cultural History of the Middle Ages – Supplementary to displays in Bryggens Museum*, Bergen, Bryggens Museum, 1978

Index

Abbo of Saint-German-des-Prés 17, 45, 79, 87, 140 n. 26, 181 n. 134
Abbot Suger 15, 42, 131, 144 n. 5
Abulcasis 12, 51, 54, 131, 132
Adam of Breman 25, 75, 83, 93, 131
African ants 51
Ahmad ibn Fadlān 16, 131, 83, 93
Ahmad ibn Rusta 83, 170
Albigensian Crusade 1, 16, 19, 78, 133, 137
alcohol 102, 109, 125
Alfanus 9, 132
Alfred, King of England (The Great) 104
aloes 19, 145 nn. 37 and 38
amputation 24, 36, 44, 53–6, 87, 92
Anglo-Saxon Chronicle 121, 129, 149 n. 8, 167 n. 5, 187 n. 94
Annals of Clonmacnoise 83, 140 n. 26
Annals of Fulda 15–16, 131, 144 n. 8
Annals of St Bertin 15, 70, 98, 112, 131, 148 n. 76
Annals of Ulster 5, 83, 93, 105
Annals of Xanten 98, 176 n. 38
armour 1, 2, 20, 21, 44, 59, 61, 64, 70, 80, 98, 109, 146 n. 50, 154 nn. 9 and 10, 157 n. 67, 160 n. 4, 165 nn. 95 and 99
army 3, 12, 14, 16, 29, 31, 37, 41, 44, 53, 72, 77, 89, 94–6, 98–9, 101, 103, 106–7, 115–16, 123, 129, 133, 137, 142 n. 50, 143 n. 66, 152 n. 49, 154 n. 85, 155 n. 17, 165 n. 99, 187 n. 94
arrows vii, 1, 3, 5, 11, 12, 17, 19, 22, 27, 39–40, 43–9, 70, 89, 94, 110, 149 n. 89, 153–4 n. 82, 154 nn. 7–10, 155 nn. 13, 14, 17, 20, 27, 156 nn. 32, 34, 37, 165 n. 97, 181 n. 134
assistants to physicians and surgeons, 32, 47, 60, 62, 63, 64, 161 n. 31, 162 n. 51

Aulus Cornelius Celsus 53
Avicenna 82, 131–2
axes vii, 1, 49, 53, 61, 63, 64, 66, 70, 114, 157 n. 63
Azerbaijan 16, 95–6, 120, 134

Bald's Leechbook 4, 6–8, 18, 47, 54–5, 61–2, 67, 71, 78, 81, 97, 103, 107, 131–2, 134, 186 n. 82
Bamberg Surgery 11, 62, 73, 132, 142 n. 58, 157 n. 53, 163 n. 65
bandages 11, 17, 31–2, 34, 47, 49, 61–2, 64, 73, 82, 108
Bannockburn, Battle of 90
barber-surgeons 3, 60, 168 n. 27
Bartholomew Anglicus 128
battle-fetter 114–15, 117
Bede 31, 132
Beowulf 17, 116, 164 n. 104
Bernard of Angers 22, 23, 136, 186 n. 83
Bernard from Auvergne 3, 122
Bertran de Born 20, 165 n. 95
Birka 5, 71, 138 n. 6
Bishop Thorlak, The Saga of 179 n. 97
blacksmiths (also metalsmiths) 37–9, 46, 72, 152–3, 155
blood-eagle 83, 170 n. 72
bloodletting (phlebotomy) 57, 84–5, 159 n. 100
Bohemond I 9, 142 n. 50
Bologna 9, 10, 12, 133, 165 n. 91
bonesetters 3, 37, 40, 59–60, 160 n. 9
Bosi and Herraud, The Saga of 2, 65, 157 n. 46
bruises (also contusions), 30, 71, 84, 85, 124, 160 n. 17
Bruno da Longoburgo 10, 51, 66, 131, 132
Budeč, Czech Republic 89

burn injuries 1, 3, 30, 31, 58, 75, 78–82, 85, 88, 92, 119, 159 n. 104, 170 nn. 56 and 57
Burnt Njal, The Story (Saga) of 17, 53, 61, 64, 66, 70, 79, 118–19, 167 n. 8, 183 n. 23

caltrop (also calthrop) 45
cannula 51–2, 157 n. 53
Carmen Widonis 89, 132, 150 n. 8, 152 n. 49, 153 n. 78, 155 n. 17, 165 n. 95
Cathars 16, 19, 133, 171 n. 77
Causcy, Roger 3, 29
cautery 14, 34, 43, 47, 54, 55, 58, 68, 72, 78, 103, 158 n. 78
Charlemagne 15, 94, 136, 137, 144 n. 8
charms (and spells) 7, 13, 18, 33, 113–15, 134, 176 n. 33
chicken (used in healing) 74, 78
Chrétien de Troyes (general) 18–19, 32, 64, 67, 88, 150–1 nn. 22 and 25
  Cligés 45, 53, 68, 142 n. 52, 157 n. 65
  Erec and Enide 37, 56, 64, 67, 69, 142 nn. 52 and 54, 145 n. 36, 151 n. 34
  The Knight of the Cart (Lancelot) 19, 67, 120
  The Knight with the Lion (Yvain) 17, 76, 164 n. 79, 168 n. 17
  The Story of the Grail (Perceval) 32, 33, 64, 88, 145 n. 34, 150 n. 22, 187 n. 101
cinnamon 67
clavicle (collarbone) 59, 63–4, 162 nn. 43, 45, 47 and 48
cleft lip 78, 168
Clontarf, Battle of 41
cold therapy (analgesic) 58, 82
compound (open) fracture 14, 62–3, 156 n. 44
Constantine the African 9, 10, 13, 103, 127, 132, 133, 142 n. 58
Cremona 74, 89, 110, 121
crossbow 44, 45, 79, 81, 110, 124, 154 n. 10, 156 n. 37
crusades
  Albigensian Crusade 1, 16, 19, 78, 133, 137

  First Crusade 9, 21, 81, 86
  Third Crusade 80–1, 126, 135, 167 n. 4, 178 n. 68
  Fifth Crusade 12, 133
  Seventh Crusade 106
  Ninth Crusade 91, 174 n. 138
cupping 57, 159 n. 100

Denmark 4, 18, 75, 123, 139 n. 19
depression 3, 111–13, 116, 123–4, 127, 182 n. 7
diet 51, 56–7, 62–3, 84–5, 103, 110, 159 nn. 96 and 97
dislocation of bones and joints (also luxation) 3, 11, 42, 59–60, 62–6, 84–5, 150 n. 12, 160 n. 11, 162–3 nn. 51, 60, 63 and 65
domestic abuse 124–5, 187 n. 107
dry healing 109–10
Dublin 5, 105, 135, 140 n. 26, 170 n. 71, 179 n. 94
Dunstable, Bedfordshire 67
dysentery vii, 3, 6, 34, 94–7, 107, 110, 175 nn. 17, 25 and 26

ears 27, 69, 86, 113, 171 n. 97
Edward I, King of England 3, 29, 40, 44, 81, 90, 91, 96–7, 173 n. 131
Edward II, King of England 40, 90
eggs (in medicine) 41, 62, 64, 66, 78, 82, 161 n. 26
Egil and Asmund 18, 58, 87
Egil's Saga 18, 150 n. 17, 156–7 n. 46
Eirik the Red's Saga 18, 65
elixir of grief 127
ergotism (also St Anthony's Fire) 55, 93, 94, 97–100, 176–7, nn. 33, 43, 44, 49 and 54
Exeter Book 116
eyes 23, 72, 77, 80, 82, 87, 90, 92, 121, 157 n. 47, 166 n. 122

face 23–4, 32, 39, 43, 47, 67, 70, 73, 75, 76, 78, 81, 86, 89, 95, 98, 103, 104, 123, 124, 147 n. 64, 163 n. 78, 164 n. 79, 167 n. 11, 168 n. 29, 170 n. 56, 172 n. 100, 176 n. 43, 179 n. 102

Fantosme, Jordan 49, 133, 142 n. 52
feet 52–3, 61, 71, 75, 82, 84–5, 87, 89, 96, 99, 117, 158 n. 69, 171 n. 77
femur 61
fingers 30, 55, 62, 64, 87, 103, 117
Flavius Vegetius Renatus 94
Florence of Worcester 96
Four Humours, The Theory of the, 57, 159 nn. 97, 98 and 100
Fragmentary Annals of Ireland 66
frankincense 11, 13, 85
Frugard, Roger (Roger of Parma) 4, 10–11, 13, 33, 47, 49, 50, 57, 62, 63, 66, 68, 73, 82, 109, 119, 127, 132, 133, 135–7, 142 nn. 55 and 56, 143 n. 63, 151 n. 29, 166 n. 129, 178–9 n. 87, 181 nn. 130 and 131
furrier's stitch 52

Galen 12, 58, 132
games 1–2, 59, 60, 65, 139 n. 8, 143–4 n. 4
Gariopontus 9–10
garlic 57, 68
Gerald of Wales 16, 44, 72, 81, 105, 127
Germany 15, 36, 76, 87, 97, 109, 133, 142 n. 54, 144 n. 8, 148 n. 75
Gilbertus Anglicus 97
Gisli Surssons Saga 118, 168–9 n. 35, 185 n. 61
Gjermundbu Helmet 71
Goirans, William 21–2
gonorrhea 100–3, 177 n. 65
Great Viking Army (also Great Heathen Army) 123, 187 n. 94
Greek fire 80–1, 169 nn. 47, 49 and 50
Greenlanders, The Saga of 18
Grettir the Strong, The Saga of (also Grettis' Saga) 79, 86, 114
Grimbald (physician to Henry I) 119
Grógaldr or *Groa's Chant* 115, 184 n. 36
Guglielmo da Brescia 128, 143 n. 70, 189 n. 140
Guibert of Nogent 26, 76, 86, 158 n. 69, 171 n. 77
Guido II of Arezzo 11, 135
Gunnlaug Serpent-Tongue, The Saga of 123–4

Guy de Chauliac 33, 60, 68, 133, 151 n. 28, 164 n. 85

Hacon, The Saga of 140 n. 29, 152 n. 48
hands 12, 24, 27, 29, 31, 46, 50, 66, 67, 75, 82, 85, 87, 89, 95, 157 n. 67, 158 n. 85, 174 n. 137, 179 n. 97
Harald Hardrada (King of Norway) 129
Harold II, King of England (Godwinson) 36, 129, 152 n. 49
hashish 127
Hastings, Battle of 36, 41, 45, 70, 132, 152 n. 49, 155 n. 17, 175 n. 25
Hávamál or *The lay of the High One (Odin)* 114–15, 176 n. 33, 184 n. 36
Hedeby 5–6, 140 n. 28
Heimskringla or *A History of the Norse Kings* 31, 35, 49, 83, 107, 136
helmet 1, 66, 67, 70–3, 145 n. 42, 160 n. 4, 163 n. 78, 164 n. 79, 165 nn. 97, 99 and 104, 166 nn. 106 and 122
hemlock 7, 54–5, 57, 100, 181 n. 134
henbane 7, 18, 24, 54–5, 57–8, 67–9, 159 n. 102
Henri de Mondeville 84–5, 109–10, 133, 137, 171 n. 91, 181 n. 133
Henrik Harpestræng 13, 155 n. 20
Henry I, King of England 121, 123
Henry II, Holy Roman Emperor 94
Henry II, King of England 2, 49, 81, 94, 102, 133, 138 n. 4, 142 n. 52
Henry III, King of England 14, 102
Henry V, Holy Roman Emperor 153 n. 82
Henry of Huntingdon 67, 133
Henry of Mâchecourt 39, 46
hernia 38, 153 n. 64, 176 n. 33
Hildegard of Bingen 10, 34, 81, 120, 133
honey 57, 67, 71, 74, 103, 159 n. 101
Hord, The Saga of 115
horses 2, 11, 18, 44–5, 50, 59–60, 63–6, 80, 84–5, 88, 96, 102, 107, 109, 111, 115, 146, 148, 154 n. 9, 162 n. 57, 163 n. 63, 170 n. 73, 172 n. 116
hospital 25, 37, 40, 55, 90–1, 99–100, 101, 105, 107, 174 n. 138, 177 n. 54, 185 n. 56
Hubert of Pierrelatte 46–7

Hugh de Gundeville 2–3, 139 n. 12, 149 n. 89
Hugo da Lucca 3, 10, 12, 29, 103, 133, 137
humerus (bone) 63, 64, 66
Hywel Dha or Howel the Good 29, 49, 62

Ibrahim ibn Yacoub al-Tartushi (also Abraham ben Jacob) 5, 140 n. 28
Iceland 15, 18, 35, 150 n. 17
infection vii, 7, 26, 39, 46–9, 52, 55, 62–3, 77, 81, 85, 93–5, 107–10, 126, 162 n. 39, 164 n. 86, 175 n. 15, 180 nn. 118 and 119, 181 nn. 128 and 134
intestines 38, 44, 49–52, 57, 95, 96, 107, 122, 157 nn. 53 and 61
Ireland 2, 5, 6, 15, 66, 72, 83, 105, 127, 135, 139 n. 121, 140 n. 26, 149 n. 89, 153 n. 79
Ishaq Ibn Imran 127
Islamic medicine 2, 5, 12, 36, 51, 82, 127, 137

Jean de Bredella 52, 122
John, King of England 14, 83, 117, 175 n. 26
Jomsviking Saga 30, 163 n. 72

King Hrolf and his Champions 168–9 n. 35
King Sigferth 121, 186 n. 80
Knight of the Two Swords, The 20, 60, 64, 73, 146 n. 44, 162 n. 48, 163 n. 78, 164 n. 88
Knights of Narbonne, The 66, 165 n. 100
Kormak's Saga 2, 18, 139 n. 10, 144 n. 25, 180 n. 115

La Chanson de la croisade contre les Albigeois (The Song of the Crusade Against the Albigensians) 1, 19, 30, 40, 53, 79, 95, 98, 129, 133, 157 n. 47, 169 n. 38, 176 n. 35
La Chanson de Guillaume or *The Song of William* 31, 42, 50, 53, 88, 134
laceration 5, 11, 30, 32, 35, 51, 66
Lacnunga 13, 54, 127, 134
lances 1, 37, 49, 50, 76, 77, 138 n. 3, 145 n. 42, 146 n. 44, 149 n. 89 *see also* spears

Lanfranchi of Milan 7, 10, 52, 57, 58, 86, 134, 137, 159 n. 98, 168 n. 29, 173 n. 126
Langton, Stephen, Archbishop of Canterbury 23, 84
Lascelles (young knight) 50, 77
laxatives (also evacuation of the bowels) 57, 84–5, 110, 159 nn. 97 and 100
Lay of the Nibelungs, The 11, 29, 138, 154 n. 85
Leechbook III 3, 7–8, 18, 50, 57, 65, 67, 71, 127, 134, 141 n. 36, 156 n. 30, 170 n. 57, 175–6 n. 29
Leopold V, Duke of Austria 62
leprosy 3, 93, 94, 103–7, 146 n. 58, 178–9, nn. 86–8, 94, 101–2 and 105
lily 81
lime (also quicklime) 80, 169 n. 39
London 34, 55, 60, 73–4, 81, 89, 96, 101, 102
Louis VI of France 15, 96, 123, 131, 175 n. 26

Macer Floridus De Viribus Herbarum 13, 67, 97, 100, 133–4, 145 n. 38, 150–1 n. 25, 158 n. 76, 176 n. 30
McIndoe, Sir Archibald 3, 139
Magh Rath, Battle of 117, 184 n. 50
magic 18, 38, 105, 127, 145 n. 28, 189 n. 129
Man in the Panther's Skin, The 5, 127
mandrake 55, 57
manure 85
Marie de France 18
marrow (bone) 55, 63
Master Wace 41, 70, 134
Mathfred 43–4, 47, 125, 154 nn. 6 and 7, 180 n. 119, 181 n. 121, 186 n. 83, 187 n. 104, 188 n. 111
Matthew Paris 14–15, 60, 78, 80, 93, 106, 134–5, 143 n. 2, 169 n. 49, 174 n. 1, 178 n. 79, 180 n. 116
Merseburg Charms 115
metalsmiths *see* blacksmiths
miracles (general) 2, 15, 21–8, 43, 65, 77, 99, 110, 147 nn. 70–1, 148 n. 76, 149 n. 89, 154 n. 5, 168 n. 21, 180 n. 119

Miskawayh 16, 96, 120, 134
monks 3, 5, 12, 15, 17, 22, 24, 25, 26, 28, 29, 39, 55, 63, 91, 122, 147 n. 63, 147 n. 70, 148 n. 75, 152 n. 62
Monte Cassino 9, 103, 127, 132
Montpellier 9–10, 20, 21, 34, 96, 128, 133, 137, 142 nn. 52–4
muscle 30, 53–4, 159 n. 101, 161 n. 27
music (as therapy) 127–8
myrrh 19, 145 nn. 37 and 38

neck 2, 12, 46, 47, 64, 67, 70, 76, 89, 148 n. 78, 156 n. 34, 162 n. 48, 165 n. 97
Nidaros (modern Trondheim, Norway) 25–6
nightmares vii, 111, 112, 116, 118–20, 123, 169 n. 37, 182 nn. 2 and 7
Norway 25–6, 37, 45, 71, 98, 105, 129, 134, 136, 166 n. 106, 168 n. 27, 169 n. 50, 176 nn. 33, 34 and 41
nose 11, 23, 55, 67, 75–7, 86, 101, 167 n. 4, 171 nn. 97 and 99
nuns 3, 5, 26, 29

Odin 93–4, 113, 115, 120, 175–6 n. 29
ointment of the three Marys 19
Olaf Haraldson, The Saga of 35
Old English Herbarium 13, 18, 119, 135, 163 n. 75
Old Icelandic Medical Miscellany 13, 62, 81, 135
olive oil 80, 82
Olöf (Icelandic Healer) 35, 56
Onund Treefoot 87, 114
opium 55, 57–8, 82, 100, 127
Orderic Vitalis 9, 16, 25, 43, 83, 87, 90, 93, 105, 108, 123, 129, 135, 143–4 n. 4, 169 n. 49, 170 n. 56, 175 n. 25
oregano 67
Owen, Wilfred 21, 92, 118, 182 n. 9

pain relief, 54, 56–8, 62, 159 n. 102
Pantegni 9
Paris 9, 15, 17, 45, 79, 87, 98, 112, 124, 131, 133, 134, 140 n. 26, 144 n. 8
Parzival 20, 33
penis 103, 171 n. 77, 178 nn. 83 and 84

People of Laxardal, The Saga of the 53
pepper 57, 67
Peter of Eboli 47
Peter of les Vaux-de-Cernay 16, 78, 84
Peverel, Pagan 21, 146 n. 50
placebo effect 24, 127
Pope Innocent III 16, 133
porpoise 127, 189 n. 129
Post Traumatic Stress Disorder (PTSD) 111, 118, 119, 123, 184 nn. 39, 44 and 48, 189 n. 144
poultice 10, 57, 65, 73
prostheses 17, 56, 75, 86–8, 144 n. 15, 164 n. 86, 171–2 nn. 99 and 107
prostitution 100–2, 178 n. 72
pus 11, 47–8, 109, 137, 181 nn. 129 and 131 *see also* dry healing

radish 127, 141 n. 40
radius (bone) 60
Ragnar Lothbrok 127
Raimon of Avignon 11, 66, 135, 143 n. 63, 166 n. 129
Raymond from Valières 23–4, 28, 147 n. 63
recovery 2, 44, 56–8, 89, 112, 128, 148 n. 75
ribs 18, 65, 83, 129, 148 n. 75
Richard I, King of England 81, 135
Rigaud 111–12, 116, 122
Rocamadour Abbey 27–8, 39, 46, 77, 117, 135, 149 n. 89
Rocmadour Miracle collection 2, 21, 27–8, 37, 39, 46, 65, 67–8, 77, 99, 109, 117, 125, 135, 148 nn. 84 and 85, 149 n. 89, 155 n. 24, 181 n. 121
Roger de Hoveden 135, 161 n. 37, 169 n. 51
Roger of Wendover 16, 80, 82, 135, 150 n. 16, 157 n. 67, 161 n. 37, 169 n. 47, 175 n. 26, 179 n. 89
Roland of Parma 10, 12, 49, 66, 82, 109, 136
Roland, Song of 52, 122, 134, 137
Rollo 98
Roman de Rou 40–1, 70
Roncevaux Pass, Battle of 137

rooster 62, 161 n. 34, 176 n. 33
rose (rosewater) 74, 82, 85, 96–7, 176 n. 30
Royal Frankish Annals 15, 95, 136, 114 n. 8

St Anthony's Fire (see ergotism)
St Foy, Abbey of 22–3, 152 n. 62, 166 n. 120
St Foy Miracle collection 23–4, 37–9, 43–4, 72, 76–7, 83, 99, 108, 121, 124, 136, 139 n. 14, 147, 177 n. 48, 186 n. 83
St Godric of Finchdale, Miracles of 50, 77
St Helen-on-the-Walls 60, 162 n. 60
St Hugh of Lincoln, Miracles of 23, 117
St Ivo, Miracles of 21, 146 n. 55, 163 n. 63
St James of Reading, Miracles of 147 n. 70
St John's wort 127, 189 n. 125
St Mary 65, 99
St Mary Magdalen 105
St Mary Spital 60, 73
St Thomas of Canterbury, Miracles of, 105–6, 136, 146 n. 58, 148 n. 76, 179 n. 102
St William of Norwich, Miracles of 84, 88, 136, 172 n. 114
Salerno 6, 8–9, 11, 13, 19–21, 34, 100, 103, 106, 132, 135, 137, 141 n. 46, 142 nn. 50 and 52
salt 41, 54, 82, 103, 107, 127, 158 n. 76, 171 n. 77
salve 4, 7, 19, 47, 55, 57, 61, 65, 71, 72, 78, 82, 85, 101, 103, 109, 161 n. 26
Saxo Grammaticus 31, 70, 76, 112, 120, 126–7, 136, 138 n. 6, 152 n. 59
scars 3, 24, 39, 76–8, 79, 81, 85, 89, 92, 112, 114, 167 n. 11, 168 nn. 12, 15, 17, 22 and 29, 170 n. 56
Scotland 5, 40, 44, 49, 90, 96, 120, 127, 133, 142 n. 52, 164 n. 83
Scottish War of Independence 44, 81, 90
Senorez from Dordogne 27–8
Sexually Transmitted Infections (STIs) 94, 100–3
shoulder 12, 17, 35, 42, 52, 53, 59, 64, 65–6, 150 n. 12, 162 nn. 45, 53, 57 and 60, 163 nn. 63 and 65, 171 n. 77
Siegfried Sassoon 21, 120, 184 n. 48, 185 n. 56

Simeon of Durham 5, 96, 136, 140 n. 23
Simon de Montfort 20, 30, 78, 133, 137, 166 n. 122
Skallagrímsson, Egil 18, 113
skull 3, 26, 43, 59, 69–74, 79, 119, 127, 129, 156 n. 44, 165 n. 100, 167 n. 133
Snorri Sturluson 31, 35, 45, 49, 83, 136, 175–6 n. 29, 183 n. 22
Solmund, Kari (also Scorched Kari), 79, 81, 119, 169 n. 36
Sonatorrek (The Loss of Sons) 113
Song of Dermot, The 42
Song of Girart of Vienne, The 64, 70, 165 n. 95
Song of Roland, The 52, 122, 134, 137
soporific sponge 55
Soutra Aisle 55, 127
spears vii, 1, 20, 27, 32, 42, 52, 61, 76, 108, 109, 113, 138 n. 4, 145 n. 42, 161 n. 22, 184 n. 34 *see also* lances
spells *see* charms
splints 61–4, 69, 161 n. 26
Stamford Bridge, Battle of 129
Stephen, King of England 91
Stiklestad, Battle of 35, 37, 45, 49
stomach 13, 36, 44, 49–52, 57, 77, 95, 96, 99, 121, 122, 125, 133, 150 n. 19, 161 n. 36
suicide vii, 16, 112, 116, 120–2, 128, 187–8 n. 107
sulphur 79–81, 109, 169 n. 38
superstition 24, 28, 94, 97, 128
surgery, medical text 4, 10–13, 33, 47, 50, 52–4, 57–8, 64, 66, 68, 84, 86, 89, 103, 109, 119, 121, 132–4, 136–7, 142–3 n. 62, 156 n. 34, 162 n. 51, 166 n. 129, 185 n. 68
surgery, treatment of the body 7, 17, 36, 39, 43–58, 63, 69, 76, 131, 151 n. 34, 162 n. 57, 180 n. 114
sutures (stitches) 5, 11, 34, 49, 51–2, 56, 78, 109, 151 n. 32, 157 n. 53
Sweden 4, 55, 60, 63, 64, 71, 75, 83, 93, 105, 138 n. 6, 161 n. 25, 162 n. 47, 165 n. 99
Switzerland 35, 87
swords vii, 1–3, 23–4, 27, 32, 49, 53, 57, 59, 61, 63, 66, 68, 69–71, 74, 78, 83, 87,

91, 94, 102, 110, 111–12, 119, 120, 126, 145 n. 42, 149 n. 89, 157 nn. 63, 65 and 67, 161 n. 22, 163 n. 78, 165 n. 104, 166 n. 129, 180 n. 115, 183 n. 19, 186 n. 85
syphilis 101, 177–8 n. 66

Taddeo Alderotti 10, 60, 165 n. 91
teeth 3, 6, 27, 47, 59, 66–9, 73, 87, 107, 163 n. 72, 164 nn. 83–5 and 87–8, 166 n. 122, 171 n. 77
testicles 171 n. 77
Theodoric 4, 10–13, 33, 48, 51, 54–7, 62–4, 68, 69, 74, 78, 82, 103, 109, 131, 133–4, 136–7, 143 n. 77, 146 n. 44, 151 n. 32, 154 n. 10, 156 n. 32, 159 nn. 100 and 101, 162 n. 43, 181 nn. 130 and 132
Thor 93–4, 175–6 n. 29
Thordar's Saga (The Story of Thórðr Hreða) 35, 56
Thordis the Prophetess 18
Thormod Kolbrunarskald 45–6
Thorstein, Viking's Son, The Saga of 105, 163 n. 72, 170 n. 72
torture 15, 16, 75, 82–6, 88, 92, 96, 98, 144 nn. 7 and 12, 146 n. 54, 170 nn. 67, 70 and 71, 171 n. 77, 177 n. 44
tournaments 1–2, 20, 36, 59, 60, 63, 76, 102, 137 nn. 4 and 6, 178 n. 79
trepanation 26, 73–4, 127, 166 n. 129
Trotula 103, 137, 141 n. 47
Tyr 114, 183 nn. 19 and 23

ulna 60
Uppsala 83, 93
Usāmah ibn Munqidh 16, 40, 59, 76, 109, 127–8, 137

valerian (common) 127, 189 n. 125
valkyries 115, 184 n. 34
Vapnfjord Men, The (Vápnfirðinga Saga) 18
Varnhem Abbey 63
Viga-Glum, The Saga of 35
Vikings
  medicine 4–6, 8, 17–18, 21, 31, 35–7, 45–6, 49, 56–8, 65, 86–8, 93–4, 152 n. 48, 159 n. 102, 176 n. 33

mental health 3, 112–16, 118–21, 123–4, 126–7, 182–3 n. 13
Rūs 16, 80, 83, 93, 95–6, 121, 131, 134, 140 nn. 26 and 27, 149–50 n. 8
slavery 5, 36, 83, 93, 96, 140 nn. 26, 28 and 29
vinegar 54–5, 58, 67, 80, 82, 109, 127
Visby, Battle of 61, 161 n. 25, 165 n. 99

Waltharius 35, 53, 66, 157 n. 64
Wanderer, The 111, 116, 118, 126, 184 nn. 40 and 44, 188 n. 118
William I, King of England (also the Conqueror) 28, 90, 143–4 n. 4, 153 n. 78, 173 n. 123, 175 n. 25
William I, King of Scotland 49
William (Guillaume) de Congenis 30, 34, 137, 150 n. 12, 180 n. 118
William of Malmesbury 89, 101
William of Saliceto 3–4, 10–12, 29, 33, 48, 51–2, 57–8, 62–3, 68, 74, 82–5, 89, 103, 110, 121–2, 134, 137, 143 n. 70, 145 n. 38, 156 n. 34, 159 nn. 101 and 102, 161 n. 31, 162 n. 51, 162–3 n. 60, 164 n. 90, 173 n. 126, 186 n. 85
William of Tudela 19, 30, 133, 145 n. 39
Wiltshire, Harold (Dr) 112, 182 n. 9, 183 n. 24
Wimborne Minster 121, 186 n. 80
wine 32, 42, 48, 52, 56, 67, 69, 74, 79, 82, 96, 103, 109, 110
Wither, George 111, 182 n. 2
Wolfram von Eschenbach 20, 33
women (as physicians, surgeons and healers) 3, 8, 10, 19, 25, 34–7, 45, 47, 49, 65, 103, 116, 133, 137, 151 n. 34, 152 n. 48

Yarm Helmet 71
yarrow 81
York 60, 63, 69, 73–4, 81, 90, 129, 173 n. 120